T0133987

BIOCHEMISTRY, BIOPHYSICS, AND MOLECULAR CHEMISTRY

Applied Research and Interactions

Innovations in Physical Chemistry: Monograph Series

BIOCHEMISTRY, BIOPHYSICS, AND MOLECULAR CHEMISTRY

Applied Research and Interactions

Edited by

Francisco Torrens, PhD
Debarshi Kar Mahapatra, PhD
A. K. Haghi, PhD

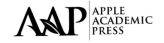

Apple Academic Press Inc.
4164 Lakeshore Road
Burlington ON L7L 1A4, Canada

Apple Academic Press, Inc.
1265 Goldenrod Circle NE
Palm Bay, Florida 32905, USA

© 2020 by Apple Academic Press, Inc.

First issued in paperback 2021

Exclusive worldwide distribution by CRC Press, a member of Taylor & Francis Group
No claim to original U.S. Government works

ISBN 13: 978-1-77463-510-0 (pbk)
ISBN 13: 978-1-77188-816-5 (hbk)

Library and Archives Canada Cataloguing in Publication

Title: Biochemistry, biophysics, and molecular chemistry : applied research and interactions /
  edited by Francisco Torrens, PhD, Debarshi Kar Mahapatra, PhD, A.K. Haghi, PhD.
Names: Torrens, Francisco (Torrens Zaragoza), editor. | Mahapatra, Debarshi Kar, editor. |
  Haghi, A. K., editor.
Series: Innovations in physical chemistry.
Description: Series statement: Innovations in physical chemistry: monographic series |
  Includes bibliographical references and index.
Identifiers: Canadiana (print) 20190239921 | Canadiana (ebook) 20190239948 |
  ISBN 9781771888165 (hardcover) | ISBN 9780429284175 (ebook)
Subjects: LCSH: Biochemistry. | LCSH: Biophysics. | LCSH: Chemistry, Physical and theoretical.
Classification: LCC QH345 .B53 2020 | DDC 572—dc23

CIP data on file with US Library of Congress

Apple Academic Press also publishes its books in a variety of electronic formats. Some content that appears in print may not be available in electronic format. For information about Apple Academic Press products, visit our website at **www.appleacademicpress.com** and the CRC Press website at **www.crcpress.com**

ABOUT THE EDITORS

Francisco Torrens, PhD
Lecturer, Physical Chemistry, Universitat de València, València, Spain

Francisco Torrens, PhD, is Lecturer in physical chemistry at the Universitat de València in Spain. His scientific accomplishments include the first implementation at a Spanish university of a program for the elucidation of crystallographic structures and the construction of the first computational-chemistry program adapted to a vector-facility supercomputer. He has written many articles published in professional journals and has acted as a reviewer as well. He has handled 26 research projects, has published two books and over 350 articles, and has made numerous presentations.

Debarshi Kar Mahapatra, PhD
Assistant Professor, Department of Pharmaceutical Chemistry, Dadasaheb Balpande College of Pharmacy, Rashtrasant Tukadoji Maharaj Nagpur University, Nagpur, Maharashtra, India

Debarshi Kar Mahapatra, PhD, is currently Assistant Professor in the Department of Pharmaceutical Chemistry at Dadasaheb Balpande College of Pharmacy, Rashtrasant Tukadoji Maharaj Nagpur University, Nagpur, Maharashtra, India. He was formerly Assistant Professor in the Department of Pharmaceutical Chemistry, Kamla Nehru College of Pharmacy, RTM Nagpur University, Nagpur, India. He has taught medicinal and computational chemistry at both undergraduate and postgraduate levels and has mentored students in their various research projects. His area of interest includes computer-assisted rational designing and synthesis of low molecular weight ligands against druggable targets, drug delivery systems, and optimization of unconventional formulations. He has published research, book chapters, reviews, and case studies in various reputed journals and has presented his work at several international platforms, for which he has received several awards by a number of bodies. He also authored the book *Drug Design*. Presently, he is serving as a reviewer and editorial board member for several journals of international repute. He is a member of a number of professional and scientific societies, such as the International Society for Infectious Diseases (ISID), the International Science Congress Association (ISCA), and ISEI.

A. K. Haghi, PhD

Professor Emeritus of Engineering Sciences, Editor-in-Chief, *International Journal of Chemoinformatics and Chemical Engineering* and *Polymers Research Journal*; Member, Canadian Research and Development Center of Sciences and Cultures (CRDCSC), Canada

A. K. Haghi, PhD, is the author and editor of 165 books, as well as 1000 published papers in various journals and conference proceedings. Dr. Haghi has received several grants, consulted for a number of major corporations, and is a frequent speaker to national and international audiences. Since 1983, he served as professor at several universities. He is the former Editor-in-Chief of the *International Journal of Chemoinformatics and Chemical Engineering* and *Polymers Research Journal* and is on the editorial boards of many international journals. He is also a member of the Canadian Research and Development Center of Sciences and Cultures (CRDCSC), Montreal, Quebec, Canada.

INNOVATIONS IN PHYSICAL CHEMISTRY: MONOGRAPH SERIES

This book series offers a comprehensive collection of books on physical principles and mathematical techniques for majors, non-majors, and chemical engineers. Because there are many exciting new areas of research involving computational chemistry, nanomaterials, smart materials, high-performance materials, and applications of the recently discovered graphene, there can be no doubt that physical chemistry is a vitally important field. Physical chemistry is considered a daunting branch of chemistry—it is grounded in physics and mathematics and draws on quantum mechanics, thermodynamics, and statistical thermodynamics.

Editors-in-Chief

A. K. Haghi, PhD
Former Editor-in-Chief, *International Journal of Chemoinformatics and Chemical Engineering* and *Polymers Research Journal*; Member, Canadian Research and Development Center of Sciences and Cultures (CRDCSC), Montreal, Quebec, Canada
E-mail: AKHaghi@Yahoo.com

Lionello Pogliani, PhD
University of Valencia-Burjassot, Spain
E-mail: lionello.pogliani@uv.es

Ana Cristina Faria Ribeiro, PhD
Researcher, Department of Chemistry, University of Coimbra, Portugal
E-mail: anacfrib@ci.uc.pt

BOOKS IN THE SERIES

- **Applied Physical Chemistry with Multidisciplinary Approaches**
  Editors: A. K. Haghi, PhD, Devrim Balköse, PhD, and Sabu Thomas, PhD

- **Biochemistry, Biophysics, and Molecular Chemistry: Applied Research and Interactions**
  Editors: Francisco Torrens, PhD, Debarshi Kar Mahapatra, PhD, and A. K. Haghi, PhD

- **Chemistry and Industrial Techniques for Chemical Engineers**
  Editors: Lionello Pogliani, PhD, Suresh C. Ameta, PhD, and
  A. K. Haghi, PhD

- **Chemistry and Chemical Engineering for Sustainable Development: Best Practices and Research Directions**
  Editors: Miguel A. Esteso, PhD, Ana Cristina Faria Ribeiro, and
  A. K. Haghi, PhD

- **Chemical Technology and Informatics in Chemistry with Applications**
  Editors: Alexander V. Vakhrushev, DSc, Omari V. Mukbaniani, DSc, and Heru Susanto, PhD

- **Engineering Technologies for Renewable and Recyclable Materials: Physical-Chemical Properties and Functional Aspects**
  Editors: Jithin Joy, Maciej Jaroszewski, PhD, Praveen K. M., Sabu Thomas, PhD, and Reza K. Haghi, PhD

- **Engineering Technology and Industrial Chemistry with Applications**
  Editors: Reza K. Haghi, PhD, and Francisco Torrens, PhD

- **High-Performance Materials and Engineered Chemistry**
  Editors: Francisco Torrens, PhD, Devrim Balköse, PhD, and Sabu Thomas, PhD

- **Methodologies and Applications for Analytical and Physical Chemistry**
  Editors: A. K. Haghi, PhD, Sabu Thomas, PhD, Sukanchan Palit, and Priyanka Main

- **Modern Physical Chemistry: Engineering Models, Materials, and Methods with Applications**
  Editors: Reza K. Haghi, PhD, Emili Besalú, PhD, Maciej Jaroszewski, PhD, Sabu Thomas, PhD, and Praveen K. M.

- **Molecular Chemistry and Biomolecular Engineering: Integrating Theory and Research with Practice**
  Editors: Lionello Pogliani, PhD, Francisco Torrens, PhD, and
  A. K. Haghi, PhD

- **Modern Green Chemistry and Heterocyclic Compounds: Molecular Design, Synthesis, and Biological Evaluation**
  Editors: Ravindra S. Shinde, and A. K. Haghi, PhD

- **Physical Chemistry for Chemists and Chemical Engineers: Multidisciplinary Research Perspectives**
  Editors: Alexander V. Vakhrushev, DSc, Reza K. Haghi, PhD, and J. V. de Julián-Ortiz, PhD
- **Physical Chemistry for Engineering and Applied Sciences: Theoretical and Methodological Implication**
  Editors: A. K. Haghi, PhD, Cristóbal Noé Aguilar, PhD, Sabu Thomas, PhD, and Praveen K. M.
- **Practical Applications of Physical Chemistry in Food Science and Technology**
  Editors: Cristóbal Noé Aguilar, PhD, Jose Sandoval Cortes, PhD, Juan Alberto Ascacio Valdes, PhD, and A. K. Haghi, PhD
- **Research Methodologies and Practical Applications of Chemistry**
  Editors: Lionello Pogliani, PhD, A. K. Haghi, PhD, and Nazmul Islam, PhD
- **Theoretical Models and Experimental Approaches in Physical Chemistry: Research Methodology and Practical Methods**
  Editors: A. K. Haghi, PhD, Sabu Thomas, PhD, Praveen K. M., and Avinash R. Pai
- **Theoretical and Empirical Analysis in Physical Chemistry: A Framework for Research**
  Editors: Miguel A. Esteso, PhD, Ana Cristina Faria Ribeiro, PhD, and A. K. Haghi, PhD

CONTENTS

CONTRIBUTORS

Vivek Asati
Department of Pharmaceutical Chemistry, NRI Institute of Pharmacy, Bhopal 462021, Madhya Pradesh, India

Sanjay B. Bari
Department of Pharmaceutical Chemistry, H. R. Patel Institute of Pharmaceutical Education and Research, Shirpur, Dist. Dhule, Maharashtra 425405, India

Sanjay Kumar Bharti
Institute of Pharmaceutical Sciences, Guru Ghasidas Vishwavidyalaya (A Central University), Bilaspur 495009, Chhattisgarh, India

Gloria Castellano
Departamento de Ciencias Experimentales y Matemáticas, Facultad de Veterinaria y Ciencias Experimentales, Universidad Católica de Valencia San Vicente Mártir, Guillem de Castro-94, E-46001 València, Spain

Chin Kang Chen
The Indonesian Institute of Sciences, Indonesia

Kishor R. Danao
Department of Pharmaceutical Chemistry, Dadasaheb Balpande College of Pharmacy, Nagpur 440037, Maharashtra, India

Sumeet Dwivedi
Department of Pharmacognosy and Biotechnology, Swami Vivekanand College of Pharmacy, Indore 452020, Madhya Pradesh, India

Ahmed A. El-Rashedy
Department of Natural and Microbial Product, Research Division of Pharmaceutical and Drug Industries, National Research Centre, Dokki, Cairo 12622, Egypt

Leu Fang-Yie
The Indonesian Institute of Sciences, Indonesia University of Brunei, Bandar Seri Begawan, Brunei

Saurabh Khadse
Department of Pharmaceutical Chemistry, R. C. Patel Institute of Pharmaceutical Education and Research, Shirpur, Dist. Dhule, Maharashtra 425405, India

Debarshi Kar Mahapatra
Department of Pharmaceutical Chemistry, Dadasaheb Balpande College of Pharmacy, Nagpur 440037, Maharashtra, India

Satyaendra K. Shrivastava
Department of Pharmacognosy and Biotechnology, Swami Vivekanand College of Pharmacy, Indore 452020, Madhya Pradesh, India

Anamika Singh
Department of Botany, Maitreyi College, University of Delhi, New Delhi

Rajeev Singh
Department of Environmental studies, Satyawati College, University of Delhi, New Delhi

Heru Susanto
The Indonesian Institute of Sciences, Indonesia Tunghai University, Taichung, Taiwan

Francisco Torrens
Institut Universitari de Ciència Molecular, Universitat de València, Edifici d'Instituts de Paterna, P. O. Box 22085, E-46071 València, Spain

Vinod G. Ugale
Department of Pharmaceutical Chemistry, R. C. Patel Institute of Pharmaceutical Education and Research, Shirpur, Dist. Dhule, Maharashtra 425405, India

Rahul Wani
Department of Pharmaceutical Chemistry, R. C. Patel Institute of Pharmaceutical Education and Research, Shirpur, Dist. Dhule, Maharashtra 425405, India

ABBREVIATIONS

ADRs	adverse drug reactions
ADs	Alzheimer's diseases
AI	artificial intelligence
AKI	acute kidney injury
ALR	aldose reductase
AMPA	α-amino-3-hydroxy-5-methyl-4-isoxazolepropionic acid
ARBs	angiotensin receptor blockers
ATM	ataxia telangiectasia-mutated
BD	big data
BZI	benzimidazole
cAMP	cyclic adenosine monophosphate
CDC	centers for disease control
CDP	cytidine diphosphate
CRG	chronic risk groups
DDBJ	DNA database of Japan
DDBM	2-(1,1-dimethyl-1,3-dihydro-benzo[e]indol-2-ylidene)-malonaldehyde
DL	deep learning
dTTP	deoxy thymidine triphosphate
EMR	electronic medical records
EVs	electric vehicles
FBS	fasting blood sugar
FGFR3	fibroblast growth factor receptor 3
FLT3	FMS-like tyrosine kinase-3
GABA	γ-amino butyric acid
GR	graphene
GSK3	glycogen synthase kinase 3
GST	glutathione-S-transferase
HA	hemagglutinin
hERG	human ether-a-go-go related gene
HTRF	homogeneous time-resolved fluorescence
I/R	ischemia–reperfusion
ICIJ	International Consortium of Investigative Journalists

IDDM	insulin-dependent DM
IFN	interferon
iGluRs	ionotropic glutamate receptors
IIoT	industrial internet of things
IR	ionizing radiation
IS	information system
KEGG	Kyoto Encyclopedia of Genes and Genomes
LBD	ligand-binding domain
NA	neuraminidase
NIDDM	non-insulin-dependent DM
NMDARs	N-methyl-D-aspartate receptors
NMR	nuclear magnetic resonance
NPPs	nuclear power plants
NPs	nanoparticles
PCP	phencyclidine
PDB	Protein Data Bank
PDGFR	platelet-derived growth factor receptors
PLK1	Polio-like kinase 1
PM	personalized medicine
PPBS	postprandial blood sugar
PTE	periodic table of the elements
PTKs	protein kinases
PTP	protein tyrosine phosphatase
QC	quantum chemistry
QSAR	quantitative structure-activity relationship
RF	random forest
RNA	ribonucleic acid
SBDD	structure-based drug design
SBML	Systems Biology Markup Language
Ser/Thr	serine/threonine kinases
SGK	serum and glucocorticoid-induced Kinase
TK	thymidylate kinase
TrkA	tropomyosin receptor kinase A
WFT	wavefunction theory
WWI	World War I

PREFACE

This book has been designed to help the postgraduate students to understand the basic concepts of biochemistry, biophysics, and molecular chemistry. This book is written mostly from the viewpoint of the basic scientist who works at the cellular and molecular level. As molecular chemistry is one of the forefront subjects in research and development these days, it has become almost necessary for the students to have a hold on this subject. This book addresses enormous advances in biochemistry, particularly in the areas of structural biology and bioinformatics, by providing a solid biochemical foundation that is rooted in chemistry to prepare students for the scientific challenges of the future. This volume will prove to be a valuable reference for those engaged in or entering the field of molecular chemistry and biology, and will provide the necessary background for those interested in setting up and using the latest molecular techniques. The book provides the background needed in biophysics and molecular chemistry and offers a great deal of advanced biophysical knowledge.

It also emphasizes the growing interrelatedness of molecular chemistry and biochemistry, and acquaints one with experimental methods of both disciplines.

CHAPTER 1

SCALING SYMMETRIES: ENVIRONMENTAL PROTECTION, CHEMISTRY, AND SOCIETY

FRANCISCO TORRENS[1*] and GLORIA CASTELLANO[2]

[1]Institut Universitari de Ciència Molecular, Universitat de València, Edifici d'Instituts de Paterna, P. O. Box 22085, E-46071 València, Spain

[2]Departamento de Ciencias Experimentales y Matemáticas, Facultad de Veterinaria y Ciencias Experimentales, Universidad Catolica de Valencia San Vicente Mártir, Guillem de Castro-94, E-46001 València, Spain

*Corresponding author. E-mail: torrens@uv.es

ABSTRACT

Faced with a new subject, one should approach it with the good luck of the beginner: Enjoying every word and thinking what every word tells him. The testimony is that of a layman that sees proofs of wonderful things. New ideas and general ontological and methodological changes are discovered. Transhumanism, new conceptions on the limits of being and its privacy or working and research methods with computational models are good examples of the philosophy. Correlations do not imply causality; nor do they indicate truthfulness. Sea dumping of industrial waste is a new form of piracy. The codes of ethics are important but, in the end, they are a personal theme. The actions should be performed in an ambit of respect and without eagerness to intimidation. The principle is noble, and the way to transmit the message and obtain its acceptance should be dignified. Demographic and environmental sustainabilities should be looked after.

1.1 INTRODUCTION

Setting the scene: Scaling symmetries in the real world, environmental protection, and chemistry and society. Faced with a new subject, one should approach it with the good luck of the beginner: Enjoying every word and thinking what every word tells him. Our testimony is that of a layman that sees proofs of wonderful things. In a more philosophical view, new concepts and general ontological and methodological changes are discovered. Transhumanism, new conceptions on the limits of being and its privacy, or working and research methods with computational models are good examples of this philosophical view.

The moral of the tale follows: Correlations do not imply causality. Nor do they indicate truthfulness. Sea dumping of industrial waste is a new form of piracy. The codes of ethics are important but, in the end, they are a personal theme. These actions should be carried out in an ambit of respect and without eagerness to intimidation. The principle is noble and the way to transmit the message and obtain its acceptance should also be dignified. Both demographic (aging) and environmental sustainabilities should be looked after.

Earlier publications reported fractals for hybrid orbitals in protein models,[1] fractal hybrid-orbital analysis of the protein tertiary structure,[2] molecular diversity classification via information theory,[3] complexity, emergence, molecular diversity via information theory,[4] molecular classification, diversity, complexity via information entropy,[5] dialectic walk on science,[6] Brownian motion, random trajectory, diffusion, fractals, chaos theory, dialectics,[7] nuclear fusion, American nuclear cover-up in Spain after Palomares (Almería) disaster (1966),[8] Manhattan Project, Atoms for Peace, nuclear weapons, accidents,[9] periodic table of the elements (PTE),[10–12] quantum simulators,[13–21] science, ethics of developing sustainability via nanosystems, devices,[22] green nanotechnology as an approach towards environment safety,[23] molecular devices, machines as hybrid organic–inorganic structures,[24] PTE, quantum biting its tail, sustainable chemistry,[25] quantum molecular spintronics, nanoscience, graphenes,[26] cancer, its hypotheses,[27] precision personalized medicine from theory to practice, cancer,[28] how human immunodeficiency virus and acquired immunodeficiency syndrome destroy immune defences, hypothesis,[29] 2014 emergence, spread, uncontrolled Ebola outbreak,[30,31] Ebola virus disease, questions, ideas, hypotheses, models,[32] metaphors that made history, reflections on philosophy, science, deoxyribonucleic acid,[33] scientific integrity and ethics, science communication and psychology.[34] The present report reviews scaling symmetries in the real world, environmental protection versus nuclear power, incineration and health, cosmetics and health, artificial ingredients and nanoingredients, science and gender. The aim of this work is to initiate a debate by suggesting a number of questions (Q), which can arise when addressing subjects of scaling symmetries in the real world, environmental protection, chemistry and society, and hypotheses on incineration and health, cosmetics and health, artificial ingredients and nanoingredients, science and gender, in different fields, and providing, when possible, answers (A) and hypotheses (H).

1.2 SCALING SYMMETRIES IN THE REAL WORLD

Jones proposed hypotheses and questions on scaling symmetries in the real world.[35]

H1. (West, 2018). Scale: Life/Growth/Death Universal Laws in Organisms/Cities/Companies.[36]

H2. (Ballesteros et al., 2018). Metabolic-scaling origin.[37]

Q1. What to do with bad data?

Q2. What is wrong with this?

Q3. Why is scaling important?

Q4. What was the sample selection criterion, constant surface brightness?

Q5. What was the sample selection criterion, constant density?

Q6. What was the sample selection criterion…?

Q7. What could possibly be the mechanism driving Zipf's law on the size of cities?

Q8. How may cities evolve?

H1. Moral of the tale: Correlations do not imply causality. Nor do they indicate truthfulness.

Q9. The presentation of the data: Can this be read?

Q10. The presentation of the data: What is the underlying cause?

Q11. The presentation of the data: What is wrong?

1.3 ENVIRONMENTAL PROTECTION

Novikov proposed questions, answer and hypotheses on environmental protection.[38]

Q1. Mountains of wastes are the monuments being raised by our civilization at end of 20th century?

Q2. Does not mankind resort to emergency with view to saving natural habitable environment?

Q3. Is nuclear holocaust prevented?

Q4. (Vernadsky). Has mankind's activity become a powerful geological force?

Q5. Was economic/industrial activity of humanity inspiring with reckless optimism still yesterday?

Q6. Was it called not else as conquering of nature?

Q7. What was it previously invisible without modern communication facilities?

Q8. What is happening to the forests of Brazil?

Q9. How do whole regions in Africa undergo desertification?

Q10. What disastrous state are the forests of Asia in?

H1. Sea dumping of industrial waste is a new form of piracy.

H2. (Edward IV, 1273). He banned the use of coal for heating dwellings in London.

Q11. What is the cause of O_3 hole?

A11. O_3 layer is destroyed by catalytic reactions with active Cl/F-atoms/substances formed from freons under ultraviolet (UV) in stratosphere.

1.4 NUCLEAR POWER

In the course of 60 years, the nuclear power plants (NPPs) are in service, heavy accidents existed: At Windscale (UK, 1957), an accident occurred in the reactor with emission of radioactive fission products; a reactor's cooling system malfunctioned to bring an accident at a unit of NPP at Three Mile Island (1979). Chernobyl (overnight April 25-26, 1986) disaster took place with large amount of radioactive fission products injected into the environment. Chernobyl accident drastically aggravated the problems of further development of NPP industry on Earth. One important lesson to be drawn from Chernobyl accident, by all those who live on Earth, concerns the danger potential inherent in technology failures that are possible not only at NPPs but also at the military bases and installations where nuclear or chemical weapons are stationed. It suffices to recall the hundreds of aircraft on routine airborne alert over the planet, carrying nuclear bombs, or the nuclear-armed ships and submarines constantly patrolling seas and oceans. The discussion so far concentrated on random events (accidents at NPPs presenting intrinsic causes). They are bound to happen solely because no technology is altogether safe and reliable, much less the sophisticated technologies that the present NPP stations result. People strive to make the reliability absolute and will continue to do so as long as NPPs developed accidents.

1.5   INCINERATION AND HEALTH

Nanoparticles (NPs) present a great ability to pass corporal-tissues membranes and involve a high grade of possible toxicity because their biodegradability is difficult and their penetration of the different animal species and humans could alter vital functions.[39] Nanotechnology is a new science in development that presents many questions, as NPs properties change versus the size that they show and nanostructures interactions with environment are not known. Some manufactured NPs could be more toxic per unit of mass than others of the same nature but of greater size. The natural enzymes that exist in environment could change NPs surface and turn them into colloids, which could transport at distance heavy metals or molecules contained in fertilizers and pesticides. Doubts are a lot.

1.6   COSMETICS AND HEALTH. ARTIFICIAL INGREDIENTS: NANOINGREDIENTS

Nowadays, nanoingredients, small particles for which a regulation is necessary, were incorporated into cosmetics. On reducing toxic-particles size with nanotechnology, one increases their penetration, especially with cold creams, that extend throughout body. Nanomaterials should be considered new chemical entities with new safety rules and their use should be specified on labels. Group Friends of the Earth makes a campaign for the products to be labeled.

1.7   SCIENCE AND GENDER

In history, the role of women in science should be put in its social context. However, one should not put this context as an excuse.

1.8   DISCUSSION

Faced with a new subject, one should approach it with the good luck of the beginner: Enjoying every word and thinking what every word tells him. Our testimony is that of a layman that sees proofs of wonderful things.

In a more philosophical view, new concepts, and general ontological and methodological changes are discovered. Transhumanism, new conceptions on the limits of being and its privacy, or working and research methods with computational models are good examples of this philosophical view.

1.9   FINAL REMARKS

From the present results and discussion, the following final remarks can be drawn.

1. Moral of the tale: Correlations do not imply causality. Nor do they indicate truthfulness.
2. Sea dumping of industrial waste is a new form of piracy.
3. The codes of ethics are important but, in the end, they are a personal theme.
4. These actions should be carried out in an ambit of respect and without eagerness to intimidation.
5. The principle is noble, and the way to transmit the message and obtain its acceptance should also be dignified.

6. In a more philosophical view, new concepts, and general ontological and methodological changes are discovered. Transhumanism, new conceptions on the limits of being and its privacy or working and research methods with computational models are good examples of this philosophical view.
7. Both demographic (aging) and environmental sustainabilities should be looked after.

ACKNOWLEDGMENTS

The authors thank support from Generalitat Valenciana (Project No. PROMETEO/2016/094) and Universidad Católica de Valencia San Vicente Mártir (Project No. 2019-217-001).

KEYWORDS

- nuclear power
- incineration
- health
- cosmetics
- artificial ingredient
- nanoingredient
- science

REFERENCES

1. Torrens, F. Fractals for Hybrid Orbitals in Protein Models. *Complexity Int.* **2001,** *8,* 1–13.
2. Torrens, F. Fractal Hybrid-orbital Analysis of the Protein Tertiary Structure. *Complexity Int.*, in press.
3. Torrens, F.; Castellano, G. Molecular Diversity Classification *via* Information Theory: A Review. *ICST Trans. Complex Syst.* **2012,** *12* (10–12), e4–1–8.
4. Torrens, F.; Castellano, G. Complexity, Emergence and Molecular Diversity via Information Theory. In *Complexity Science, Living Systems, and Reflexing Interfaces:*

New Models and Perspectives; Orsucci, F., Sala, N., Eds.; IGI Global: Hershey, PA, 2013; pp 196–208.

5. Torrens, F.; Castellano, G. Molecular Classification, Diversity and Complexity via Information Entropy. In *Chaos and Complex Systems*; Stavrinides, S. G., Banerjee, S., Caglar, H., Ozer, M., Eds.; Springer: Berlin, Germany, in press.

6. Torrens, F.; Castellano, G. Dialectic Walk on Science. In *Sensors and Molecular Recognition*; Laguarda Miro, N., Masot Peris, R., Brun Sánchez, E., Eds.; Universidad Politécnica de Valencia: València, Spain, 2017; Vol. 11, pp 271–275.

7. Torrens, F.; Castellano, G. Brownian Motion, Random Trajectory, Diffusion, Fractals, Theory of Chaos, and Dialectics. In *Modern Physical Chemistry: Engineering Models, Materials, and Methods with Applications*; Haghi, R., Besalú, E., Jaroszewski, M., Thomas, S., Praveen, K. M., Eds.; Apple Academic–CRC: Waretown, NJ, in press.

8. Torrens, F.; Castellano, G. Nuclear Fusion and the American Nuclear Cover-Up in Spain: Palomares Disaster (1966). In *Engineering Technology and Industrial Chemistry with Applications*; Haghi, R., F. Torrens, F., Eds.; Apple Academic–CRC: Waretown, NJ, in press.

9. Torrens, F.; Castellano, G. Manhattan Project, Atoms for Peace, Nuclear Weapons and Accidents. In *Molecular Chemistry and Biomolecular Engineering: Integrating Theory and Research with Practice*; Pogliani, L., Torrens, F., Haghi, A. K., Eds.; Apple Academic–CRC: Waretown, NJ, in press.

10. Torrens, F.; Castellano, G. Reflections on the Nature of the Periodic Table of the Elements: Implications in Chemical Education. In *Synthetic Organic Chemistry*; Seijas, J. A., Vázquez Tato, M. P., Lin, S. K., Eds.; MDPI: Basel, Switzerland, 2015; Vol. 18, pp 1–15.

11. Torrens, F.; Castellano, G. Nanoscience: From a Two-Dimensional to a Three-Dimensional Periodic Table of the Elements. In *Methodologies and Applications for Analytical and Physical Chemistry*; Haghi, A. K., Thomas, S., Palit, S., Main, P., Eds.; Apple Academic–CRC: Waretown, NJ, 2018; pp 3–26.

12. Torrens, F.; Castellano, G. Periodic Table. In: *New Frontiers in Nanochemistry: Concepts, Theories, and Trends*; Putz, M. V., Ed.; Apple Academic–CRC: Waretown, NJ, in press.

13. Torrens, F.; Castellano, G. Ideas in the History of Nano/Miniaturization and (Quantum) Simulators: Feynman, Education and Research Reorientation in Translational Science. In *Synthetic Organic Chemistry*; Seijas, J. A., Vázquez Tato, M. P., Lin, S. K., Eds.; MDPI: Basel, Switzerland, 2015; Vol. 19, pp 1–16.

14. Torrens, F.; Castellano, G. Reflections on the Cultural History of Nanominiaturization and Quantum Simulators (Computers). In *Sensors and Molecular Recognition*; Laguarda Miró, N., Masot Peris, R., Brun Sánchez, E., Eds.; Universidad Politécnica de Valencia: València, Spain, 2015; Vol. 9, pp 1–7.

15. Torrens, F.; Castellano, G. Nanominiaturization and Quantum Computing. In *Sensors and Molecular Recognition*; Costero Nieto, A. M., Parra Álvarez, M., Gaviña Costero, P., Gil Grau, S., Eds.; Universitat de València: València, Spain, 2016; Vol. 10, pp 31–1–5.

16. Torrens, F.; Castellano, G. Nanominiaturization, Classical/Quantum Computers/Simulators, Superconductivity, and Universe. In *Methodologies and Applications for*

Analytical and Physical Chemistry; Haghi, A. K., Thomas, S., Palit, S., Main, P., Eds.; Apple Academic–CRC: Waretown, NJ, 2018; pp 27–44.

17. Torrens, F.; Castellano, G. Superconductors, Superconductivity, BCS Theory and Entangled Photons for Quantum Computing. In *Physical Chemistry for Engineering and Applied Sciences: Theoretical and Methodological Implication*; Haghi, A. K., Aguilar, C. N., Thomas, S., Praveen, K. M., Eds.; Apple Academic–CRC: Waretown, NJ, 2018; pp 379–387.

18. Torrens, F.; Castellano, G. EPR Paradox, Quantum Decoherence, Qubits, Goals and Opportunities in Quantum Simulation. In *Theoretical Models and Experimental Approaches in Physical Chemistry: Research Methodology and Practical Methods*; Haghi, A. K., Ed.; Apple Academic–CRC: Waretown, NJ, 2018; Vol. 5, pp 317–334.

19. Torrens, F.; Castellano, G. Nanomaterials, Molecular Ion Magnets, Ultrastrong and Spin–Orbit Couplings in Quantum Materials. In *Physical Chemistry for Chemists and Chemical Engineers: Multidisciplinary Research Perspectives*; Vakhrushev, A. V., Haghi, R., de Julián-Ortiz, J. V., Allahyari, E., Eds.; Apple Academic–CRC: Waretown, NJ, in press.

20. Torrens, F.; Castellano, G. Nanodevices and Organization of Single Ion Magnets and Spin Qubits. In *Chemical Science and Engineering Technology: Perspectives on Interdisciplinary Research*; Balköse, D., Ribeiro, A. C. F., Haghi, A. K., Ameta, S. C., Chakraborty, T., Eds.; Apple Academic–CRC: Waretown, NJ, in press.

21. Torrens, F.; Castellano, G. Superconductivity and Quantum Computing via Magnetic Molecules. In *New Insights in Chemical Engineering and Computational Chemistry*; Haghi, A. K., Ed.; Apple Academic–CRC: Waretown, NJ, in press.

22. Torrens, F.; Castellano, G. Developing Sustainability via Nanosystems and Devices: Science–Ethics. In *Chemical Science and Engineering Technology: Perspectives on Interdisciplinary Research*; Balköse, D., Ribeiro, A. C. F., Haghi, A. K., Ameta, S. C., Chakraborty, T., Eds.; Apple Academic–CRC: Waretown, NJ, in press.

23. Torrens, F.; Castellano, G. Green Nanotechnology: An Approach towards Environment Safety. In *Advances in Nanotechnology and the Environmental Sciences: Applications, Innovations, and Visions for the Future*; Vakhrushev, A. V.; Ameta, S. C.; Susanto, H., Haghi, A. K., Eds.; Apple Academic–CRC: Waretown, NJ, in press.

24. Torrens, F.; Castellano, G. Molecular Devices/Machines: Hybrid Organic–Inorganic Structures. In *Research Methods and Applications in Chemical and Biological Engineering*; Pourhashemi, A., Deka, S. C., Haghi, A. K., Eds.; Apple Academic–CRC: Waretown, NJ, in press.

25. Torrens, F.; Castellano, G. The Periodic Table, Quantum Biting its Tail, and Sustainable Chemistry. In *Chemical Nanoscience and Nanotechnology: New Materials and Modern Techniques*; Torrens, F., Haghi, A. K., Chakraborty, T., Eds.; Apple Academic–CRC: Waretown, NJ, in press.

26. Torrens, F.; Castellano, G. Quantum Molecular Spintronics, Nanoscience and Graphenes. In *Molecular Physical Chemistry*; Haghi, A. K., Ed.; Apple Academic–CRC: Waretown, NJ, in press.

27. Torrens, F.; Castellano, G. Cancer and Hypotheses on Cancer. In *Molecular Chemistry and Biomolecular Engineering: Integrating Theory and Research with Practice*;

Pogliani, L., Torrens, F., Haghi, A. K., Eds.; Apple Academic–CRC: Waretown, NJ, in press.

28. Torrens, F.; Castellano, G. Precision Personalized Medicine from Theory to Practice: Cancer. In *Molecular Physical Chemistry*; Haghi, A. K., Ed.; Apple Academic–CRC: Waretown, NJ, in press.

29. Torrens, F.; Castellano, G. AIDS Destroys Immune Defences: Hypothesis. *New Front. Chem.* **2014**, *23*, 11–20.

30. Torrens-Zaragozá, F.; Castellano-Estornell, G. Emergence, Spread and Uncontrolled Ebola Outbreak. *Basic Clin. Pharmacol. Toxicol.* **2015**, *117* (Suppl. 2) 38–38.

31. Torrens, F.; Castellano, G. 2014 Spread/Uncontrolled Ebola Outbreak. *New Front. Chem.* **2015**, *24*, **81–91**.

32. Torrens, F.; Castellano, G. Ebola virus disease: Questions, Ideas, Hypotheses and Models. *Pharmaceuticals* **2016**, *9*, 14–6–6.

33. Torrens, F.; Castellano, G. Metaphors That Made History: Reflections on Philosophy/Science/DNA. In *Molecular Physical Chemistry*; Haghi, A. K., Ed.; Apple Academic–CRC: Waretown, NJ, in press.

34. Torrens, F.; Castellano, G. Scientific Integrity/Ethics: Science Communication and Psychology. In *Molecular Physical Chemistry*; Haghi, A. K., Ed.; Apple Academic–CRC: Waretown, NJ, in press.

35. Jones, B. J. T. Personal Communication.

36. West, G. *Scale: The Universal Laws of Life, Growth, and Death in Organisms, Cities, and Companies*; Penguin: London, UK, 2018.

37. Ballesteros, F. J.; Martinez, V. J.; Luque, B.; Lacasa, L.; Valor, E.; Moya, A. On the Thermodynamic Origin of Metabolic Scaling. *Sci. Rep.* **2018**, *8*, 1448–1–10.

38. Novikov, Y. *Environmental Protection*; MIR: Moscow, USSR, 1990.

39. Valls-Llobet, C. *Medio Ambiente y Salud: Mujeres y Hombres en un Mundo de Nuevos Riesgos*; Feminismos No. 131, Cátedra–Universitat de València: Madrid, Spain, 2018.

CHAPTER 2

SCIENTIFIC INTEGRITY AND ETHICS: SCIENCE COMMUNICATION AND PSYCHOLOGY

FRANCISCO TORRENS[1*] and GLORIA CASTELLANO[2]

[1]*Institut Universitari de Ciència Molecular, Universitat de València, Edifici d'Instituts de Paterna, P. O. Box 22085, E-46071 València, Spain*

[2]*Departamento de Ciencias Experimentales y Matemáticas, Facultad de Veterinaria y Ciencias Experimentales, Universidad Catolica de Valencia San Vicente Martir, Guillem de Castro-94, E-46001 València, Spain*

Corresponding author. E-mail: torrens@uv.es

ABSTRACT

Ethics versus moral was informed in a report on an apology of immorality. The syllabus of the Course/Workshop on Scientific Integrity/Ethics is reported. What can people expect if the scientific community forms an integral part of that same society? In peer evaluation systems, who does he teach people to practice a good refereeing? The objective of the Course/Workshop is that the student body obtain a general view on the integrity and ethics of science, fundamental for those who desire to begin science careers in a competitive world. Author contributions in the journal PLoS ONE are published in the periodical. Science communication in the 21st century, between naïveté and cynicism, is presented from a sociological perspective. A study on knowledge psychology was carried out, with the objective of analyzing the relationship between scientific production, knowledge spreading and psychological characteristics of the authors of at least one scientific publication. The study belongs to the Generalitat Valenciana Research Project Sitting of the Flows of Academic Knowledge, Transference Channels and Personality Traits of Researchers. The work includes a questionnaire on the physiological characteristics of the authors of one or more scientific articles.

2.1 INTRODUCTION

Setting the scene: Ethics versus moral, scientific integrity and ethics, communicating science in the 21st century between naïveté and cynicism, psychology of knowledge and psychological characteristics of authors of at least one scientific publication are fundamental, in particular, for those students who desire to begin science careers. Ethics versus moral was informed in a publication on an apology of immorality. Aluja Schuneman Hofer directed the Course/Workshop on Scientific Integrity/Ethics. Table 2.1 gives the syllabus of the Course/Workshop. The following two questions were raised.

Q1.   What can people expect if the scientific community forms an integral part of that same society?

Q2.   In peer evaluation systems, who does he teach people to practice a good refereeing?

The objective of this Course/Workshop was that the student body obtain a general view on the integrity and ethics of science, which is fundamental for those persons who desire to begin science careers in a so competitive and complex world. Author contributions in the journal PLoS ONE were published in this periodical publication.

TABLE 2.1   Syllabus of Course/Workshop on Scientific Integrity/Ethics.

Syllabus
1. Conceptual framework and review of forced/suggested references and Web pages.
2. Ethics versus moral (group analysis/discussion of Rivero Weber, 2004).
3. Analysis of general values crisis in all societies. What can people expect if scientific community forms integral part of that same society?
4. Importance of establishing a culture of respect for values and ethics from primary education to university.

TABLE 2.1 *(Continued)*

5. Abilities of the scientific community in 21st century (intellectual versus emotional intelligence).

6. Ethically unacceptable and questionable conducts (gray area in which many people shelter).

Scientific integrity applied to

7. Processes of publication.

8. Processes of financing of the science activity.

9. Peer evaluation systems (who does he teach people to practice a good refereeing?).

10. Conflicts of interest and effort.

11. Training of human resources.

12. Structuring a curriculum vitae.

13. Writing letters of recommendation.

14. Studies of environmental impact.

15. General considerations and conclusions.

Science communication in the 21st century, between naïveté and cynicism, is presented from a sociological perspective. A study on psychology of knowledge was carried out, with the objective of analyzing the relationship existing between scientific production, knowledge spreading, and psychological characteristics of the authors of at least one scientific publication. This study belonged to the Research Project of Generalitat Valenciana Sitting of the Flows of Academic Knowledge, Transference Channels and Personality Traits of Researchers. This work included a knowledge-psychology questionnaire, on the physiological characteristics of the authors of one or more scientific articles.

Earlier publicartions reported the periodic table of the elements (PTE),[1–3] quantum simulators,[4–12] science, ethics of developing sustainability via nanosystems, devices,[13] green nanotechnology as an approach towards environment safety,[14] molecular devices, machines as hybrid organic–inorganic structures,[15] PTE, quantum biting its tail, sustainable chemistry,[16] quantum molecular spintronics, nanoscience, and graphenes,[17] it was informed cancer, its hypotheses,[18] precision personalized medicine from theory to practice, cancer,[19] how human immunodeficiency virus/acquired immunodeficiency syndrome (HIV/AIDS) destroy immune defences, hypothesis,[20] 2014 emergence, spread, uncontrolled Ebola outbreak,[21,22] Ebola virus disease, questions, ideas, hypotheses, models,[23] metaphors that made history, and reflections on philosophy, science, and DNA.[24] In the present report, some reflections on ethics versus moral, scientific integrity, ethics, communicating science in the 21st century between naïveté and cynicism, psychology of knowledge, scientific production, knowledge spreading and physiological characteristics of authors of at least one scientific publication are reviewed. The aim of this work is to initiate a debate by suggesting a number of questions (Q), which can arise when addressing subjects of ethics, moral, scientific integrity, communicating science in 21st century, naïveté, cynicism, knowledge psychology, scientific production, knowledge spreading, physiological characteristics, and authors of one or more scientific publication, and providing, when possible, answers (A) and hypotheses (H).

2.2 ETHICS VERSUS MORAL

Rivero Weber informed ethics versus moral in a publication on an apology of immorality in the journal Este País (México).[25]

2.3 SCIENTIFIC INTEGRITY/ETHICS

Aluja Schuneman Hofer proposed questions and hypotheses on scientific integrity/ethics.[26–28]

Q1.   What can people expect if the scientific community forms an integral part of that same society?

Q2.   In peer evaluation systems, who does he teach people to practice a good refereeing?

Q3.   Is a fraudulent scientific a black sheep or a product of the institutional circumstances?

H1.   Figure 2.1 shows error impact in research truthfulness in case of random/systematic errors/fraud.

Q4.   Fraud?

Q5.   Truthfulness?

H2.   (Goleman, 2000). He wrote the book Working with Emotional Intelligence.[29]

H3.   Intellectual versus emotional intelligence.

H4.   Science→knowledge→power→corruption.

H5.   Ethically unacceptable and questionable conducts: Gray area in which many people shelter.

Q6.   What to do in the case of refereeing when time is pressing?

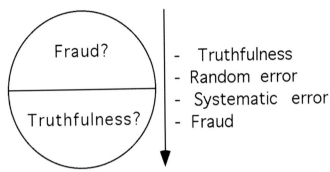

FIGURE 2.1   Impact of error in the truthfulness of research in case of error, systematic error and fraud.

Table 2.2 lists author contributions in the journal PLoS ONE: Conceptualization, formal analysis, funding acquisition, investigation, methodology, project administration, resources, supervision, visualization, writing (original draft) and writing (review and editing).[30]

TABLE 2.2   Author Contributions in the Journal PLoS ONE.

Author contributions
Conceptualization
Formal analysis
Funding acquisition
Investigation
Methodology
Project administration
Resources
Supervision
Visualization
Writing—original draft
Writing—review and editing

He proposed the following additional hypotheses on scientific integrity/ethics.[31–35]

H6. Ethics codes are important but, in the end, they are a personal subject.

H7. Actions above should be carried out in a sphere of respect and with no desire for intimidation.

He proposed the following conclusions (Cs).

C1. Ethical codes and personal implication should be promoted; the formers are a personal subject.

C2. Actions above should be carried out in a sphere of respect and with no desire for intimidation.

C3. The principle is noble and way of transmitting message/achieving acceptance should be noble.

2.4 COMMUNICATING SCIENCE IN 21ST CENTURY: BETWEEN NAÏVETÉ AND CYNICISM

Ariño Villarroya proposed the following hypotheses on the social invention of science.[36]

H1. (Bacon, 1620). New method: Novum Organum.[37]

H2. (Descartes, 1637). Discourse on the Method.[38]

He revised the following Lamo de Espinosa (LE)'s paradoxes (Pas) of science.

Pa1. (LE). Ontologic Pa: All science develops with an autonomous logic out of ethics.

Pa2. (LE). Science is not neutral; it is subordinated to an interest.

Pa3. (LE). Science, when it is applied, generates unexpected results, for example, nuclear waste.

Pa4. (LE). Pragmatic H: People do not know what to do with what they know.

Pa5. (LE). Ethical H: There is a distance between knowledge and wisdom.

He proposed a hypothesis on the resistances to science.

H3. Two critiques of science: Distrust and cynicism.

He proposed question and hypotheses on proposals to spread science in the 21st century.

Q1.   Are we pachyderms that expect people to come or should we go to inform them scientifically?

H4.   Principle of caution about science: It is caused by a reflexive critique.

H5.   People should reject fundamentalisms (Islamic, catholic, etc.) and cynicism.

H6.   Societies are in continuous evolution. Science should also be.

He proposed the following consequences (Cos).

Co1. People cannot simplify science. People cannot obviate the paradoxes of science.

Co2. People cannot ignore the social context of science.

Co3. People cannot ignore public; available/rights shift of time; ethical science consequences.

Co4. People must move in/no exit exists from Pas. Ends question has no exit. Exit is social/political.

2.5   KNOWLEDGE PSYCHOLOGY: CHARACTERISTICS OF ONE-PUBLICATION AUTHORS

Azagra Caro carried out a study on psychology of knowledge, with the objective of analyzing the relationship between scientific production, knowledge spreading, and psychological characteristics of the authors of at least one scientific publication.[39] This study belonged to the Research Project of Generalitat Valenciana Sitting of the Flows of Academic Knowledge, Transference Channels, and Personality Traits of Researchers. This work included a knowledge-psychology questionnaire, on the physiological characteristics of the authors of at least one scientific article (cf. Fig. 2.2).

Table 2.3 collects the knowledge-psychology questionnaire, on the physiological characteristics of the authors of one or more scientific reports. The questionnaire section Physiological Characteristics deals with one's personality and behavior. In general, it should be answered with spontaneity and without devoting too much time to every question and with the confidence that there are neither good nor bad answers. In particular, in the question of how one sees himself, it should be indicated until that point one identifies himself with every pair of adjectives, although one identify him better than the other.

B. CARACTERÍSTICAS PSICOLÓGICAS

Esta sección versa sobre su personalidad y su comportamiento. Por favor, responda con espontaneidad y sin dedicar demasiado tiempo a cada pregunta, y con la confianza de que no hay respuestas buenas ni malas.

¿Por qué realiza su trabajo?

	Totalmente en desacuerdo	Muy en desacuerdo	En desacuerdo	Ni de acuerdo ni en desacuerdo	De acuerdo	Muy de acuerdo	Totalmente de acuerdo
Porque quiero ayudar a los otros/as a través de mi trabajo	○	○	○	○	○	○	○
Porque me gusta el trabajo en sí mismo	○	○	○	○	○	○	○
Porque con mi trabajo tendré un reconocimiento social	○	○	○	○	○	○	○
Porque encuentro el trabajo interesante	○	○	○	○	○	○	○
Porque trabajo mejor si obtengo algún beneficio económico	○	○	○	○	○	○	○
Porque me preocupo por beneficiar a los otros/as a través de mi trabajo	○	○	○	○	○	○	○
Porque el trabajo hace que los demás tengan una buena percepción sobre mí	○	○	○	○	○	○	○
Porque lo disfruto	○	○	○	○	○	○	○
Porque con mi trabajo los demás sabrán lo bueno que soy	○	○	○	○	○	○	○
Porque para mí es importante hacer el bien a los demás a través de mi trabajo	○	○	○	○	○	○	○
Porque es divertido	○	○	○	○	○	○	○
Porque quiero tener impacto positivo en los demás	○	○	○	○	○	○	○

¿Trabaja usted fuera del horario laboral?

	Nunca	Casi nunca	A veces	Frecuentemente	Muy frecuentemente
En fin de semana	○	○	○	○	○
En vacaciones	○	○	○	○	○
En días laborables, pero fuera del horario laboral	○	○	○	○	○

FIGURE 2.2   Questionnaire on physiological characteristics of authors of at least one scientific publication (fragment).

TABLE 2.3   Questionnaire on Physiological Characteristics of Authors of at Least One Scientific Publication.

Physiological characteristics
Why do you carry out your work?
Do you work out of the labor hour?
Why do you work out of the labor hour?
How do you see yourself?
How do you think what you are in relation to your emotions and feelings?
How do you think that you confront situations?
With which frequency are you in the following states of mind?
What do you think about your ceative capacity?
In the last two years, have you created any artistic work in the following areas?
Till what point would you say that you behave so?

2.6 FINAL REMARKS

From the present results, the following final remarks can be drawn.

1. On a par, ethical codes and personal implication should be promoted. Ethical codes are important but, in the end, they are a personal subject. Actions above should be carried out in a sphere of respect and with no desire for intimidation. The principle is noble, and the way of transmitting the message and achieving its acceptance should also be noble.

2. People cannot simplify science. People cannot obviate the paradoxes of science. People cannot ignore the social context of science. People cannot ignore public and consider them as clients. People cannot ignore the shift of time between available and rights. People cannot ignore the ethical consequences of science. People should move in paradoxes. No exit exists from paradoxes. The question of ends has no exit. The exit is social and political.

3. It is important to know the physiological characteristics of the authors of one or more scientific publications, for the sitting of the flows of academic knowledge, transference channels and personality traits of researchers.

4. Chemistry is immersed in cultural values, which matter for science public acceptance. Signs of prejudice should not exist in a literary work. Science is seen as experimental but another theoretical one exists and classification is part of this. The artificial/natural dilemma comes from alchemy: Cause is the lack of spreading. Need for communicating is a creativity secondary effect. To create a critical conscience in people who must speak is more important than to know science.

5. People live in a fragile world and forget that economic growth is a means to a sustainable present of all humanity. Living on earth, believing that no need of concepts of enough and equity exists, is risky. People should take way of ethics based on resource conservation, etc. The knowledge of the factors hindering the translation of science education research to teaching practice remains to be solved. As educators of the professionals of tomorrow, professors have the ethical duty of providing them an integral training, where teachers should include environment protection.

ACKNOWLEDGMENTS

The authors thank support from Generalitat Valenciana (Project No. PROMETEO/2016/094) and Universidad Católica de Valencia San Vicente Mártir (Project No. 2019-217-001).

KEYWORDS

- moral
- communicating science
- nanveté
- cynicism
- knowledge psychology
- psychological characteristic
- one-publication author

REFERENCES

1. Torrens, F.; Castellano, G. Reflections on the Nature of the Periodic Table of the Elements: Implications in Chemical Education. In *Synthetic Organic Chemistry*; Seijas, J. A., Vázquez Tato, M. P., Lin, S. K., Eds.; MDPI: Basel, Switzerland, 2015; Vol. 18, pp 1–15.
2. Torrens, F.; Castellano, G. Nanoscience: From a Two-Dimensional to a Three-Dimensional Periodic Table of the Elements. In *Methodologies and Applications for Analytical and Physical Chemistry*; Haghi, A. K., Thomas, S., Palit, S., Main, P., Eds.; Apple Academic–CRC: Waretown, NJ, 2018; pp 3–26.
3. Torrens, F.; Castellano, G. Periodic Table. In: *New Frontiers in Nanochemistry: Concepts, Theories, and Trends*; Putz, M. V., Ed.; Apple Academic–CRC: Waretown, NJ, in press.
4. Torrens, F.; Castellano, G. Ideas in the History of Nano/Miniaturization and (Quantum) Simulators: Feynman, Education and Research Reorientation in Translational Science. In *Synthetic Organic Chemistry*; Seijas, J. A., Vázquez Tato, M. P., Lin, S. K., Eds.; MDPI: Basel, Switzerland, 2015; Vol. 19, pp 1–16.
5. Torrens, F.; Castellano, G. Reflections on the Cultural History of Nanominiaturization and Quantum Simulators (Computers). In *Sensors and Molecular Recognition*; Laguarda Miró, N., Masot Peris, R., Brun Sánchez, E., Eds.; Universidad Politécnica de Valencia: València, Spain, 2015; Vol. 9, pp 1–7.
6. Torrens, F.; Castellano, G. Nanominiaturization and Quantum Computing. In *Sensors and Molecular Recognition*; Costero Nieto, A. M., Parra Álvarez, M., Gaviña Costero, P., Gil Grau, S., Eds.; Universitat de València: València, Spain, 2016; Vol. 10, pp 31–1–5.

7. Torrens, F.; Castellano, G. Nanominiaturization, Classical/Quantum Computers/ Simulators, Superconductivity, and Universe. In *Methodologies and Applications for Analytical and Physical Chemistry*; Haghi, A. K., Thomas, S., Palit, S., Main, P., Eds.; Apple Academic–CRC: Waretown, NJ, 2018; pp 27–44.

8. Torrens, F.; Castellano, G. Superconductors, Superconductivity, BCS Theory and Entangled Photons for Quantum Computing. In *Physical Chemistry for Engineering and Applied Sciences: Theoretical and Methodological Implication*; Haghi, A. K., Aguilar, C. N., Thomas, S., Praveen, K. M., Eds.; Apple Academic–CRC: Waretown, NJ, 2018; pp 379–387.

9. Torrens, F.; Castellano, G. EPR Paradox, Quantum Decoherence, Qubits, Goals and Opportunities in Quantum Simulation. In *Theoretical Models and Experimental Approaches in Physical Chemistry: Research Methodology and Practical Methods*; Haghi, A. K., Ed.; Apple Academic–CRC: Waretown, NJ, 2018; Vol. 5, pp 317–334.

10. Torrens, F.; Castellano, G. Nanomaterials, Molecular Ion Magnets, Ultrastrong and Spin–Orbit Couplings in Quantum Materials. In: *Physical Chemistry for Chemists and Chemical Engineers: Multidisciplinary Research Perspectives*; Vakhrushev, A. V., Haghi, R., de Julián-Ortiz, J. V., Allahyari, E., Eds.; Apple Academic–CRC: Waretown, NJ, in press.

11. Torrens, F.; Castellano, G. Nanodevices and Organization of Single Ion Magnets and Spin Qubits. In *Chemical Science and Engineering Technology: Perspectives on Interdisciplinary Research*; Balköse, D., Ribeiro, A. C. F., Haghi, A. K., Ameta, S. C., Chakraborty, T., Eds.; Apple Academic–CRC: Waretown, NJ, in press.

12. Torrens, F.; Castellano, G. Superconductivity and Quantum Computing via Magnetic Molecules. In *New Insights in Chemical Engineering and Computational Chemistry*; Haghi, A. K., Ed.; Apple Academic–CRC: Waretown, NJ, in press.

13. Torrens, F.; Castellano, G. Developing Sustainability via Nanosystems and Devices: Science–Ethics. In *Chemical Science and Engineering Technology: Perspectives on Interdisciplinary Research*; Balköse, D., Ribeiro, A. C. F., Haghi, A. K., Ameta, S. C., Chakraborty, T., Eds.; Apple Academic–CRC: Waretown, NJ, in press.

14. Torrens, F.; Castellano, G. Green Nanotechnology: An Approach Towards Environment Safety. In *Advances in Nanotechnology and the Environmental Sciences: Applications, Innovations, and Visions for the Future*; Vakhrushev, A. V.; Ameta, S. C.; Susanto, H., Haghi, A. K., Eds.; Apple Academic–CRC: Waretown, NJ, in press.

15. Torrens, F.; Castellano, G. Molecular Devices/Machines: Hybrid Organic–Inorganic Structures. In *Research Methods and Applications in Chemical and Biological Engineering*; Pourhashemi, A., Deka, S. C., Haghi, A. K., Eds.; Apple Academic– CRC: Waretown, NJ, in press.

16. Torrens, F.; Castellano, G. The Periodic Table, Quantum Biting its Tail, and Sustainable Chemistry. In *Chemical Nanoscience and Nanotechnology: New Materials and Modern Techniques*; Torrens, F., Haghi, A. K., Chakraborty, T., Eds.; Apple Academic–CRC: Waretown, NJ, in press.

17. Torrens, F.; Castellano, G. Quantum Molecular Spintronics, Nanoscience and Graphenes. In *Molecular Physical Chemistry*; Haghi, A.VK., Ed.; Apple Academic– CRC: Waretown, NJ, in press.

18. Torrens, F.; Castellano, G. Cancer and Hypotheses on Cancer. In *Molecular Chemistry and Biomolecular Engineering: Integrating Theory and Research with Practice*; Pogliani, L., Torrens, F., Haghi, A. K., Eds.; Apple Academic–CRC: Waretown, NJ, in press.

19. Torrens, F.; Castellano, G. Precision Personalized Medicine from Theory to Practice: Cancer. In *Molecular Physical Chemistry*; Haghi, A. K., Ed.; Apple Academic–CRC: Waretown, NJ, in press.

20. Torrens, F.; Castellano, G. AIDS Destroys Immune Defences: Hypothesis. *New Front. Chem.* **2014**, *23*, 11–20.

21. Torrens-Zaragozá, F.; Castellano-Estornell, G. Emergence, Spread and Uncontrolled Ebola Outbreak. *Basic Clin. Pharmacol. Toxicol.* **2015**, *117* (Suppl. 2), 38–38.

22. Torrens, F.; Castellano, G. 2014 Spread/Uncontrolled Ebola Outbreak. *New Front. Chem.* **2015**, *24*, 81–91.

23. Torrens, F.; Castellano, G. Ebola Virus Disease: Questions, Ideas, Hypotheses and Models. *Pharmaceuticals* **2016**, *9*, 14–6-6.

24. Torrens, F.; Castellano, G. Metaphors That Made History: Reflections on Philosophy/Science/DNA. In *Molecular Physical Chemistry*; Haghi, A. K., Ed.; Apple Academic–CRC: Waretown, NJ, in press.

25. Rivero Weber, P. Apología de la inmoralidad. *Este País (México)* **2004**, *2004* (8), 46–50.

26. Aluja, M., Birke, A., Eds. *El Papel de la Ética en la Investigación Científica y la Educación Superior*; Academia Mexicana de Ciencia: México, México, 2003.

27. Aluja, M., Birke, A. Eds. *El Papel de la Ética en la Investigación Científica y la Educación Superior*; Fondo de Cultura Económica: México, México, 2004.

28. Aluja Schuneman Hofer, M. R. *Curso/Taller sobre Integridad/Ética Científica*, València, Spain, May 17-18, 2018; Universitat de València: València, Spain, 2018.

29. Goleman, D. *Working with Emotional Intelligence*; Bantam: New York, NY, 2000.

30. Tscharntke, T.; Hochberg, M. E.; Rand, T. A.; Resh, V. H.; Krauss, J. Author Sequence and Credit for Contributions in Multiauthored Publications. *PLoS Biol.* **2007**, *5*, e18–13–14.

31. Scanlon, P. M.; Neumann, D. R. Internet Plagiarism Among College Students. *J. Coll. Stud. Dev.* **2002**, *43*, 374–385.

32. Martinson, B. C.; Anderson, M. S.; de Vries, R. Scientists Behaving Badly. *Nature (London)* **2005**, *435*, 737–738.

33. Errami, M.; Garner, H. A Tale of Two Citations. *Nature (London)* **2008**, *451*, 397–399.

34. Fanelli, D. How Many Scientists Fabricate and Falsify Research? A Systematic Review and Meta-analysis of Survey Data. *PLoS ONE* **2009**, *4*, e5738–1–11.

35. Elliott, K. C.; Resnik, D. B. Scientific Reproducibility, Human Error, and Public Policy. *BioScience* **2015**, *65*, 5–6.

36. Arino Villarroya, A. Entre la candidesai el cinisme: Comunicar la ciencia en el segle XXI. *Metode* **2019**, *100* (1), 38–45

37. Bacon, F. *Novum Organum*; John Bill: London, UK, 1620.

38. Descartes, R. *Discours de la Méthod: Pour Bien Conduire sa Raison, et Chercher la Vérité dans les Sciences*; Ian Maire: Leyde, The Netherlands, 1637.

39. Azagra Caro, J. M. Personal Communication.

CHAPTER 3

LOLIOLIDE, LACTONES, BUDLEIN A, CALEIN C: PROTECTION AND PHYTOTHERAPY

FRANCISCO TORRENS[1*] and GLORIA CASTELLANO[2]

[1]*Institut Universitari de Ciència Molecular, Universitat de València, Edifici d'Instituts de Paterna, P. O. Box 22085, E-46071 València, Spain*

[2]*Departamento de Ciencias Experimentales y Matemáticas, Facultad de Veterinaria y Ciencias Experimentales, Universidad Catolica de Valencia San Vicente Mártir, Guillem de Castro-94, E-46001 València, Spain*

Corresponding author. E-mail: torrens@uv.es

ABSTRACT

Loliolide is a monoterpenoid hydroxylactone found in many algae, for example, freshwater green algae *Prasiola japonica*. Loliolide and compounds in *P. japonica* were not studied systematically with respect to skin pharmacology. In Asteraceae, the presence of sesquiterpene lactones, the taxonomic characteristic of the family, is related to many bioactivities. The major compounds credited to the pharmacological effects are germacranolides and chromenes. The cytotoxic activities of the germacranolides present in *Calea uniflora* are effective versus leukemia cell line U937. Antileishmanial activity of chromenes isolated from *C. pinnatifida* is effective versus *Leishmania amazonensis*, and antitrypanosomal activity, versus *Trypanosoma cruzi*. The 10 characteristics of a phytomedicine, and the procedures and observances for Good Manufacturing Practices from raw material to product is proposed.

Budlein A may interfere with inflammasome assembly given signal 1 already occurred. A sesquiterpene lactone, calein C, was isolated from *Calea pinnatifida*, and its chemical structure, characterized by spectroscopic and spectrometric analysis. The neurodegenerative diseases are usually distinguished as disorders with loss of neurones. Since the history of mankind, plants not only provided shelter, fuel, and food but also they were always a vital source of folk medicine imparting health benefits.

3.1 INTRODUCTION

In Asteraceae, the presence of sesquiterpene lactones (STLs), the taxonomic characteristic of the family, is related to many bioactivities (e.g., antiparasitic, antiinflammatory, antileishmanial, antitrypanosomal, antimicrobial, cytotoxic activities). The major compounds credited to the pharmacological effects are germacranolides and chromenes. Previous studies showed that the cytotoxic activities of the germacranolides present in *Calea uniflora* are effective versus leukemia cell line U937. Antileishmanial activity of chromenes isolated from *C. pinnatifida* is effective versus *Leishmania amazonensis*, and antitrypanosomal activity, versus *Trypanosoma cruzi*.

Ganoderma was reviewed as a cancer immunotherapy.[1]

Earlier publications classified 31 STLs.[2,3] It was informed the tentative mechanism of action, resistance of artemisinin (ART) derivatives (ARTDs),[4] reflections, proposed molecular mechanism of bioactivity, resistance,[5] chemical and biological screening approaches, phytopharmaceuticals,[6] chemical components from *Artemisia austro-yunnanensis*, antiinflammatory effects, lactones,[7] information entropy-based classification of triterpenoids and steroids from *Ganoderma*,[8] cultural interbreeding in indigenous and scientific ethnopharmacology,[9] ethnobotanical studies of medicinal plants, underutilized wild edible plants, food, medicine,[10] and biodiversity as a source of drugs: *Cordia, Echinacea, Tabernaemontana,* and *Aloe*.[11] The aim of this work is to review the oxidative stress (OS)-protective and antimelanogenic effects of loliolide from *Prasiola japonica*, budlein A, a *Viguiera robusta* STL, which alleviates pain and inflammation in goat, calein C (from *Calea pinnatifida*), which inhibits mitotic progression and induces apoptosis, neuroprotective roles of phytochemicals, the

10 characteristics of a phytomedicine and Good Manufacturing Practices from raw material to product.

3.2 OS-PROTECTIVE/ANTIMELANOGENIC EFFECTS OF LOLIOLIDE FROM *P. japonica*

Green algae are considered as one of the representative biosources to be applied for preparation of pharmaceutical, nutraceutical, and cosmoceutical products. *Prasiola japonica* is freshwater green algae with a lot of compounds, for example, (–)-loliolide (Fig. 3.1), methylpyrazine, 1-hydroxy-2-propanone, diisopropylamine, 1,6-dihydro-6-oxo-3-pyridinecarboxamide, mannitol, mannose, and glucitol, according to gas chromatography/mass spectrometric (GC/MS) analysis. Of them, loliolide results as an active component in green algae with a number of bioroles (e.g., antiaging, antiviral, antiinflammatory activities). However, the effects of freshwater green algae components, loliolide and *P. japonica* ethanol (EtOH) extract (PjEE), on the skin were not studied extensively. The OS-protective effects of loliolide and PjEE were investigated in human keratinocyte HaCaT cells.[12] To do this, the effects of loliolide and PjEE on the expression of antioxidant protein nuclear factor (erythroid-derived 2)-like 2 (NRF2)-Kelch-like ECH-associated protein 1 (KEAP1) signalling pathway proteins were confirmed by Western blot. The expression of genes encoding matrix metalloproteinases (MMPs) was confirmed by reverse transcription-polymerase chain reaction (RT-PCR) and real-time PCR analyses, and cell viability was determined by 3-(4,5-dimethylthiazol-2-yl)-2,5-diphenyltetrazolium bromide (MTT) assay. Mouse melanoma B16F10 cells were used to assess the antimelanogenic effects of loliolide and PjEE measuring level of melanin content and secretion. The expression of melanocortin-1 receptor (MC1R) proteins related to melanogenesis was confirmed by Western blot.

3.3 BUDLEIN A, A *Viguiera robusta* STL, ALLEVIATES PAIN/ INFLAMMATION IN GOAT

Budlein A (Fig. 3.2), an SQL from *Viguiera robusta*, alleviates pain and inflammation in a model of acute gout arthritis in mice.[13]

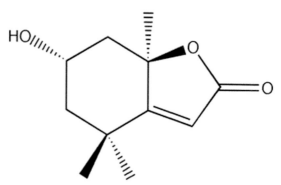

FIGURE 3.1   Molecular structure of loliolide.

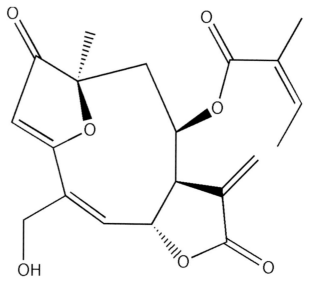

FIGURE 3.2   Chemical structure of Budlein A.

3.4   CALEIN C (*C. pinnatifida*) INHIBITS MITOTIC PROGRESSION/INDUCES APOPTOSIS

Calein C, an STL isolated from *aruca*, *cipó cruz* or *quebra-tudo Calea pinnatifida* (Asteracee), inhibits mitotic progression and induces apoptosis in MCF-7 cells. It was proposed that the isolated compound presents the structure of calein C (Fig. 3.3).[14]

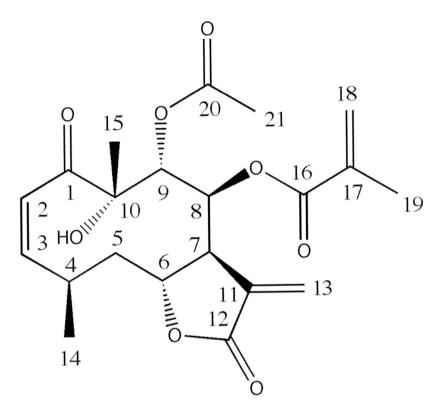

FIGURE 3.3 Calein C chemical structure isolated from *Calea pinnatifida*.

3.5 NEUROPROTECTIVE ROLES OF PHYTOCHEMICALS

It is necessary to develop new and more effective therapeutic strategies to combat devastating neurodegenerative diseases (NDs). Fighting chronic disease by phytochemicals or herbal medicine became a hot topic, and numerous studies via phytochemicals for treating NDs were published. The neuroprotective roles of phytochemicals were reviewed, emphasizing the importance of phytochemicals (Fig. 3.4) in Alzheimer's (AD) and Parkinson's (PD) diseases, in particular the potential mechanism of action of the natural compounds.[15]

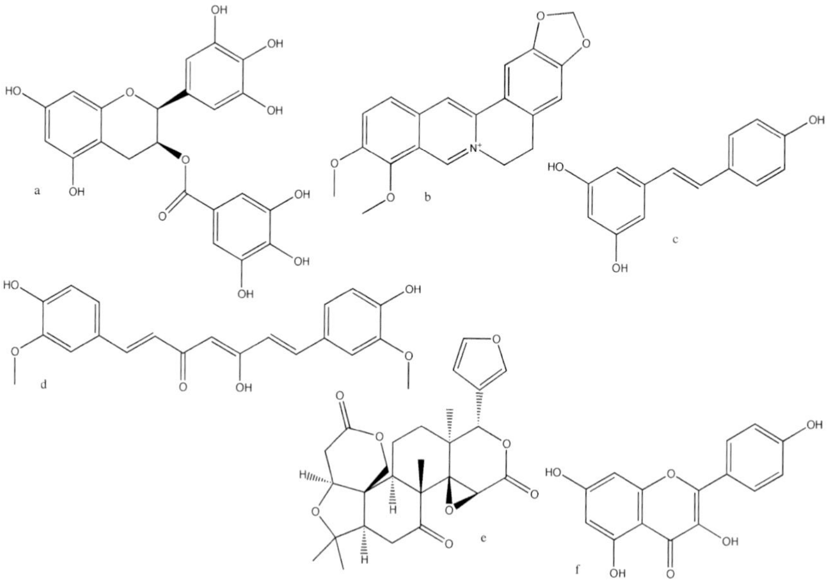

FIGURE 3.4 (a) Epigallocatechin-3-galate, (b) berberin, (c) resveratrol, (d) curcumin, (e) limonoid, and (f) quercetin.

3.6   THE 10 CHARACTERISTICS OF A PHYTOMEDICINE

Lozoya Legorreta proposed the 10 characteristics of a phytomedicine.[16]

1. They are elaborated from medicinal plants that were used in an empirical way, for a long time, in the framework of the so called Traditional or Popular Medicines and count with a case history of ethnomedical information that supports the security of their use and low toxicity.
2. They conform a new category of medicines elaborated from complex natural extracts and products obtained from plants, without combinations with other active compounds from chemical synthesis origin and with the minimum of excipients required for their formulation.
3. They are elaborated with extracts that contain numerous biologically active components that, frequently, present synergic effects on several systems of the human body.

4. The extracts with which they are elaborated were previously subjected to chimiopharmacological studies that generated new scientific information, or that validate the properties and actions described in the traditional use of the plants from which they come.

5. They are products standardized in their quantity of active principle, which allows suitably establishing their suitable dosage and pharmaceutical presentation, and were reason of controlled and randomized clinical studies that guarantee their security and therapeutic effectiveness.

6. They count with the methods of quality control demanded for all medicines, which are applied throughout their process of elaboration and commercialization.

7. Mostly are products that are used in the symptomatological handling of chronic ailments or dysfunctions that require lengthy treatments, frequently accompanied by other therapeutic measures, for example, diet, exercise, hygienic regimens, etc.

8. Their administration is carried out oral or topically in schemes of treatment established in traditional phytotherapy and aromatherapy.

9. Generally, they lack toxicity and collateral effects in comparison to chimiopharmaceutical and specialities medicines.

10. They count with registry before the regulating authority, in a specific category of medicine according with the rules of every country, and are of free sale without prescription of the type over-the-counter (OTC).

3.7   GOOD MANUFACTURING PRACTICES FROM RAW MATERIAL TO PRODUCT

Barroso proposed procedures and observances of Good Manufacturing Practices, including[17]:

1. Validation of equipments and processes.

2. Procedures undertaking all aspects of manufacturing.

3. Registers of cleaning and calibration of equipments.

4. Control of the atmosphere of the factory, air, and water.

5. Identification of all materials and tests of raw materials.

6. Identification confirmed by comparison with a reference material.

7. Traceability (identification of batch, batch registers).

8. Reconciliation (raw materials, products, packings, and labels).

9. Analyses.

10. Procedures of release.

11. Stability tests of finished products.

12. Complaints procedures and registers.

13. Microbiological tests and dispersion of contaminants.

3.8 DISCUSSION

Budlein A may interfere with inflammasome assembly given signal 1 already occurred. Mechanistically, STLs inhibit nuclear factor κ-light-chain-enhancer of activated B-cells (NF-κB) activation by either targeting amino acid residue Cys38 of NF-κB p65 subunit or by targeting the upstream enzyme inhibitor of κB (IκB) kinase. Concerning inflammasome assembly, treatment with parthenolide [an α-methylene-γ-lactones (ML)] reduces interleukin (IL)-1β maturation by alkylating cysteinyl-directed aspartate-specific protease (caspase)-1 in the cysteine (Cys) amino acid (AA) residue at position 285 (active site of caspase-1). It is suggested that α-methylene-γ-lactone with an α,β-unsaturated carbonyl structure might share mechanisms of action. Budlein A is an α-methylene-γ-lactone with an α,β-unsaturated carbonyl structure, which is a possible explanation by which budlein A targeted inflammasome assembly. Direct targeting of inflammasome and reduction of NFκB activation is likely to explain the in vitro and in vivo effects of budlein A over tumor necrosis factor (TNF)-α production and IL-1β production/maturation. The reduction of monosodium urate (MSU)-induced IL-1β and TNF-α production, and the inhibition of inflammasome components of messenger ribonucleic acid (mRNA) expression are crucial to the analgesic effect of budlein A.

An STL, calein C, was isolated from *Calea pinnatifida*, and its chemical structure, characterized by spectroscopic and spectrometric analysis. It effectively inhibited the proliferation of MCF-7 cells, an oestrogen (OES)⁺ breast cancer (BC) cell line, via mitotic arrest. The antimitotic effect of calein C was associated with its capacity for reducing aurora

AURB and polo-like kinase *PLK-1* expression levels. The proapoptotic activity of calein C was evident because of its ability to reduce B-cell lymphoma type-2 (BCL-2)/BCL-2-associated X protein (BAX) *BCL-2/ BAX* ratio. The NDs are usually distinguished as disorders with loss of neurones. A number of compounds were tested to treat NDs, but they possess solitary symptomatic advantages with numerous side effects. Accumulative studies were conducted to validate the benefit of phyto-chemicals to treat NDs, for example, AD and PD. The potential efficacy of phytochemicals, for example, epigallocatechin-3-galate (EGCG), berberin, curcumin, resveratrol, quercetin, and limonoids versus the most common NDs, for example, AD and PD was explored. The benefi-cial potentials of the phytochemicals were shown by evidence-based, but more extensive investigation needs to be conducted for reducing the progression of AD and PD.

Since the history of mankind, plants not only provided shelter, fuel, and food but also they were always a vital source of folk medicine imparting health benefits. Because of the high cost and safety of pharmaceutical medicine, renewed interest exists in the use of plants/ herbs as a food and medicine. The medicinal products obtained from a number of plants are considered safer. Eighty percent of the world's population, especially in Africa and South Asia, depends on tradi-tional medicine, mainly the plant-derived natural products (NPs) and phytomedicines, to accomplishing their basic healthcare needs. Many food and medicinal plants, especially aromatic herbs and spices, were evaluated for nutrapharmaceutical potential because of containing a wide array of natural bioactive compounds (NBCs) and new chemical entities (NCEs).

3.9 FINAL REMARKS

From the present results and discussion, the following final remarks can be drawn:

1. Challenges of algae follow: a) improvement in the systems of search and detection of algae species and active compounds; b) improvement in the knowledge of algae genome to know production routes of different compounds; c) rational use

of information with objective of a sustainable production of foods, health, and energy; d) optimization of the processes of production of biomass (via design of efficient bioreactors); e) process optimization of algae-compounds recovery/ purification (via environmentally friendly processes/solvents); f) design of biorefineries that allow the rational use of all produced resources, for example, residues reuse; g) search for applications in which algae (or residues) be economically profitable beside tradition; h) design of economic/ecological strategies that allow improving the joint work of different species.

2. Budlein A reduced pain and inflammation in a model of acute gout arthritis in mice. It is likely that molecules with the ability of targeting nuclear factor κ-light-chain-enhancer of activated B-cells activation and inflammasome assembly, for example, budlein A, are interesting approaches to treat gout flares.

3. Calein C is a promising antimitotic agent that should be considered for further in vivo studies.

4. Some most commonly used naturally available phytochemicals that can be used to treat neurodegenerative diseases were reviewed. The phytochemicals protect versus neuronal damage and a number of pathways via which the phytochemicals protect versus neurodegenerative diseases were explained. The potential benefits of the phytochemicals were studied, but more extensive studies need to be conducted in order to establish the long-term effects and efficacy of using phytochemicals as therapeutics for neurodegenerative diseases.

ACKNOWLEDGMENTS

The authors acknowledge support from Generalitat Valenciana (Project No. PROMETEO/2016/094) and Universidad Católica de Valencia *San Vicente Mártir* (Project No. 2019-217-001).

KEYWORDS

- antioxidant
- antimelanogenesis
- *Prasiola japonica*
- knee pain
- joint pain
- gout treatment
- rheumatic disease

REFERENCES

1. Cao, Y.; Xu, X.; Liu, S.; Huang, L.; Gu, J. *Ganoderma*: A Cancer Immunotherapy Review. *Front. Pharmacol.* **2018,** *9*, 1217–1-14.

2. Castellano, G.; Redondo, L.; Torrens, F. QSAR of Natural Sesquiterpene Lactones as Inhibitors of Myb-Dependent Gene Expression. *Curr. Top. Med. Chem.* **2017,** *17*, 3256–3268.

3. Torrens, F.; Redondo, L.; León, A.; Castellano, G. Structure–Activity Relationships of Cytotoxic Lactones as Inhibitors and Mechanisms of Action. *Curr. Drug Discov. Technol.*, in press.

4. Torrens, F.; Redondo, L.; Castellano, G. Artemisinin: Tentative Mechanism of Action and Resistance. *Pharmaceuticals* **2017,** *10*, 20–4-4.

5. Torrens, F.; Redondo, L.; Castellano, G. Reflections on Artemisinin, Proposed Molecular Mechanism of Bioactivity and Resistance. In *Applied Physical Chemistry with Multidisciplinary Approaches*; Haghi, A. K., Balköse, D., Thomas, S., Eds; Apple Academic–CRC: Waretown, NJ, 2018, pp 189–215.

6. Torrens, F.; Castellano, G. Chemical/Biological Screening Approaches to Phytopharmaceuticals. In *Research Methods and Applications in Chemical and Biological Engineering*; Pourhashemi, A., Deka, S. C., Haghi, A. K., Eds; Apple Academic–CRC: Waretown, NJ, 2018, pp 189–215.

7. Torrens, F.; Castellano, G. Chemical Components from Artemisia Austro-yunnanensis: Antiinflammatory Effects and Lactones. In *Molecular Chemistry and Biomolecular Engineering: Integrating Theory and Research with Practice*; Pogliani, L., Torrens, F., Haghi, A. K., Eds; Apple Academic–CRC: Waretown, NJ, in press.

8. Castellano, G.; Torrens, F. Information Entropy-based Classification of Triterpenoids and Steroids from *Ganoderma*. *Phytochemistry* **2015**, *116*, 305–313.

9. Torrens, F.; Castellano, G. Cultural Interbreeding in Indigenous/Scientific Ethnopharmacology. In *Research Methods and Applications in Chemical and Biological Engineering*; Pourhashemi, A., Deka, S. C., Haghi, A. K., Eds; Apple Academic–CRC: Waretown, NJ, in press.

10. Torrens, F.; Castellano, G. Ethnobotanical Studies of Medicinal Plants: Underutilized Wild Edible Plants, Food, and Medicine. In *Molecular Chemistry and Biomolecular Engineering: Integrating Theory and Research with Practice*; Pogliani, L., Torrens, F., Haghi, A. K., Eds; Apple Academic–CRC: Waretown, NJ, in press.

11. Torrens, F.; Castellano, G. Biodiversity as a Source of Drugs: Cordia, Echinacea, Tabernaemontana and Aloe. In: *Green Chemistry and Biodiversity: Principles, Techniques, and Correlations*; Aguilar, C. N., Ameta, S. C., Haghi, A. K., Eds. Apple Academic–CRC: Waretown, NJ, in press.

12. Park, S. H.; Choi, E.; Kim, S.; Kim, D. S.; Kim, J. H.; Chang, S.; Choi, J. S.; Park, K. J.; Roh, K. B.; Lee, J.; Yoo, B. C.; Cho, J. Y. Oxidative Stress-protective and AntiMelanogenic Effects of Loliolide and Ethanol Extract from Fresh Water Green Algae, *Prasiola japonica*. *Int. J. Mol. Sci.* **2018**, *19*, 2825–1-15.

13. Fattori, V.; Zarpelon, A. C.; Staurengo-Ferrari, L.; Borghi, S. M.; Zaninelli, T. H.; Da Costa, F. B.; Alves-Filho, J. C.; Cunha, T. M.; Cunha, F. Q.; Casagrande, R.; Arakawa, N. S.; Verri,W. A., Jr. Budlein A, A Sesquiterpene Lactone from *Viguiera robusta*, Alleviates Pain and Inflammation in a Model of Acute Gout Arthritis in Mice. *Front. Pharmacol.* **2018**, *9*, 011076.

14. Caldas, L. A.; Horvath, R. O.; Ferreira-Silva, G. Á.; Ferreira, M. J. P.; Ionta, M.; Sartorelli, P. Calein C, A Sesquiterpene Lactone Isolated from *Calea pinnatifida* (Asteraceae), Inhibits Mitotic Progression and Induces Apoptosis in MCF-7 cells. *Front. Pharmacol.* **2018**, *9*, 01191.

15. Velmurugan, B. K.; Rathinasamy, B.; Lohanathan, B. P.; Thiyagarajan, V.; Weng, C. F. Neuroprotective Role of Phytochemicals. *Molecules* **2018**, *23*, 2485–1-15.

16. Lozoya Legorreta, X. Personal Communication.

17. Barroso, C. Produtos de Saúde à Base de Plantas: Boas Práticas de Fabrico Desde a Matéria-Prima Até Ao Produto Acabado. *Revista de Fitoterapia* **2009**, *9* (S1), 39–41.

CHAPTER 4

CLINICAL TRANSLATIONAL RESEARCH: CANCER, DIABETES, CARDIOVASCULAR DISEASE

FRANCISCO TORRENS[1*] and GLORIA CASTELLANO[2]

[1]*Institut Universitari de Ciència Molecular, Universitat de València, Edifici d'Instituts de Paterna, P. O. Box 22085, E-46071 València, Spain*

[2]*Departamento de Ciencias Experimentales y Matemáticas, Facultad de Veterinaria y Ciencias Experimentales, Universidad Catolica de Valencia San Vicente Mártir, Guillem de Castro-94, E-46001 València, Spain*

Corresponding author. E-mail: torrens@uv.es

ABSTRACT

After *European Society for Medical Oncology Congress*, Lluch Hernández organized *I Day on Clinical Translational Research Post-ESMO 2018*. The post-congress resulted in an update on digestive, melanoma, lung, genitourinary, gynecological, head and neck, breast, and miscellany tumors. Navarro Pérez organized *III Day* on Research in prediabetes, diabetes, and cardiovascular disease. Obesity, genes, and age could cause diabetes that could produce cancer. There are more diabetic men than women but diabetic women have more obesity index. Is a gender perspective needed? The main studies of prevention of diabetes were not performed with a gender focus. An egalitarian participation by sexes is needed in any type of studies and a differentiated analysis. The treatment of diabetes should be global, early, and pursues to prevent, delay, or avoid chronic complications.

Certain hypoglycemiants can, besides preventing, delay or avoid chronic complications.

4.1 INTRODUCTION

After *European Society for Medical Oncology* (ESMO) *Congress* (Munich, Germany, 2018), Lluch Hernández organized *I Day on Clinical Translational Research Post-ESMO 2018*. The post-congress resulted in an update on digestive, melanoma, lung, genitourinary, gynecological, head and neck (HNTs), breast, and miscellany tumors.

Navarro Pérez organized *III Day* on Research in prediabetes (PD), diabetes, and cardiovascular disease (CVD). Hypotheses were proposed.

H1.   (Pomares). Obesity, genes, age → diabetes → cancer.

H2.   (Pomares). More diabetic men than women exist but diabetic women have more obesity index.

In PD, is a gender perspective necessary? The main studies of prevention of diabetes have not been carried out with a gender focus. An egalitarian participation by sexes in any type of studies and a differentiated analysis would be necessary. The treatment of diabetes should be global, early, and pursues to prevent, delay, or avoid chronic complications. Certain hypoglycemiants can, besides preventing, delay or avoid chronic complications.

In earlier publications, the modeling of complex multicellular systems and tumor-immune cells competition,[1] information theoretic entropy for molecular classification of oxadiazolamines as potential therapeutic agents,[2] molecular classification of 5-amino-2-aroylquinolines and 4-ar oyl-6,7,8-trimethoxyquinolines as highly potent tubulin polymerization inhibitors,[3] polyphenolic phytochemicals in cancer prevention, therapy, bioavailability versus bioefficacy,[4] molecular classification of antitubulin agents with indole ring binding at colchicine-binding site,[5] molecular classification of 2-phenylindole-3-carbaldehydes as potential antimitotic agents in human breast cancer cells,[6] cancer, its hypotheses,[7] precision personalized medicine (PPM) from theory to practice and cancer[8] was informed. It was reported how human immunodeficiency virus/acquired immunodeficiency syndrome (HIV/AIDS) destroy immune defences, hypothesis,[9] 2014 emergence, spread, uncontrolled Ebola outbreak,[10,11] and Ebola virus disease, questions, ideas, hypotheses, and models.[12]

The present report reviews clinical translational research on cancer, and research on PD, diabetes, and CVD. The aim of this chapter is to initiate a debate by suggesting a number of questions (Q), which can arise when addressing subjects of digestive, melanoma, lung, genitourinary, gynecological, NHTs, breast, and miscellany tumors, PD, gender perspective, diabetes, aging CVD, and hypotheses on updating, cancer and diabetes, in different fields, and providing, when possible, answers (A) and hypotheses (H).

4.2 UPDATING ON DIGESTIVE, MELANOMA, LUNG, AND GENITOURINARY TUMORS

Lluch Hernández organized *I Day on Clinical Translational Research Post-ESMO 2018*.[13] In Round Table 1 on updating on digestive/melanoma/lung/genitourinary tumors, Richart Aznar proposed Q/A on digestive tumors.[14]

Q1. Immunotherapies in metastatic colorectal cancer (mCRC): Changing the landscape?

Q2. Can physicians really make a cold tumor hot?

Q3. Are people in view of a new standard of first-line treatment of advanced anal cancer?

A3. Obtained results seem that yes.

Soriano raised the following question on updating on melanoma.

Q4. Who did they discontinue study therapy?

Insa proposed the following questions and answers on updating on lung tumors.

Q5. Why not to measure protein IHC?

Q6. Mesenchymal-epithelial transition (MET) growth factor receptor?

Q7. Crizotinib?

Q8. What is the role of Bevacizumab?

Q9. Is the mutational charge of peripheral blood determinant?

A9. It will be answered.

Caballero proposed questions and answers on updating on genitourinary tumors.

Q10. Does not it increase the complications of radical cystectomy?

Q11. Is pembrolizumab good enough to beat the 25–35% pathologic complete response (pCR) rate?

Q12. What is new in adjuvancy?

Q13. Do these results support Avelumab + Axitinib therapy?

Q14. Renal cancer: What is new in adjuvancy?

Q15. Benefit of surgical and ablative metastasectomy for results?

Q16. What do you mean by risk or volume?

Q17. Does low-risk metastatic hormone-naïve prostate cancer (mHNPC) benefit from Abiraterone?

A17. All patients should benefit from Abiraterone/Enzalutamide.

Q18. Abiraterone + androgen deprivation therapy (ADT), should physicians offer it to patients?

4.3 UPDATING ON GYNECOLOGICAL/HEAD AND NECK/ BREAST/MISCELLANY TUMORS

In Round Table 2 on updating on gynecological, HNTs, breast, and miscellany tumors, Corbellas Aparicio raised Qs on gynecological tumors.[18]

Q1. Hyperthermic intraperitoneal chemotherapy (HIPEC): Is there a role in ovarian cancer (OC)?

Q2. What is new in the management of OC?

Q3. Trial SOLO1: Has it a good control arm?

Q4. Does tumor remain after the operation?

Q5. Why do physicians continue to treat patients with more toxic schemes?

Q6. Pegylated liposomal doxorubicina (PLD) or carboplatin (CBDCA)-PLD, possible biomarker (BM)?

Q7. ARID1A, a predictive BM?

García Sánchez raised Qs on HNTs. He raised Qs on locally advanced (LA) HNTs.

Q8. Human papillomavirus-positive oropharyngeal carcinoma (HPV⁺OC), different clinical entity?

Q9. *Cis*platin + radiotherapy (RT) versus Cetuximab + RT, lower toxicity?

Q10. Has the patient ever smoked?

Q11. Comparable toxicities given the low compliance?

Q12. Can people say that Cetuximab is worse than *Cis*platin (CDDP) in HPV⁺OC?

Q13. Are the differences between Cetuximab and CDDP kept on adjusting?

Q14. Test De-ESCALANTE, does it change physicians clinical practice?

He raised the following questions on recurrent/metastatic (R/M) HNTs.

Q15. What does it happen to patients with 1–20% expression of programed death-ligand (PD-L)1 cancer prevention study (CPS)?

Q16. What does it contribute KeyNote-048 test to clinical practice in R/M HNTs in first line?

Escoín raised the following hypothesis on updating on miscellany tumors.

H1. To evaluate general visceral afferent fibers (GVA) tumor as glioblastoma (GBM).

4.4 PREDIABETES: IS A GENDER PERSPECTIVE NEEDED?

Navarro Pérez organized *III Day* on Research in PD/Diabetes/CVD. The Hs were proposed.

H1. (Pomares). Obesity, genes, age → diabetes → cancer.

H2. (Pomares). More diabetic men than women exist but diabetic women have more obesity index.

In Round Table 1 on PD/gender perspective, Sangrós proposed Q/A/H on PREDAPS test.[22]

Q1. PD, is a gender perspective needed?

H3. (Frame and Carlson, 1975). Criteria: prevention-policies conditions for early disease detection.

Q2. Questions to solve?

A2. PD.

H4. PD risk factors (RFs): family history; type (hypoglycemia/metabolic syndrome/both); abdominal obesity; daily fruit consumption.

H5. Abdominal obesity is more important than general obesity as PD RF.

H6. Fatty liver index (FLI) is related to PD.

Millaruelo proposed hypotheses, questions and As on need of a gender perspective.

H7. Importance of PD: rise in total and CV mortality; rise in cancer risk; progression to diabetes.

Q3. (DECODE/European Diabetes Epidemiology Group, 2003). Is diabetes relevant to all-causes and non/CVDs mortality risk ?

H8. PD: affects CVDs; does not affect mortality; affects cancer depending on PD definition.

H9. PD does not affect mortality because it is a pre-disease.

Q4. Does PD affect cancer?

A4. It depends on PD definition.

H10. The effect of PD in cancer is small because it is a pre-disease.

H11. (Huang, 2014). Prediabetes and the risk of cancer: A meta-analysis.

Q5. (Huang, Cai, Qiu, Chen, Tang, Hu and Huang, 2014). Which does it give cancer to prediabetics?

A5. It is better to have changes in lifestyle.

Q6. Are there changes?

A6. Diet plus physical activity reduce or delay the incidence of type-2 diabetes (TD2).

Q7. Are there more studies?

H12. [Diabetes Prevention Program Research Group (DPPRG), 2009]. Diabetes incidence/weight loss.

H13. (Glechner, 2015). Sex-specific differences in diabetes prevention: A review/meta-analysis.

H14. PD men lose weight but women do not.

H15. Valencian women weigh more but have less diabetes.

H16. Impaired fasting glycemia (IFG) in women is not adequate because men muscle weighs more.

H17. (DPPRG, 2009). Regression from prediabetes to normal glucose regulation.

H18. Women with glucose intolerance respond better than men with glucose intolerance.

H19. RFs in men are different from women.

H20. (Welch, 2018). Mediterranean diet reduces stroke risk in a population with CVD risks.[29]

H21. (Welch, 2018). Mediterranean diet reduces stroke risk in women because they have more atherogenic effects.

H22. (Donahue, 2007). Sex differences in endothelial function biomarkers (BMs) before PD.

Q8. (Donahue, 2007). Does the clock start ticking earlier among women?

H23. (Chen, 2014). Evaluation of Finnish diabetes risk score in screening diabetes/PD.

H24. (Goldberg, 2017). Effect of long-term Metformin and lifestyle in coronary artery calcium.

H25. Women have less coronary calcium, which is good but it is not the final result.

H26. (Giráldez-García, 2015). Modifiable risk factors associated with PD in men and women.

H27. Diabetes RFs: obesity; abdominal obesity; low high-density lipoprotein (HDL) cholesterol (CHOL); hypertension; alcohol consumption in men; stronger results in men.

H28. (Rojo, 2018). Lower development of diabetes from normoglycaemia.

H29. (Rojo, 2018). Greater incidence of diabetes from impaired glucose tolerance (IGT)/IFG/both.

H30. (Rojo, 2018). Lower importance of obesity/weight maintenance/gain during observation period.

He raised the following questions without answer.

Q9. Is any PD definition different in development prediction of diabetes/complications in women?

A9. No.

Q10. Are diet and exercise effects (even Metformin) similar in women?

He provided the following conclusions (Cs).

C1.   The main studies of prevention of diabetes have not been carried out with a gender focus.

H30. One should not trust in the first results of prevention studies.

C2.   It would be necessary in any study an egalitarian participation by sexes/differentiated analysis.

H31. (Navarro Pérez). Affected women have more social vulnerability (poverty).

H32. (Millaruelo). Men treat women badly; women have no alternative than eating.

H33. (Millaruelo). It is more important the postal code than the genetic code.

H34. (Woolcott, 2018). Relative fat mass (RFM) as estimator of whole-body fat percentage.

H35. (Sangrós). RFM index of whole-body fat.

Q11. (Sangrós). Have physicians a perfect parameter of obesity?

A11. (Sangrós). No, parameters vary with age.

4.5 DIABETES AND AGING

In Round Table 2 on diabetes and aging, the following hypotheses were proposed.

H1.   Multimorbidity: From 60 to 65 years, changes of more than 16 diseases go off.

H2.   (Guthrie, 2012). Multimorbidity epidemiology: healthcare/research/ medical-education.

H3.   (Guthrie, 2015). The rising tide of polypharmacy and drug–drug interactions.

H4.   In addition, the number of drugs (10–15) goes off.

H5.   Besides, the number of interactions between drugs goes off.

H6.   Clinical risk groups (CRGs): from only diabetes to diabetes plus many comorbidities.

H7.   One disease costs €592 per year: imagine 16 diseases.

H8.   Cluster of different diseases: CVD, Parkinson's, etc.

H9.   Hypoglycemia is related to falls and frailty.

From geriatrics, Rodríguez Mañas proposed Q/A/H on tackling diabetes in elderly.

Q1. How to tackle diabetes in elderly?

H10. From unique disease to polypharmacy and polymedication.

Q2. (McCracken and Grossman, 2013). Can Google solve death (Fig. 4.1)?

Q3. Is immortality what people want?

A3. Constant longevity of 84/88 years for men/women; people are not going to live more.

H11. Medical researchers showed that continual annoyance imposes mental stresses on humans.

H12. To pursue an impossible objective causes melancholy.

H13. The objective is not immortality but life quality: lifestyle produces function.

H14. More people die because they have a disability; it is not disease but disability.

H15. Disease (Charlson index) does not explain risk of entering a hospital but functionality does.

H16. Aging causes related frailty.

H17. (Studenski, 2009). Target population for clinical trials.

H18. Strength → (reversible) Frailty → (irreversible) Disability.

H19. Physicians should act on frailty, not disability.

H20. In cancer, oncologists should act before metastasis (disability-like).

Q4. To age… but, at what price?

Q5. Frailty?

Q6. What to do?

A6. Lifestyle and asocial chronic disease (function arrest).

H21. Diabetes is not only a model that explains mortality but also aging (function arrest).

H22. 70% of diabetics are old people.

H23. Diabetes does not kill when old but at 30–35 years.

Q7. Then, what does diabetes do?

A7. To arrest functionally in 3.5 years.

H24. If mortality is measured, the program is worthless.

H25. However, function should be measured!

H26. Diabetes –impairs↔Function.

Q8. (Keynes). When the facts change, I change my mind. What do you do, Sir?

H27. (WHO, 2016). Global Report on Diabetes.

H28. (Thomas, 2017). Assessing investment return of NHS diabetes prevention program .

H29. (Thomas, 2017). Clinical challenge: Improving accuracy and subgroup-effectiveness estimates.

Q9. Lack of evidence-based principle?

Q10. Do disease and loss of function obey the same underlying causes?

Q11. What to measure?

A11. March speed; weight; frailty indices; sittings; diet.

Q12. How long does the patient take to sit and stand up?

Q13. What does the patient eat?

H30. That the patients do not live a lot but well! Remove tablets.

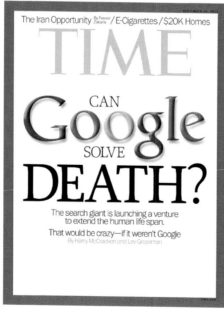

FIGURE 4.1   Can Google solve death?
Source: Ref. 38.

Viña proposed Hs/Q on diabetes, aging, frailty, and role of free radicals (FRs)/disease.

H31. FRs have two functions: signals and damage.

H32. Minimum detectable activity (MDA) in whole cell: It is not mitochondrial.

H33. Diabetes causes damage and inflammation: vascular damage.

H34. There are gender differences in longevity.

H35. Females are more protected versus FRs because oestrogens (OESTs) stimulate antioxidant enzymes production.

H36. Female rats have oxidative stress (OS) similar to males.

Q14. (Viña, 2005). Why females live longer than males ?

H37. Ovariectomized (OVX) rats have the same longevity as males.

H38. Physicians cannot administer phytoestrogens that bind feminizing α-receptor.

H39. Physicians can administer phytoestrogens that bind non-feminizing β-receptor.

H40. Physicians can administer wine and genistein (soya).

He proposed the following hypotheses, questions and answers on FRs in aging and frailty.

H41. (Harman, 1956). Ageing: A theory based on FR and radical chemistry.

H42. (Harman, 1956). Delayed aging in Frenchmen is because of wine.

H43. (Wei, 2001). Mitochondrial theory of ageing matures.

Q15. (Richardson, 2009). Is OS theory of aging dead?

Q16. (Ristow and Zarse, 2010). How increased OS promotes longevity and metabolic health ?

H44. (Kelly, 2011). Unified aging theories.

H45. (Viña, 2014). OS is related to frailty, not to age or sex, in a geriatric population.

H46. Lipid peroxidation is not related to age but frailty.

H47. (Viña, Borras and Gomez-Cabrera, 2018). An FR theory of frailty.

H48. Physiological stress: OS or damage.

H49. Reactive oxygen species (ROSs): Acting as signals increase longevity; OS decreases longevity.

H50. Exercise induces antioxidant enzymes: Administer exercise like a medicine.

H51. Exercise causes a little damage (like a vaccine) followed by a beneficial effect.

H52. People should not take antioxidants for improving performance.

H53. Exercise reverts frailty.

H54. Exercise should be multicomponent.

H55. To revert frailty will delay dependence: economic impact.

H56. If frailty halves, spending halves: do exercise (not walk).

Q17. What is the effect of antioxidants?

A17. (Viña). Antioxidants are bad for health, for example, vitamin (Vit)-C can cause cancer, etc.

Q18. (Viña). Metformin like antiageing?

A18. (Rodríguez-Mañas). It has problems of authorization.

H57. (Rodríguez-Mañas). The hypothesis is that Metformin improves ageing.

4.6   DIABETES AND CARDIOVASCULAR DISEASE

In Round Table 3 on diabetes and CVD, Redón proposed Hs and Qs on diabetes and CVD.

H1. Diabetes increases ×2 coronary heart disease (CHD), ×3 stroke; ×3 congestive heart failure (CHF); chronic kidney disease (CKD) risks.

Q1. Cluster of comorbidity after 55 years: How to diagnose?

Q2. Cluster of comorbidity after 55 years: How to act?

H2. American Diabetes Association (ADA) recommendations are for old, not young/middle-aged!

H3. (FDA, 2008). It is necessary that diabetes treatment decrease CVD (not cancer).

Real proposed hypotheses, question and answer on diabetes concept and mechanisms.

H4. Diabetes → (50% asymptomatic) atherosclerosis: multivessel; aggressive; hard to handle; early.

H5. Atherogenic dyslipidemia (AD): Triglycerides (TGs) rise; high-density lipoprotein (HDL) CHOL decays.

Q3. Why?

A3. Insulin resistance!

He provided the following conclusions.

C1. Treatment should be global/early and pursues to prevent/delay/avoid chronic complications.

C2. Certain hypoglycemiants can, besides preventing, delay or avoid chronic complications.

Górriz proposed hypotheses, Qs and As on handling diabetic kidney disease (DKD).[53]

H6. Better DKD versus worse diabetic nephropathy (DN): from DN to DKD.

H7. Necessity to decrease CV and renal residual risks.

H8. (Górriz, 2015). Nephroprotection by hypoglycemic agents.

Q4. (Górriz, 2015). Do we have supporting data?

Q5. (Górriz, 2015). Are there renal benefits beyond glycemia control in hypoglycemiants?

A5. However, in many patients CKD does not provide neuroprotection.

H9. Renal structures in the kidney: Glomerulus should be protected from inflammation!

H10. An excess of glucose accumulates in tubular cells: This excess is toxic.

H11. Glycemia control improves because it decreases glucose concentration in glomerulus.

Q6. What is the benefit of albuminuria?

A6. Glycemia control produces regression of albuminuria.

Q7. Reversibility with sodium-dependent glucose transport (SGLT)2 protein?

Q8. What problems can sclerotics have besides candidiasis in women with tendency to candidiasis?

Q9. What is the state of volume?

Q10. What is the level of arterial pressure?

Q11. Possible effects of glucagon-like peptide-1 receptor (GLP1R) agonists?

Q12. Indirect effects: improvement of microbiota?

Q13. Direct effects: effect on glomerular heamodynamics?

4.7 FINAL REMARKS

From the present results, the following final remarks can be drawn.

1. The main studies of prevention of diabetes have not been carried out with a gender focus.
2. It would be necessary an egalitarian participation by sexes in any type of studies and a differentiated analysis.
3. The treatment of diabetes should be global, early, and pursues to prevent, delay, or avoid chronic complications.
4. Certain hypoglycemiants can, besides preventing, delay or avoid chronic complications.

ACKNOWLEDGMENTS

The authors thank support from Generalitat Valenciana (Project No. PROMETEO/2016/094) and Universidad Católica de Valencia *San Vicente Mártir* (Project No. 2019-217-001).

KEYWORDS

- oncology
- breast cancer
- research in a comic style
- cancer hypothesis
- computational systems biology
- mathematical oncology
- association

REFERENCES

1. Torrens, F; Castellano, G. Modelling of Complex Multicellular Systems: Tumour-Immune Cells Competition. *Chem. Central J.* **2009,** *3* (Suppl. I), 75–1-1.

2. Torrens, F.; Castellano, G. Information Theoretic Entropy for Molecular Classification: Oxadiazolamines as Potential Therapeutic Agents. *Curr. Comput.-Aided Drug Des.* **2013,** *9,* 241–253.

3. Torrens, F.; Castellano, G. Molecular Classification of 5-amino-2-aroylquinolines and 4-aroyl-6,7,8-trimethoxyquinolines as Highly Potent Tubulin Polymerization Inhibitors. *Int. J. Chemoinf. Chem. Eng.* **2013,** *3* (2), 1–26.

4. Estrela, J. M.; Mena, S.; Obrador, E.; Benlloch, M.; Castellano, G.; Salvador, R.; Dellinger, R. W. Polyphenolic Phytochemicals in Cancer Prevention and Therapy: Bioavailability *Versus* Bioefficacy. *J. Med. Chem.* **2017,** *60,* 9413–9436.

5. Torrens, F.; Castellano, G. Molecular Classification of Antitubulin Agents with Indole Ring Binding at Colchicine-Binding Site. In *Molecular Insight of Drug Design*; Parikesit, A. A., Ed.; InTechOpen: Vienna, 2018, pp 47–67.

6. Torrens, F.; Castellano, G. Molecular Classification of 2-Phenylindole-3-carbaldehydes as Potential Antimitotic Agents in Human Breast Cancer Cells. In *Theoretical Models and Experimental Approaches in Physical Chemistry: Research Methodology and Practical Methods*; Haghi, A. K., Thomas, S., Praveen, K. M., Pai, A. R., Eds; Apple Academic–CRC: Waretown, NJ, in press.

7. Torrens, F.; Castellano, G. Cancer and Hypotheses on Cancer. In *Molecular Chemistry and Biomolecular Engineering: Integrating Theory and Research with Practice*; Pogliani, L., Torrens, F., Haghi, A. K., Eds.; Apple Academic–CRC: Waretown, NJ, In press.

8. Torrens, F.; Castellano, G. Precision Personalized Medicine from Theory to Practice: Cancer. In *Green Chemistry and Biodiversity: Principles, Techniques, and Correlations*; Aguilar, C. N., Ameta, S. C., Haghi, A. K., Eds; Apple Academic–CRC: Waretown, NJ, in press.

9. Torrens, F.; Castellano, G. AIDS Destroys Immune Defences: Hypothesis. *New Front. Chem.* **2014,** *23,* 11–20.

10. Torrens-Zaragozá, F.; Castellano-Estornell, G. Emergence, Spread and Uncontrolled Ebola Outbreak. *Basic Clin. Pharmacol. Toxicol.* **2015,** *117* (Suppl. 2), 38–38.

11. Torrens, F.; Castellano, G. 2014 Spread/Uncontrolled Ebola Outbreak. *New Front. Chem* **2015,** *24,* 81–91.

12. Torrens, F.; Castellano, G. Ebola Virus Disease: Questions, Ideas, Hypotheses and Models. *Pharmaceuticals* **2016,** *9,* 14–6-6.

13. Lluch Hernández, A., Ed. Book of Abstracts, I Jornada de Investigación Clínica Traslacional Post-ESMO 2018, València, Spain, October 30, 2018; Instituto de Investigación Sanitaria: València, Spain, 2018.

14. Richart Aznar, P. Book of Abstracts, I Jornada de Investigación Clínica Traslacional Post-ESMO 2018, València, Spain, October 30, 2018; Instituto de Investigación Sanitaria: València, Spain, 2018; RT-1.

15. Soriano, V. Book of Abstracts, I Jornada de Investigación Clínica Traslacional Post-ESMO 2018, València, Spain, October 30, 2018; Instituto de Investigación Sanitaria: València, Spain, 2018; RT-1.

16. Insa, A. Book of Abstracts, I Jornada de Investigación Clínica Traslacional Post-ESMO 2018, València, Spain, October 30, 2018; Instituto de Investigación Sanitaria: València, Spain, 2018; RT-1.

17. Caballero, C. Book of Abstracts, I Jornada de Investigación Clínica Traslacional Post-ESMO 2018, València, Spain, October 30, 2018; Instituto de Investigación Sanitaria: València, Spain, 2018; RT-1.

18. Corbellas Aparicio, M. Book of Abstracts, I Jornada de Investigación Clínica Traslacional Post-ESMO 2018, València, Spain, October 30, 2018; Instituto de Investigación Sanitaria: València, Spain, 2018; RT-2.

19. García Sánchez, J. Book of Abstracts, I Jornada de Investigación Clínica Traslacional Post-ESMO 2018, València, Spain, October 30, 2018; Instituto de Investigación Sanitaria: València, Spain, 2018; RT-2.

20. Escoín, C. Book of Abstracts, I Jornada de Investigación Clínica Traslacional Post-ESMO 2018, València, Spain, October 30, 2018; Instituto de Investigación Sanitaria: València, Spain, 2018; RT-2.

21. Navarro Pérez, J., Ed. Book of Abstracts, III Jornada de Investigación en Prediabetes, Diabetes y Enfermedad Cardiovascular, València, Spain, November 5, 2018; Instituto de Investigación Sanitaria: València, Spain, 2018.

22. Sangrós, J., Book of Abstracts, III Jornada de Investigación en Prediabetes, Diabetes y Enfermedad Cardiovascular, València, Spain, November 5, 2018; Instituto de Investigación Sanitaria: València, Spain, 2018; RT-1.

23. Millaruelo, J. M., Book of Abstracts, III Jornada de Investigación en Prediabetes, Diabetes y Enfermedad Cardiovascular, València, Spain, November 5, 2018; Instituto de Investigación Sanitaria: València, Spain, 2018; RT-1.

24. DECODE Study Group; European Diabetes Epidemiology Group. Is the Current Definition For Diabetes Relevant To Mortality Risk From All Causes and Cardiovascular and Noncardiovascular Diseases? *Diabetes Care* **2003**, *26*, 688–696.

25. Huang, Y.; Cai, X.; Qiu, M.; Chen, P.; Tang, H.; Hu, Y.; Huang, Y. Prediabetes and the Risk of Cancer: A Meta-analysis. *Diabetologia* **2014**, *57*, 2261–2269.

26. Diabetes Prevention Program Research Group. 10-year Follow-up of Diabetes Incidence and Weight Loss in the Diabetes Prevention Program Outcomes Study. *Lancet* **2009**, *374*, 1677–1686.

27. Glechner, A.; Harreiter, J.; Gartlehner, G.; Rohleder, S.; Kautzky, A.; Tuomilehto, J.; van Noord, M.; Kaminski-Hartenthaler, A.; Kautzky-Willer, A. Sex-specific Differences in Diabetes Prevention: A Systematic Review and Meta-analysis. *Diabetologia* **2015**, *58*, 242–254.

28. Perreault, L.; Kahn, S. E.; Christophi, C. A.; Knowler, W. C.; Hamman, R. F.; the Diabetes Prevention Program Research Group. Regression from Pre-diabetes to Normal Glucose Regulation in the Diabetes Prevention Program. *Diabetes Care* **2009**, *32*, 1583–1588.

29. Paterson, K. E.; Myint, P. K.; Jennings, A.; Bain, L. K. M.; Lentjes, M. A. H.; Khaw, K. T.; Welch, A. A. Mediterranean Diet Reduces Risk of Incident Stroke in a Population with Varying Cardiovascular Disease Risk Profiles. *Stroke* **2018**, *49*, 2415–2420.

30. Donahue, R. P.; Rejman, K.; Rafalson, L. B.; Dmochowski, J.; Stranges, S.; Trevisan, M. Sex Differences in Endothelial Function Markers Before Conversion

to Pre-Diabetes: Does the Clock Start Ticking Earlier Among Women? The Western New York Study. *Diabetes Care* **2007**, *30*, 354–359.

31. Zhang, L.; Zhang, Z.; Zhang, Y.; Hu, G.; Chen, L. Evaluation of Finnish Diabetes Risk Score in Screening Undiagnosed Diabetes and Prediabetes Among U.S. Adults by Gender and Race: NHANES 1999–2010. *PLoS ONE* **2014**, *9*, e97865–1-9.

32. Goldberg, R. B.; Aroda, V. R.; Bluemke, D. A.; Barrett-Connor, E.; Budoff, M.; Crandall, J. P.; Dabelea, D.; Horton, E. S.; Mather, K. J.; Orchand, T. J.; Schade, D.; Watson, K.; Temprosa, M.; Diabetes Prevention Program Research Group. Effect of Long-term Metformin and Lifestyle in the Diabetes Prevention Program and its Outcome Study on Coronary Artery Calcium. *Circulation* **2017**, *136*, 52–64.

33. Díaz-Redondo, A.; Giráldez-García, C.; Carrillo, L.; Serrano, R.; García-Soidán, F. J.; Artola, S.; Franch, J.; Díez, J.; Ezkurra, P.; Millaruelo, J. M.; Seguí, M.; Sangrós, J.; Martínez-Candela, J.; Muñoz, P.; Goday, A.; Regidor, E. Modifiable Risk Factors Associated with Prediabetes in Men and Women: A Cross-Sectional Analysis of the Cohort Study in Primary Health Care on the Evolution of Patients with Prediabetes (PREDAPS-Study). *BMC Family Practice* **2015**, *16*, 5–1-9.

34. Woolcott, O. O.; Bergman, R. N. Relative Fat Mass (RFM) as a New Estimator of Whole-Body Fat Percentage—A Cross-Sectional Study in American Adult Individuals. *Sci. Rep.* **2018**, *8*, 10980.

35. Barnett, K.; Mercer, S. W.; Norbury, M.; Watt, G.; Wyke, S.; Guthrie, B. Epidemiology of Multimorbidity and Implications for Health Care, Research, and Medical Education: A Cross-Sectional Study. *Lancet* **2012**, *380*, 37–43.

36. Guthrie, B.; Makubate, B.; Hernandez-Santiago, V.; Dreischulte, T. The Rising Tide of Polypharmacy and Drug–Drug Interactions: Population Database Analysis 1995–2010. *BMC Med.* **2015**, *13*, 74–1-10.

37. Rodríguez Mañas, L., Book of Abstracts, III Jornada de Investigación en Prediabetes, Diabetes y Enfermedad Cardiovascular, Val̀encia, Spain, November 5, 2018; Instituto de Investigación Sanitaria: Val̀encia, Spain, 2018; RT-2.

38. McCracken, H.; Grossman, L. Google *vs.* Death. *Time* **2013**, *2013*, 1.

39. Studenski, S. Target Population for Clinical Trials. *J. Nutr. Health Aging* **2009**, *13*, 729–732.

40. World Health Organization (WHO). *Global Report on Diabetes*; WHO: Geneva, Switzerland, 2016.

41. Thomas, C.; Sadler, S.; Breeze, P.; Squires, H.; Gillett, M.; Brennan, A. Assessing the Potential Return on Investment of the Proposed UK NHS Diabetes Prevention Programme in Different Population Subgroups: An Economic Evaluation. *BMJ Open* **2017**, *7*, e014953.

42. Viña, J., Book of Abstracts, III Jornada de Investigación en Prediabetes, Diabetes y Enfermedad Cardiovascular, Val̀encia, Spain, November 5, 2018; Instituto de Investigación Sanitaria: Val̀encia, Spain, 2018; RT-2.

43. Viña, J.; Borrás, C.; Gambini, J.; Sastre, J.; Pallardó, F. V. Why Females Live Longer Than Males? Importance of the Upregulation of Longevity-Associated Genes by Oestrogenic Compounds. *FEBS Lett.* **2005**, *579*, 2541–2545.

44. Harman, D. Aging: A Theory Based on Free Radical and Radical Chemistry. *J. Gerontol.* **1956**, *11*, 298–300.

45. Wei, Y. H.; Ma, Y. S.; Lee, H. C.; Lee, C. F.; Lu, C. Y. Mitochondrial Theory of Aging Matures—Roles of mtDNA Mutation and Oxidative Stress in Human Aging. *Zhonghua Yi Xue Za Zhi (Taipei)* **2001,** *64,* 259–270.

46. Pérez, V. I.; Bokov, A.; van Remmen, H.; Mele, J.; Ran, Q.; Ikeno, Y.; Richardson, A. Is the Oxidative Stress Theory of Aging Dead? *Biochem. Biophys. Acta* **2009,** *1790,* 1005–1014.

47. Ristow, M.; Zarse, K. How Increased Oxidative Stress Promotes Longevity and Metabolic Health: The Concept of Mitochondrial Hormesis (Mitohormesis)? *Exp. Gerontol.* **2010,** *45,* 410–418.

48. Kelly, D. P. Ageing Theories Unified. *Nature (London)* **2011,** *470,* 342–343.

49. Inglés, M.; Gambini, J.; Carnicero, J. A.; García-García, F. J.; Rodríguez-Mañas, L.; Olaso-González, G.; Dromant, M.; Borrás, C.; Viña, J. Oxidative Stress is Related to Frailty, Not to Age or Sex, in a Geriatric Population: Lipid and Protein Oxidation as Biomarkers of Frailty. *J. Am. Geriatr. Soc.* **2014,** *62,* 1324–1328.

50. Viña, J.; Borras, C.; Gomez-Cabrera, M. C. A Free Radical Theory of Frailty. *Free Radic. Biol. Med.* **2018,** *124,* 358–363.

51. Redón, J., Book of Abstracts, III Jornada de Investigación en Prediabetes, Diabetes y Enfermedad Cardiovascular, València, Spain, November 5, 2018; Instituto de Investigación Sanitaria: València, Spain, 2018; RT-3.

52. Real, J. T., Book of Abstracts, III Jornada de Investigación en Prediabetes, Diabetes y Enfermedad Cardiovascular, València, Spain, November 5, 2018; Instituto de Investigación Sanitaria: València, Spain, 2018; RT-3.

53. Górriz, J. L., Book of Abstracts, III Jornada de Investigación en Prediabetes, Diabetes y Enfermedad Cardiovascular, València, Spain, November 5, 2018; Instituto de Investigación Sanitaria: València, Spain, 2018; RT-3.

54. Górriz, J. L.; Nieto, J.; Navarro-González, J. F.; Molina, P.; Martínez-Castelao, A.; Pallardó, L. M. Nephroprotection by Hypoglycemic Agents: Do We Have Supporting Data? *J. Clin. Med.* **2015,** *4,* 1866–1889.

CHAPTER 5

SWINE, AVIAN, AND HUMAN FLU, AND ORIGINS OF A (H1N1) FLU PANDEMIC STRAIN

FRANCISCO TORRENS[1*] and GLORIA CASTELLANO[2]

[1]Institut Universitari de Ciència Molecular, Universitat de València, Edifici d'Instituts de Paterna, P.O. Box 22085, E-46071 València, Spain.

[2]Departamento de Ciencias Experimentales y Matemáticas, Facultad de Veterinaria y Ciencias Experimentales, Universidad Catolica de Valencia San Vicente Mártir, Guillem de Castro-94, E-46001 València, Spain.

*Corresponding author. E-mail: torrens@uv.es

ABSTRACT

Evolution is a dynamical process, which shapes the genomes of viruses and their hosts. We present patterns in mutations and reassortments, selection and pathogenesis, in the context of type-A (H1N1) influenza pandemic strain. The 1918–1919 flu pandemic killed more people than World War I. It was the most devastating epidemic in recorded world history. Known as Spanish Flu or La Grippe, the 1918–1919 flu was a global disaster. Why was it so virulent? Since 1918 and, with the discovery of the causative agent, the flu virus, a great deal of research was done to explain why it was so virulent. Could a new flu pandemic happen soon? Huge gaps exist in people knowledge and careful plans should be made to deal with a new flu pandemic, which could happen soon, within the context of an international net.

5.1 INTRODUCTION

Setting the scene: swine, avian, and human influenza, and the origins of type-A (H1N1) influenza pandemic strain. Evolution is a dynamical process, which shapes the genomes of viruses and their hosts. We shall talk about patterns in mutations and reassortments, selection and pathogenesis, in the context of type-A (H1N1) influenza pandemic strain.

The flu pandemic of 1918–1919 killed more people than World War I (WWI): 20–40 million people. It was the most devastating epidemic in recorded world history. Known as *Spanish Flu* or *La Grippe*, the 1918–1919 flu was a global disaster. Why was it so virulent? Since 1918 and, with the discovery of the causative agent, the flu virus, a great deal of research was done to explain why it was so virulent. Could a new flu pandemic happen soon? Huge gaps exist in people knowledge and careful plans should be made to deal with a new flu pandemic, which could happen soon, within the context of an international net.

In earlier publications, it was informed the modelling of complex multicellular systems and tumor-immune cells competition,[1] information theoretic entropy for molecular classification of oxadiazolamines as potential therapeutic agents,[2] molecular classification of 5-amino-2-aroylquinolines and 4-aroyl-6,7,8-trimethoxyquinolines as highly potent tubulin polymerization inhibitors,[3] polyphenolic phytochemicals in cancer prevention, therapy, bioavailability *vs.* bioefficacy,[4] molecular classification of antitubulin agents with indole ring binding at colchicine-binding site,[5] molecular classification of 2-phenylindole-3-carbaldehydes as potential antimitotic agents in human breast cancer cells,[6] cancer, its hypotheses,[7] precision personalized medicine from theory to practice, cancer[8] and clinical translational research in cancer, diabetes and cardiovascular.[9] It was reported how human immunodeficiency virus and acquired immunodeficiency syndrome destroy immune defences, hypothesis,[10] 2014 emergence, spread, uncontrolled Ebola outbreak,[11,12] Ebola virus disease, questions, ideas, hypotheses and models.[13] The present report reviews a predictive fitness model for influenza, the 1918 influenza virus in search for its origins, the history of the 1918 *Spanish Influenza* pandemic, the badly called *Spanish Influenza* a hundred years later, the avian influenza as a challenge of public health, swine, avian, and human flu, the origins of type-A virus pandemic strain and North American Flu (2009). The aim of this work is to initiate a debate by suggesting a number of questions (Q), which can arise when addressing subjects of influenza pandemics and their virulence, and hypotheses on their origins, in different fields, and providing, when possible, answers (A) and hypotheses (H).

5.2   A PREDICTIVE FITNESS MODEL FOR INFLUENZA

Luksza and Lässig created a model to predict successfully flu-virus evolution from one year to the next.[14] They proposed H/Q/A on their predictive flu fitness model.

H1.   Predictive fitness model for flu is a new, systematic way to select flu vaccine strains.

Q1.   How to infect successfully humans?

Q2.   Can one predict which of the influenza-strains competitors will win the race?

Q3.   How to reach into the future?

Q4.   Which part of the system can be actually predicted and which are random?

H2.   Ideas from physics and computer science might be used.

H3.   (Darwin). Darwin's principle: survival of the fittest.

Q5.   However, what does determine how fit an influenza virus is?

H4.   Consideration (Co)1. Innovation: virus had to keep a high mutation rate in order to escape from human immune response.

H5.   Co2. Conservation: mutations should not compromise essential virus functions (e.g., protein folding).

Q6.   Which viral strains have the optimal combination of innovation and conservation?

Q7.   Would the method lead to improved vaccines?

H6.   The approach is a principled method for vaccine selection.

H7.   More comprehensive epidemiology of flu/fast-evolving pathogens that integrates antigenic phenotypes with other viral functions coupled by genetic linkage is possible.

Q8.   How does fitness depend on genotype and host environment?

H8. Flu HA-evolution predictions inform vaccine selection if they are accurate from year to next.

H9. Coupled dynamics is captured by fitness model that predicts flu evolution from genomic data.

Q9. What does one want to predict from one year to the next?

Q10. How does vaccination affect the course of influenza evolution?

H10. (Smith, 2004; Russell, 2008; Bloom and Glassman, 2009; Bhatt, 2011). Predictions are improved integrating geno/phenotypic data (e.g., specific-mutations free-energy effects, haemagglutination inhibition, neuraminidase (NA) genomics, strains geographical distribution).

H11. Antigenic adaptation–functions conservation coupling is not limited to flu but fast-adapting-pathogens generic.

H12. Systems epidemiology is based on the ensemble of phenotypes linked to the adaptive process.

Q11. Fundamental Q. How predictable is biological evolution?

A11. There is clearly no general answer to this question.

H13. The analysis shows under what auspices limited predictions are successful.

5.3   THE 1918 INFLUENZA VIRUS: SEARCH FOR ORIGINS

In search for the keys of the origin of 1918 virus hemagglutinin (HA), the gene sequences of HA subtype H1 of several strands of influence virus were analyzed.[15–20] With these data, its phylogenetic tree was built. 1918-strand samples are inscribed in that family of the flu virus adapted to man (Figs. 5.1–5.3). The distance that results between gene H1 1918 and the known avian family reflects that it was originated in an avian-flu virus strand, although it evolved in an unidentified host before emerging in 1918. It supports the statement the fact that an avian strand of the same period conserved in a brant goose (Alaska, 1917) be, in evolutionary terms, far from 1918 strand and approach the viruses of modern avian flu.

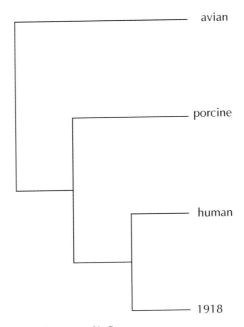

FIGURE 5.1   Familiar dendrogram of influenza.

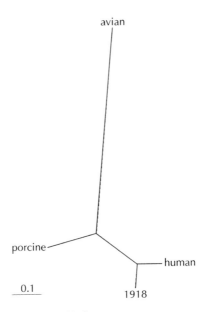

FIGURE 5.2   Familiar radial tree of influenza.

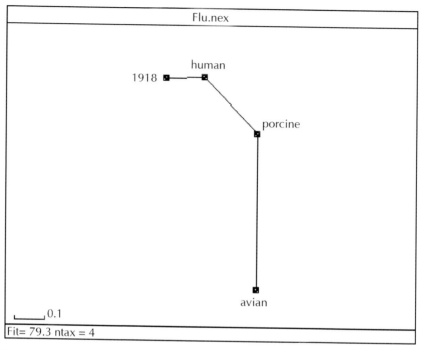

FIGURE 5.3 Familiar splits graph of influenza.

5.4 HISTORY OF THE 1918 SPANISH INFLUENZA PANDEMIC

1918–1919 flu pandemic killed more people than WWI: 20–40 million people. It was the most devastating epidemic in recorded world history. Known as *Spanish Flu* or *La Grippe*, 1918–1919 flu was a global disaster. Since then and, with the discovery of the causative agent, the flu virus, a great deal of research was done to explain why it was so virulent. Huge gaps exist in people knowledge and careful plans should be made to deal with a new flu pandemic, which could happen soon, within the context of an international net. García-Robles and Ruigrok proposed Q/H.[21]

Q1.   Why was it so virulent?

Q2.   Could a new flu pandemic happen soon?

H1.   Pigs are a basic place for mixing human/bird flu strains resulting hybrids that could infect men.

H2. Wild aquatic birds maintain the reservoir of the influence viruses for birds and mammals.

H3. Viral subtype appearance with HA different from species' proper implies that acquired immunity does not protect.

Q3. Were Has-causing pandemics able to adapt themselves fast or has any subtype the same risk?

H4. Most were in 20–40 years while in other pandemics children/old people were the most affected.

H5. Old people presented some type of immunity acquired from some previous infection.

H6. 20–40y recruitment for WWI in places with low hygiene/nutrition favored distribution.

H7. People is near that a new influenza pandemic could spread.

Q4. Why was the 1918 influenza so virulent?

Q5. Why was the 1918 influenza so devastating?

H8. Poor life conditions at soldiers fields; absence of medicines to treat secondary infections.

H9. The oldest people presented some type of immunity acquired from some previous outbreak.

H10. Virus A of the 1918 influenza presented unique pathogenic properties related to its HA.

H11. The 1918 virus was genetically uniform and was well adapted to its human host.

H12. Flu viruses causing pandemics show great virulence because they present antigenic novelties.

H13. If HA/NA were replaced pandemic responsible strain will be more virulent than if only one were.

H14. Both proteins HA and NA were antigenically new in 1918 strain.

H15. Extreme virulence of 1918 strain was due to interferon (IFN) I inhibition by viral protein NS1.

Q6. Which genomic fragments were new in the 1918 second wave with regard to the first wave?

Q7. Till wich point was the 1918 pandemic like other pandemics?

Q8. What did it make the 1918 influenza different from the others?

Q9. Are people ready for a new pandemic?

Q10. When will a new pandemic occur?

H15. The appearance of a new pandemic could be imminent.

H16. The decay of the transmission between species can avoid the emergence of the influenza virus.

Martínez Pons informed the social impact of 1918 flu epidemic in València (Spain).[22]

Journal *Mètode* reviewed 100 years of *Spanish Flu* (Fig. 5.4).[23] They proposed Q.

Q11. How did poor life conditions at soldiers fields and absence of medicines favor fatal results?

Q12. What was the origin of the pandemic?

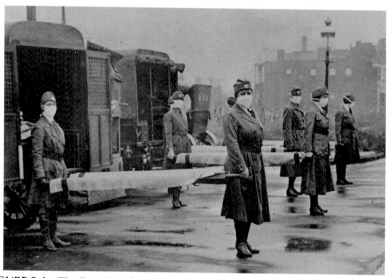

FIGURE 5.4   The *Spanish influenza.*

5.5   THE BADLY CALLED SPANISH INFLUENZA: A HUNDRED YEARS LATER

Moya organized Round Table *The Badly Called* Spanish Flu proposing Hs (Fig. 5.5).[24]

H1. In Spain, the badly called *Spanish influenza* was called *Naples Soldier*.

H2. The badly called *Spanish influenza* should be called *American flu* because it started in Kansas.

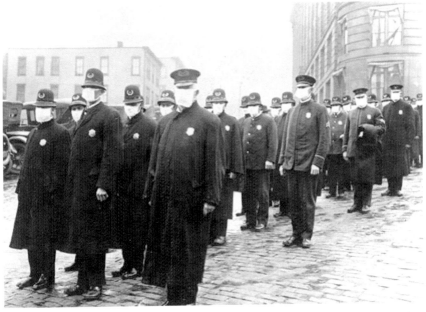

FIGURE 5.5   The badly called *Spanish influenza*.

Bernabeu-Mestre proposed questions, answers and Hs on 1918 flu pandemic lessons.[25]

Q1. What do people know about the 1918–1919 influenza pandemic?

A1. *Major health catastrophe of* 20th *century:* 25–50 millions deaths; greatest in 25–40y workers.

Q2. Why was it so aggressive?

A2. It coincided with WWI demilitarization.

Q3. How do people explain the magnitude of the catastrophe?

H3. (Gualde, 2006). *To Understand Epidemics: The Co-evolution of Microbes and Men.*[26]

Q4. What was the origin of the pandemic?

A4. The reservoir of influenza is wild migratory birds.

Q5.   Why the name of *Spanish influence?*

A5.   As Spain was neutral in WWI, it had a free press that could present without censure epidemic.

Q6.   How did people reacted *vs.* the pandemic?

Q7.   Are people ready for a new pandemic?

H4.   (WHO, 2012). *Pandemic Influenza Preparedness Framework.*[27]

H5.   Poverty is the breeding ground of infectious epidemics.

H6.   (Infante, 2015). *Ebola.*[28]

Q8.   (Infante, 2015). Ebola: Beginning and end?

      He provided the following conclusion (C).

C1.   The best way to face the danger of a new pandemic is to correct inequality.

5.6   THE AVIAN INFLUENZA: A CHALLENGE OF PUBLIC HEALTH

Grisolía edited *Avian Influenza* as a challenge of public health.[21] Conclusions were proposed

C1.   Avian flu is neither a new disease, nor has suffered substantial variations with regard to the way of manifesting in birds: H5N1 virus affected both birds and humans of Hong Kong in 1997.

C2.   By first time (July 7, 2006) a case of the disease was detected in Spain in a bird great crested grebe *somormujo lavanco Podiceps cristatus* in Salburua Park (Vitoria, Álava).

C3.   The fact above increases in Spain the risk of infection of both wild and domestic birds.

C4.   At the moment, avian flu is only a veterinary problem in Europe, which presents no repercussion in persons. In spite of that, the consumption of chicken and other edible birds, adequately prepared as food, supposes no risk of infection for persons.

C5.   It should be expected in the time an outbreak of avian flu, which would affect the humans if the person-to-person transmission of the virus occur, causing an epidemic and a pandemic as it happened in former occasions in the world. Present studies do to think that a massive reordering of H5N1 virus could cause a pandemic, but it is not possible to know when.

C6. Nowadays, people have more information, more technical and human means than ever, so that facing the future they should be positive and know that in Spain people is prepared with Response Plans and Protocols *vs.* a Flu Pandemic.

C7. In spite of that above, one should have present the different steps to adopt and deepen in their realization.

5.7   SWINE/AVIAN/HUMAN FLU AND A-PANDEMIC-STRAIN ORIGINS: NA FLU (2009)

Swine influenza is a pigs acute respiratory disease caused by type-A flu virus (Table 5.1). The affliction is transmitted *via* respiratory route. Swine influenza A/H1N1 is an H1N1-strain variant. Type-A swine influenza does not usually affect humans, but a recombination of different flu viruses could allow its propagation among humans. When viruses from other species infect pigs, they can interchange their genes. Coughing, sneezing or touching something infected, and carrying the hands to the mouth or nose transmit type-A swine influenza. Strain virulence depends on the changes in two proteins: HA and NA. The HA is responsible for the virus attack cells of one or other tissue. The NA allows the virus to diffuse from cell to cell. Pigs are like the goalkeepers of the virus: they pick it up from birds and transfer it to humans and vice versa, with the further difficulty that inside the pig the virus perfects itself to attack mammals. Common antivirals are effective and should be administered as soon as possible. The avian component of this *hybrid virus* (porcine, human, avian) is the most worrying one, since it makes the virus more contagious.

5.8   FINAL REMARKS

From the present results, the following final remarks can be drawn:

1. Innovation: virus had to keep high mutation rate to escape from human immune response.

2. Conservation: mutations should not compromise essential virus functions.
3. The appearance of a new viral subtype with a hemagglutinin different from the proper of the species implies that the immunity acquired in the past does not confer protection *vs.* new virus.
4. The best way to face the danger of a new pandemic is to correct inequality.
5. Avian flu is neither a new disease, nor has suffered substantial variations with regard to the way of manifesting in birds: H5N1 virus affected both birds and humans of Hong Kong in 1997.
6. A case of the disease was detected in Spain in a bird great crested grebe in Salburua Park.
7. The fact above increases in Spain the risk of infection of both wild and domestic birds.
8. At the moment, avian flu is only a veterinary problem in Europe, which presents no repercussion in persons. In spite of that, the consumption of chicken and other edible birds, adequately prepared as food, supposes no risk of infection for persons.
9. It should be expected in the time an outbreak of avian flu, which would affect the humans if the person-to-person transmission of the virus occur, causing an epidemic and a pandemic as it happened in former occasions in the world. Present studies do to think that a massive reordering of H5N1 virus could cause a pandemic, but it is not possible to know when.
10. Nowadays, people have more information, more technical and human means than ever, so that facing the future they should be positive and know that in Spain people is prepared with Response Plans and Protocols *vs.* a Flu Pandemic.
11. In spite of that above, one should have present the different steps to adopt and deepen in their realization.

ACKNOWLEDGMENTS

The authors acknowledge support from Generalitat Valenciana (Project No. PROMETEO/2016/094) and Universidad Católica de Valencia *San Vicente Mártir* (Project No. 2019-217-001).

TABLE 5.1 Pandemics of the 20th–21st Centuries.

Influenza	Spanish	Asiatic	Hong Kong	Hong Kong	North American	China
Year	**1918–1920**	**1956–1958**	**1968–1969**	**1997–2003**	**2009**	**2013–2017**
Deaths	45,000,000, especially young and healthy	1,000,000–2,000,000, especially children and elderly	700,000, extended in only a month	341 (considered the future pandemic of human flu, 180,000,000 foreseen)	8768 (63,000 foreseen in UK). It is possible that swine flu be the substitute of avian flu	
Virus	H1N1	H2N2	H3N2	A/H5N1	A/H1N1	A/H7N9
Origin	Avian flu adapted to human flu by mutation	Human and avian flu recombination	Human and avian flu recombination	Avian flu	Swine flu	Avian flu

KEYWORDS

- predictive fitness model
- human influenza
- avian influenza
- public health
- swine influenza
- 1918 influenza
- Spanish influenza

REFERENCES

1. Torrens, F; Castellano, G. Modelling of Complex Multicellular Systems: Tumour–Immune Cells Competition. *Chem. Central J.* **2009**, *3* (Suppl. I), 75–1-1.
2. Torrens, F.; Castellano, G. Information Theoretic Entropy for Molecular Classification: Oxadiazolamines as Potential Therapeutic Agents. *Curr. Comput.-Aided Drug Des.* **2013**, *9*, 241–253.
3. Torrens, F.; Castellano, G. Molecular Classification of 5-amino-2-aroylquinolines and 4-aroyl-6,7,8-trimethoxyquinolines as Highly Potent Tubulin Polymerization Inhibitors. *Int. J. Chemoinf. Chem. Eng.* **2013**, *3* (2), 1–26.
4. Estrela, J. M.; Mena, S.; Obrador, E.; Benlloch, M.; Castellano, G.; Salvador, R.; Dellinger, R. W. Polyphenolic Phytochemicals in Cancer Prevention and Therapy: Bioavailability Versus Bioefficacy. *J. Med. Chem.* **2017**, *60*, 9413–9436.
5. Torrens, F.; Castellano, G. Molecular Classification of Antitubulin Agents with Indole Ring Binding at Colchicine-Binding Site. In *Molecular Insight of Drug Design*; Parikesit, A. A., Ed.; InTechOpen: Vienna, 2018; pp 47–67.
6. Torrens, F.; Castellano, G. Molecular Classification of 2-Phenylindole-3-carbaldehydes as Potential Antimitotic Agents in Human Breast Cancer Cells. In *Theoretical Models and Experimental Approaches in Physical Chemistry: Research Methodology and Practical Methods*; Haghi, A. K., Thomas, S., Praveen, K. M., Pai, A. R., Eds.; Apple Academic–CRC: Waretown, NJ, in press.
7. Torrens, F.; Castellano, G. Cancer and Hypotheses on Cancer. In *Molecular Chemistry and Biomolecular Engineering: Integrating Theory and Research with Practice*; Pogliani, L., Torrens, F., Haghi, A. K., Eds.; Apple Academic–CRC: Waretown, NJ, in press.
8. Torrens, F.; Castellano, G. *Precision Personalized Medicine from Theory to Practice: Cancer*. In *Green Chemistry and Biodiversity: Principles, Techniques, and Correlations*; Aguilar, C. N., Ameta, S. C., Haghi, A. K., Eds.; Apple Academic–CRC: Waretown. NJ, in press.

9. Torrens, F.; Castellano, G. Clinical Translational Research: Cancer, Diabetes, Cardiovascular. In *Physical Chemistry and Chemical Engineering*; Haghi, A. K., Ed.; Apple Academic–CRC: Waretown, NJ, in press.

10. Torrens, F.; Castellano, G. AIDS Destroys Immune Defences: Hypothesis. *New Front. Chem.* **2014**, *23*, 11–20.

11. Torrens-Zaragozá, F.; Castellano-Estornell, G. Emergence, Spread and Uncontrolled Ebola Outbreak. *Basic Clin. Pharmacol. Toxicol.* **2015**, *117*(Suppl. 2) 38–38.

12. Torrens, F.; Castellano, G. 2014 Spread/Uncontrolled Ebola Outbreak. *New Front. Chem.* **2015**, *24*, 81–91.

13. Torrens, F.; Castellano, G. Ebola Virus Disease: Questions, Ideas, Hypotheses and Models. *Pharmaceuticals* **2016**, *9*, 14-6-6.

14. M. Luksza ; M. Lässig, A Predictive Fitness Model for Influenza, *Nature (London)* **2014**, *507*, 57–61.

15. Crosby, A. W. *America's Forgotten Pandemic: The Influenza of 1918*; Cambridge University: Cambridge, UK, 2003.

16. Reid, A. H.; Taubenberger, J. K. The Origin of the 1918 Pandemic Influenza Virus: A Continuing Enigma. *J. Gen. Virol.* **2003**, *84*, 2285–2292.

17. Kash, J. C.; Basler, C. F.; García-Sastre, A.; Cartera, V.; Billharz, R.; Swayne, D. E.; Przygodzki, R. M.; Taubenberger, J. K.; Katze, J. G.; Tumpey, T. M. Global Host Immune Response: Pathogenesis and Transcriptional Profiling of Type A Influenza Viruses Expressing The Hemagglutinin And Neuraminidase Genes from the 1918 Pandemic Virus. *J. Virol.* **2004**, *78*, 9499–9511.

18. Tumpey, T. M.; Basler, C. F.; Aguilar, P. V.; Zeng, H.; Solórzano, A.; Swayne, D. E.; Cox, N. J.; Katz, J. M.; Taubenberger, J. K.; Palese, P.; García-Sastre, A. Characterization of the Reconstructed 1918 Spanish Influenza Pandemic Virus. *Science.* **2005**, *310*, 77–79.

19. Taubenberger, J. K.; Reid, A. H.; Lourens, R. M.; Wang, R.; Jin, G.; Fanning, T. G. Characterization of the 1918 Influenza Virus Polymerase Genes. *Nature (London)* **2005**, *437*, 889–893.

20. Taubenberger, J. K.; Reid, A. H.; Fanning, T. G. El Virus de la Gripe de 1918. *Temas (Barcelona)* **2007**, *2007* (48), 60–70.

21. García-Robles, I.; Ruigrok, R. W. Història de la Pandèmia de la Grip Espanyola del 1918. *Mètode* **2005**, *2005* (45), 73–83.

22. Martínez Pons, M. *València al Límit: La Ciutat davant l'Epidèmia de Grip de 1918*; La Xara: Simat de la Valldigna, València, Spain, 1999.

23. Mètode. Cent Anys de la Grip Espanyola: Es Compleix el Centenari D'una de les Pitjors Pandèmies que ha Patit la Humanitat. *Mètode* **2018**, *2018* (98), 1–1.

24. Moya, C.; (Ed.), La Mal Anomenada Grip Espanyola: Cent Anys després. In *Book of Abstracts*, Institut Mèdic Valencià: València, Spain, November 14, 2018.

25. Bernabeu-Mestre, J., La Mal Anomenada Grip Espanyola: Cent Anys després In *Book of Abstracts*, Institut Mèdic Valencià, València (Spain), November 14, 2018; RT-1.

26. Gualde, N. *Comprendre les Épidémies: La Coévolution des Microbes et des Hommes*, Les Empêcheurs de Penser en Rond, Le Seuil, France, 2006.

27. World Health Organization (WHO). *Pandemic Influenza Preparedness Framework: For the Sharing of Influenza Viruses and Access to Vaccines and Other Benefits*, WHO, Geneva, Switzerland, 2012.

28. Infante, A. *Ébola: Principio y Final*, Nostrum: Barcelona, Spain, 2015.
29. Grisolía, S., Ed., *La Gripe Aviaria: Un Reto de Salud Pública*; Universidad de Castilla–La Mancha: Cuenca, Spain, 2006.

CHAPTER 6

BIG DATA IN ARTIFICIAL KNOWLEDGE: MODELS FOR HEALTH AND HEALTHCARE

FRANCISCO TORRENS[1*] and GLORIA CASTELLANO[2]

[1]Institut Universitari de Ciència Molecular, Universitat de València, Edifici d'Instituts de Paterna, P.O. Box 22085, E-46071 València, Spain

[2]Departamento de Ciencias Experimentales y Matemáticas, Facultad de Veterinaria y Ciencias Experimentales, Universidad Catolica de Valencia San Vicente Mártir, Guillem de Castro-94, E-46001 València, Spain

*Corresponding author. E-mail: torrens@uv.es

ABSTRACT

Connectivity is one of the key components of competitiveness. Technology and *big data* are important for health. Relevant information *vs.* data present significant in healthcare. *Big data* is significant in health and personalized medicine. Using conventional deep learning algorithms, to build quantitative structure-activity relationship models, adds little extra intelligence compared to random forest and other commonly used algorithms. The present healthcare system is untenable. People should innovate and transform the present sanatorium into the hospital of the future: innovation in care processes, innovation in purchase processes, innovation in the way of paying, and technological innovation.

6.1   INTRODUCTION

Setting the scene: *big data* (BD) in artificial knowledge and their medical applications, for example, health and healthcare models, and their future. Here the term *artificial knowledge* is preferred to *artificial intelligence* (AI). On the one hand, *knowledge* is a term in epistemology, which is a branch of philosophy concerned with the *theory of knowledge* (Leibniz); on the other, *intelligence* comes from *military intelligence.*

Connectivity is one of the key components of competitiveness. Technology and BD are important for health and healthcare. Relevant information *vs.* data present significance in health and healthcare. The BD is significant in health, healthcare, and personalized medicine (PM). Using conventional deep learning (DL) algorithms, to build quantitative structure-activity relationship (QSAR) models, adds little extra intelligence compared to random forest (RF) and other commonly used algorithms. The present healthcare system is untenable. People should innovate and transform the present sanatorium into the hospital of the future: innovation in care processes, innovation in purchase processes, innovation in the way of paying, and technological innovation.

In earlier publications, it was informed the empirical didactics of molecular shape,[1] the phylogenesis of anthropoid apes,[2] the fractal analysis of the tertiary structure of proteins,[3] fractal hybrid orbitals in biopolymer chains,[4] fractals for hybrid orbitals in protein models,[5] the fractal hybrid orbitals analysis of the tertiary structure of protein molecules,[6] resonance in interacting induced-dipole polarizing force fields, application to force-field derivatives,[7] the modelling of complex multicellular systems, tumor-immune cells competition,[8] molecular diversity classification *via* information theory,[9] a tool for the interrogation of macromolecular structure,[10] a new tool for the study of resonance in chemical education,[11] dialectic walk on science,[12] Brownian motion, random trajectory, diffusion, fractals, chaos theory, dialectics,[13] the work with nanomaterials, reductionism/positivism philosophical, and ethical considerations.[14] The present report reviews BD in AI and their medical applications, for example, health and healthcare models, and their future. The aim of this work is to initiate a debate by suggesting a number of questions (Q), which can arise when addressing subjects of BD, who BD owner is, human behavior modeling from BD data, supercomputing being the future of genomics research, BD/open (OD)/small data in health, ethical, legal, and management aspects of research with humans, BD, and data management in technology and industry, for example, factory 4.0, OD and AI as a disruptive change, BD and health, BD opening new avenues for genomics research, AI advancing healthcare research, processes, and technology innovation in search for the health model for the future, and hypotheses on the future of health and healthcare models, in different fields, and providing, when possible, answers (A) and hypotheses (H).

6.2   BIG DATA

The relationship existing between the massive exploitation of corporative data *via* potent, delocalized and parallelized computational technologies (Fig. 6.1), and the use of the information discovered *via* AI is real, and of an extraordinary value to guarantee the survival and improve the competitiveness of enterprises, as it was not known till BD breaking (Fig. 6.2).[15] Analytics of BD in biometrics and healthcare was informed.[16]

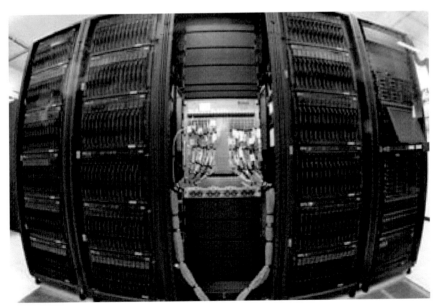

FIGURE 6.1   Universitat de València's *Tirant* supercomputer.

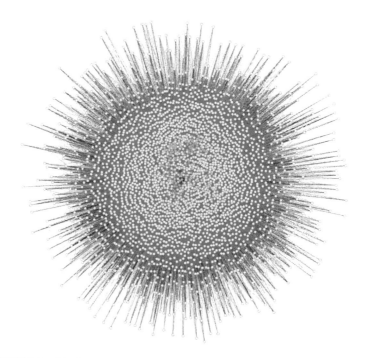

FIGURE 6.2   Big data: creating new professionals.

The following questions and hypothesis were proposed on BD:

Q1. How did International Consortium of Investigative Journalists (ICIJ) get to process information 2,600,000 TB and uncover Panama Papers case?

Q2. How can data help to fight money laundering and tax evasion?

Q3. Or to revolutionize the therapies against cancer?

Q4. How is data science transforming the market of videogames for mobile phones?

Q5. Mobile games: How did data transform the industry?

Q6. How are games built?

Q7. How are games maintained?

Q8. How do the players interact with the game?

Q9. What do they like?

Q10. What makes them quit?

Q11. How do people validate software quality in BD projects?

Q12. Are you confident that results generated by BD process are reliable/realistic/deterministic?

Q13. How data are produced, analyzed, and used in industry?

Q14. How to make money with BD?

Q15. How big is *big*?

H1. Connectivity is one of the key components of competitiveness.

6.3 WHO IS THE OWNER OF BIG DATA?

Lorenz proposed the following questions, answers, and hypotheses on BD and their ownership[17]:

Q1. What will the trends in technology and education be?

Q2. What challenges will people have to face in the next 20 or 30 years?

A2. Technological landmarks with regard to power electronics components; paradigm change in power-electronics-systems development; *Smart Factory*; future mobility.

H1. Change of paradigm in the development of power electronics systems.

Q3. Who is the owner of BD or massive data storage that are gathered anywhere?

H2. BD is a synonym of political power.

6.4 HUMAN BEHAVIOR MODELING FROM (BIG) DATA

Human Behavior Modeling and Understanding is a key challenge in intelligent-systems development. Oliver described projects that she performed over 20 years to address the challenge.[18] She gave an overview of her work on Smart Rooms (real-time facial expression recognition, visual surveillance), Smart Cars (driver manoeuvre recognition), Smart Offices (multi-modal office activity recognition), Smart Mobile Phones (boredom inference) and a Smart World (crime prediction). She highlighted opportunities, challenges, and learned lessons that could be helpful to researchers and practitioners in the area.

6.5   SUPERCOMPUTING IS THE FUTURE OF GENOMICS RESEARCH

Today, the data deluge is impacting scientists and researchers in genomics and other life sciences organizations in a profound way: (1) they are unable to manage an avalanche of data generated by more and more sources; (2) the situation is compounded because they lack the computing capacity and power to turn all the data into real scientific insights.[19] Broner proposed Q/A.

Q1.   Why is data storage crucial?

A1.   The datasets need to be stored, analyzed, and then, stored again.

6.6   BIG/OPEN/SMALL DATA IN HEALTH

Soria organized the Day BD/OD/Small Data in Health proposing the following hypotheses[20]:

H1.   In God we trust.

H2.   (W. Edwards Deming). In God we trust, all others bring data.

H3.   Volume, velocity, variety, and veracity (4Vs) model.

Peiró proposed the following questions and answer on use of data in public health[21]:

Q1.   What to do?

Q2.   To whom?

Q3.   By whom?

Q4.   Where?

Q5.   When?

Q6.   How?

Q7.   What are people talking about?

Q8.   Where are people now?

Q9.   What do people expect from BD/MEDLINE/PubMed Baseline Repository (MRB) in future?

A9.   Population stratification in chronic risk groups (CRGs); treatment monitoring; local/cloud storage; build a common database: Health-university-…

6.7 ETHICAL, LEGAL, AND MANAGEMENT ASPECTS OF RESEARCH WITH HUMANS

I Day on Ethical, Legal, and Management Aspects of Research with Humans proposed Q/H.[22]

Q1.   The ethics of research, either obstacle or guarantee?

H1.   Principle of data protection by default and from design.

   Marcos Muñoz proposed Qs/As on how to submit a project to the Ethics Committee.

Q2.   How to submit a project to the Ethics Committee?

Q3.   What are people talking about?

A3.   (1) Human beings; (2) animals; (3) biological agents.

Q4.   Why?

A4.   (1) Law; (2) protect the research; (3) necessity of being granted, published, etc.

Q5.   Who should submit a project to the Ethics Committee?

Q6.   Who is in charge of the Ethical Investigation?

A6.   The Ethics Committee of Investigation.

Q7.   How do the Ethics Committees evaluate the ethics of research?

Q8.   What to do?

A8.   Social value.

Q9.   How to do it?

A9.   Methodology, training of the research team, and adequacy of the plant.

Q10. What consequences can it have?

A10. Risks and benefits.

Q11. What should people do research into and not?

Q12. How is training justified?

Q13. What should an Ethics Committee require?

6.8   BIG DATA AND DATA MANAGEMENT IN TECHNOLOGY/ INDUSTRY: FACTORY 4.0

Automated-processes use in industry generates a great amount of information that could be expressed in useful-data form, for machines involved in productive processes, humans and the proper companies that work jointly.[23] However, despite people relying on the huge information flow, the *amount of information rises exponentially* as technology advances, and devices and *things* are connected with net. Data management is commonly known as BD, which is nothing but the capacity of *adequately picking up, analyzing, interpreting, and answering all the information*. There is one who can think that the data, despite being there, beyond the most important, constitute a diffuse and exaggerated information amalgam, which does not need to be taken into account when improving industrial processes. However, data use allows amply improving goods and services production, and sales expectations in all industries in which they were applied. Utilization of BD allows *better recognizing the weaknesses* of any industry and *better identifying their forte*, which means the possibility of significantly improving the efficiency of every one of the phases of the diverse productive processes, and all elements associated with them, from raw-materials obtaining till the moment in which the product is delivered to the consumers. Data management *via* BD and the use of Industrial Internet of Things (IoT) (IIoT) constitute the directors that allow Industry 4.0 be the most efficient industry with which people could work till now.

6.9   OPEN DATA AND ARTIFICIAL KNOWLEDGE: A DISRUPTIVE CHANGE

Soria Olivas organized II Day OD *OD and AI: A Disruptive Change*[24] proposing H on OD/AI.

H1.   (Clive Humby). Data is the new oil (comparison of BD to *Big Oil*).

H2.   (MCKINSEY, 2018). Information is the oil of 21st century and analytics, combustion engine.

H3.   (O'Reilly, 2017). *WTF: What's the Future and why it's up to Us?*[25]

H4.   (Meier, 2015). *Digital humanitarians: How is BD changing humanitarian-response face?*[26]

Puncel Chornet proposed the following hypothesis on OD and AI in the public sector:[27]

H5.   (Harari, 2018). *21 Lessons for the 21st Century*.[28]

H6.   The Trump experience has transformed liberal democracies.

6.10   BIG DATA AND HEALTH

What do Facebook, a supermarket, a bank and a hospital have in common? All generate and process BD, turning them into useful information that allows knowing better how their clients result or predicting necessity situations. All this is BD. The methods and tools can be used to improve health services and act on diseases. How? Better knowing why some pathologies appear, fitting personal and precisely diagnostics (PM), reinforcing health areas with greater risks, etc. People's life is plenty of BD. García-García presented BD keys and, especially, their health applications.[29] He proposed conclusions (Cs).

C1.   Technology and BD.

C2.   Relevant information *vs*. data.

C3.   BD in health and PM.

6.11   BIG DATA OPENS NEW AVENUES FOR GENOMICS RESEARCH

Sansom proposed questions, As and Hs on BD opening new avenues for genomics research.[30]

Q1.   What was the earliest example of digital data?

A1.   Some 30,000 years ago, in the Palaeolithic era, someone put 57 scratches on a wolf bone.

Q2.   Therefore, people are now in an age of BD, but what makes it big?

H1.   (Laney, 2001). Volume–velocity–variety (3Vs) of the growing complexity of data.

H2.   Volume–velocity–variety–veracity–value (5Vs) of the growing complexity of data.

Q3.   What is now possible?

A3.   Raw sequence data for a single genome occupies 30 GB of storage and the processed data, 1 GB.

H3.   PM: To discover or re-purpose the right drug for the right patient at the right time.

H4.   Datasets with genomic data are so rich that it becomes possible to track down an individual.

Q4.   However, whose data are they anyway?

Q5.   How are willing people to donate and share their genomic and other biomedical data?

A5.   People are willing to share data if they understand what they mean/ trust scientists using them.

6.12   ARTIFICIAL KNOWLEDGE ADVANCES HEALTHCARE RESEARCH

Ktori proposed the following hypotheses and questions on AI advancing healthcare research[31]:

H1.   (Segall). Using conventional DL algorithms, to build QSAR models, adds little extra intelligence compared to RF and other commonly used algorithms.

Q1.   (Segall). What do we have already?

Q2.   (Segall). What does our customers have?

Q3.   (Segall). Which compounds can scientists test?

Q4.   Who has the expertise to understand?

Q5.   Which phenotypes are important for the assay in development?

Q6.   Which drugs do they impact on subsets of patients?

Q7.   How do drugs impact on subsets of patients?

H2.   (Sirendi). We aim to transform the emergency medicine paradigm from rapid response to PM.

Q8.   To act on a machine-derived prediction?

6.13   PROCESSES/TECHNOLOGY INNOVATION: IN SEARCH FOR FUTURE HEALTH MODEL

Aurín Pardo proposed Q/A/H on processes/technology innovation in search for future health.[32]

Q1.   Which is the present situation?

A1.   2061: Ageing with 16.7% greater than 65 years.

Q2.   What can people do?

A2.   The three pillars of innovation: processes, technology, and value.

Q3.   To innovate in processes?

A3.   Organization by processes of a hospital: Emergency→Hospitalizati on→Tests→Examinations.

Q4.   (Porter, 2010). *What is value in healthcare?*[33]

A4.   (Porter, 2010):

$$\text{Patient value} = \frac{\text{Health outcomes}}{\text{Cost}} \tag{1}$$

Q5.   To innovate in technology?

Q6.   Which technologies are there?

A6.   Virtual/augmented reality; IoT; Smart intensive care unit (ICU); Box illumination according day hour; red/blue code; patient experience; three-dimensional (3D) printing; BD; AI.

H1.   BD-AI effects: transforming data into knowledge; improving information use; jump in clinical research.

H2.   BD-AI: personalization–prevention–participation–population–prediction (5Ps) medicine.

Q7.   Is AI new?

A7.   No, for example, *Deep Blue* won chess *vs.* Gary Kasparov; *Watson* won the quiz show Jeopardy!

She provided the following conclusions:(Cs).

C1.   The present system is untenable.

C2.   People should innovate and transform into the hospital of the future: innovation in care processes; innovation in purchase processes; innovation in the way of paying; technological innovation.

6.14   FINAL REMARKS

From the preceding results, the following final remarks can be drawn:

1. Connectivity is one of the key components of competitiveness.
2. Technology and *big data*.
3. Relevant information *vs*. data.
4. *Big data* in health and personalized medicine.
5. Using conventional deep learning algorithms, to build quantitative structure-activity relationship models, adds little extra intelligence compared to random forest and other commonly used algorithms.
6. The present healthcare system is untenable.
7. People should innovate and transform into the hospital of the future: innovation in care processes; innovation in purchase processes; innovation in the way of paying; technological innovation.

ACKNOWLEDGMENTS

The authors acknowledge support from Generalitat Valenciana (Project No. PROMETEO/2016/094) and Universidad Católica de Valencia *San Vicente Mártir* (Project No. 2019-217-001).

KEYWORDS

- artificial intelligence
- data ownership
- human behavior modeling
- supercomputing
- genomics research
- open data
- small data

REFERENCES

1. Torrens, F.; Sánchez-Pérez, E.; Sánchez-Marín, J. Didáctica Empírica de la Forma Molecular. *Enseñanza de las Ciencias* **1989**, Número Extra (III Congreso) (1), 267–268.
2. Torrens, F. Filogénesis de los Simios Antropoides. *Encuentros en la Biología* **2000**, *8* (60), 3–5.
3. Torrens, F. Análisis Fractal de la Estructura Terciaria de las Proteínas. *Encuentros en la Biología* **2000**, *8* (64), 4–6.
4. Torrens, F. Fractal Hybrid Orbitals in Biopolymer Chains. *Russ. J. Phys. Chem. (Engl. Transl.)* **2000**, *74*, 115–120.
5. Torrens, F. Fractals for Hybrid Orbitals in Protein Models. *Complexity Int.* **2001**, *8*, torren01-1-13.
6. Torrens, F. Fractal Hybrid Orbitals Analysis of the Tertiary Structure of Protein Molecules. *Molecules* **2002**, *7*, 26–37.
7. Torrens, F.; Castellano, G. Resonance in Interacting Induced-Dipole Polarizing Force Fields: Application to Force-Field Derivatives. *Algorithms* **2009**, *2*, 437–447.
8. Torrens, F.; Castellano, G. Modelling of Complex Multicellular Systems: Tumour–Immune Cells Competition. *Chem. Central J.* **2009**, *3* (Suppl. I), 75–1-1.
9. Torrens, F; Castellano, G. Molecular Diversity Classification *via* Information Theory: A Review. *ICST Trans. Complex Syst.* **2012**, *12* (10–12), e4-1-8.
10. Torrens, F.; Castellano, G. A Tool for Interrogation of Macromolecular Structure. *J. Mater. Sci. Eng. B* **2014**, *4* (2), 55–63.
11. Torrens, F.; Castellano, G. Una Nueva Herramienta Para el Estudio de la Resonancia en Docencia Química. *Avances en Ciencias e Ingeniería* **2014**, *5* (1), 81–91.
12. Torrens, F.; Castellano, G. Dialectic Walk on Science. *In Sensors and Molecular Recognition*; Laguarda Miro, N., Masot Peris, R., Brun Sánchez, E., Eds.; Universidad Politécnica de Valencia: València, Spain, in press; Vol. 11, pp 271–275.
13. Torrens, F.; Castellano, G, Brownian Motion, Random Trajectory, Diffusion, Fractals, Theory of Chaos, and Dialectics. In *Modern Physical Chemistry: Engineering Models, Materials, and Methods with Applications*; Haghi, R., Besalú, E., Jaroszewski, M., Thomas, S., Praveen, K. M., Eds.; Apple Academic-CRC: Waretown, NJ, in press.
14. Torrens, F.; Castellano, G. *El* Trabajo con Nanomateriales: Consideraciones Filosóficas: Reduccionismo/Positivismo y Éticas. In *Tecnología e Innovación Social: Hacia un Desarrollo Inclusivo y Sostenible*; Feltrero, R., Ed.; Desafíos Intelectuales del Siglo XXI No. 1, Global Knowledge Academics: Cantoblanco, Madrid, Spain, 2018; pp 11–35.
15. De la Barra Aguirre, M. Personal Communication.
16. Wang, L.; Alexander, C. A. Big Data Analytics in Biometrics and Healthcare. *J. Comput. Sci. Appl.* **2016**, *6*, 48–55.
17. Lorenz, L. *Discurs d'Investidura com a Doctor 'Honoris Causa' per la* Universitat de València: València, Spain, *February 17,* 2017.
18. Oliver, N. Personal Communication.
19. Broner, G. Supercomputing is the Future of Genomics Research. *Genet. Eng. Biotechnol. News* **2017**, *37* (3), 18–19.

20. Book of Abstracts, Big/Open/Small Data en Salud, Universitat de València: València, Spain, September 21, 2017.

21. Peiró, S. Book of Abstracts, Big/Open/Small Data en Salud, Universitat de València: València, Spain, September 21, 2017; RT-1.

22. Marcos Muñoz, M. J. Book of Abstracts, I Jornada de Aspectos Éticos, Legales y de Gestión en la Investigación con Humanos, Universitat de València: València, Spain, September 29, 2017; O-1.

23. INFAIMON. *Tecnología e Industria: La Fábrica 4.0*; INFAIMON: Barcelona, Spain, 2017.

24. Soria Olivas, E. Book of Abstracts, II Day Open Data. Open Data and AI: A Disruptive Change, Universitat de València: València, Spain, September 20, 2018; O-1.

25. O'Reilly, T. *WTF: What's the Future and Why it's up to Us*; Harper Collins: New York, NY, 2017.

26. Meier, P. *Digital Humanitarians: How BIG DATA is Changing the Face of Humanitarian Response*; CRC: Boca Raton, FL, 2015.

27. Puncel Chornet, A. Personal Communication.

28. Harari, Y. N. *21 Lessons for the 21st Century*; Jonathan Cape: London, UK, 2018.

29. García-García, F. Personal Communication.

30. Sansom, C. Big Data Opens New Avenues for Genomics Research. *Sci. Comput. World* **2018**, *2018* (162), 18–20.

31. Ktori, S. AI Advances Healthcare Research. *Sci. Comput. World* **2018**, *2018* (162), 21–23.

32. Aurín Pardo, E. Personal Communication.

33. Porter, M. E. What is Value in Health Care? *N. Engl. J. Med.* **2010**, *363*, 2477–2481.

CHAPTER 7

THEORY AND SIMULATION: PRESENT AND FUTURE OF QUANTUM TECHNOLOGIES

FRANCISCO TORRENS[1*] and GLORIA CASTELLANO[2]

[1]*Institut Universitari de Ciència Molecular,
Universitat de València, Edifici d'Instituts de Paterna,
P. O. Box 22085, E-46071 València, Spain*

[2]*Departamento de Ciencias Experimentales y Matemáticas,
Facultad de Veterinaria y Ciencias Experimentales,
Universidad Catolica de Valencia San Vicente Mártir,
Guillem de Castro-94, E-46001 València, Spain*

Corresponding author. E-mail: torrens@uv.es

ABSTRACT

The things are as they are because the rationalization and production of theoretical representation provide intellectual satisfaction. Theoretician's triangular home consists of theory, computer simulation, and understanding. It is necessary an intensive dialogue between methodologists, experimentalists, and society. It is needed to realize and notice untrue hypotheses. In the computation of graphene (GR), models are important as case studies. Applications of GR catalysis are solar cells, Li^+ batteries, fuel cells, and supercapacitors. Pyrolized chitosan and alginate are more exfoliable than GR because of their greater interlayer distances. GRs are photocatalysts for solar fuels production. Aluja Schuneman Hofer directs the *Course/Workshop on Scientific Integrity/Ethics*. The objective of the *Course* is that the student body obtains a general view on the integrity and ethics of science, fundamental for those persons who desire to begin science careers in a so competitive and complex world. Moral is an imposed theme; ethics, whereas, does not vary. Science is a delicate theme because one is creating tools that will be used by other persons. The process became aggressive, competitive and this obviously causes high risks. Accumulation of small faults is more pernicious and harmful to science system than scandals. Universal definition to justify an authorship is intellectual contribution. Editors' and referees' problems are avoided generating a scientific-integrity culture. People should institutionalize workshops to train new teams of scientific referees. Scientists should regulate themselves from laboratory and root a scientific-integrity culture. Insights into publishing enable to be more confident in science publishing helping authors get reports published easily.

7.1   INTRODUCTION

Setting the scene: theory, simulation, understanding, the present and future of quantum technologies and quantum chemistry (QC). The things are as they are because the rationalization and the production of theoretical representation provide intellectual satisfaction. A theoretician's triangular home consists of theory, computer simulation, and understanding. It is necessary an intensive dialogue between methodologists, experimentalists, and society. It is needed to realize and notice untrue hypotheses. In the computation of graphene (GR), models are important as case studies. The applications of GR catalysis are solar cells, Li^+ batteries, fuel cells, and supercapacitors. Pyrolized chitosan and alginate are more exfoliable than GR because of their greater interlayer distances. GRs are photocatalysts for solar fuels production.

Aluja Schuneman Hofer directed the *Course/Workshop on Scientific Integrity/Ethics*. Moral is an imposed theme; ethics, whereas, does not vary. Science is not a neutral instrument to obtain knowledge but a delicate theme because one is creating tools that will be used by other persons. The process of ultraquantification, ultracompetitiveness, working precariousness, and so on became aggressive, competitive, and this obviously also causes high risk of ethical faults. The accumulation of small ethical faults is more pernicious and harmful to the science system than scandalous ones. The universal definition to justify an authorship is the intellectual contribution. Editors' and referees' problems could be avoided generating a culture of scientific integrity. People should institutionalize workshops to train the new teams of scientific referees. Scientists should regulate themselves from laboratory and root a culture of scientific integrity. These insights into the publishing process will enable people to be more confident as an author in the world of science publishing and so should help them get their reports published more easily. Transmembrane but not soluble helices fold inside the ribosome tunnel.[1]

In earlier publications, it was reported the periodic table of the elements (PTE)[2–4], quantum simulators[5–13], science, ethics of developing sustainability *via* nanosystems, devices[14], *green nanotechnology* as an approach toward environment safety[15], molecular devices, machines as hybrid organic–inorganic structures[16], PTE, quantum biting its tail, sustainable chemistry[17], quantum molecular *spintronics*, nanoscience and GRs.[18] It was informed cancer, its hypotheses[19], precision personalized medicine from theory to practice, cancer[20], how human immunodeficiency virus/acquired immunodeficiency syndrome (HIV/AIDS) destroy immune defenses, hypothesis[21], 2014 emergence, spread, uncontrolled Ebola outbreak[22,23], Ebola virus disease, questions, ideas, hypotheses, models[24], metaphors that made history, reflections on philosophy, science, and deoxyribonucleic acid (DNA)[25], scientific integrity and ethics, science communication and psychology.[26] In the present report, it is reviewed some reflections on theory, simulation and understanding, the survival of QC, the triangular home of a theoretician, artificial knowledge (intelligence, AI), GR as the material of 21st century, the present and future of quantum technologies and QC, Li$^+$ revolution as the start of a new energy world, scientific integrity and ethics. The aim of this work is to initiate a debate by suggesting a number of questions (Q), which can arise when addressing subjects of QC, survival, GR, quantum technologies, Li$^+$, integrity, ethics, ultraquantification, ultracompetitiveness and working precariousness, and providing, when possible, answers (A) and hypotheses (H).

7.2 THEORY/SIMULATION/UNDERSTANDING: WILL QUANTUM CHEMISTRY SURVIVE?

In ICMol Science Day[27], Malrieu proposed Q/A/H on theory/simulation/understanding.[28]

Q1. Will QC survive to neural networks (NNs)?[29,30]

Q2.   Is QC a theoretical instrument or a computational spectrometer?

Q3.   Relation between numbers and understanding?

Q4.   Will QC survive to NNs?

Q5.   Have I something more to establish or say, or enjoy the world?

Q6.   Many new technical progresses make QC obsolete?

Q7.   Why are the things as they are?

A7.   Rationalization, production of theoretical representation: intellectual satisfaction.

Q8.   Why not to image this new design?

Q9.   (Weisberg). How will a system behave in the future?

Q10. (Weisberg). Why does it behave the way it does?

Q11. QC as a science?

Q12. What is the Universe?

H1.   The triangular home of a theoretician (*cf.* Fig. 7.1).

Q13. Who do we speak with?

A13. Intensive dialogue between methodologists, experimentalists, and society (minimal).

Q14. Explain, identify, leading effects, provide a *causal chain*?

Q15. QC victim of its success?

Q16. Experimentalists more in quest of numbers than of explanation?

Q17. QC as a computational spectrometer?

Q18. *Black-box* algorithms, iterative, 10^N variables, no access to interpretation?

Q19. Return to *ab-initio* wavefunction theory (WFT) methods, but for how long?

Q20. Mighty power drunkenness?

Q21. Prohibits the access to an identification of results?

H2.   Untrue H. (Mulliken). The more precise the computation, the more the concepts vanish in air.

Q22. The electrons (e^-) in two magnetic orbitals in a triplet or singlet spin arrangement?

Q23. What happens between these 2 e^- in the singly occupied orbitals (direct, kinetic exchange)?

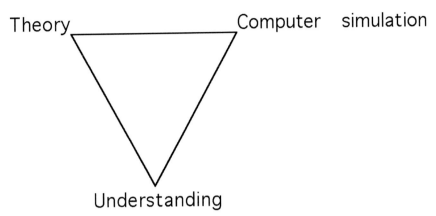

FIGURE 7.1   The triangular home of a theoretician.

He raised the following questions on AI.

Q24. Why do you recognize?

Q25. Will it be used to predict quantities (to control people, to help them, to kill them, etc.)?

Q26. This will be the end of our minor science: should we leave it?

Q27. Is science itself threatened by AI?

7.3   GRAPHENE: THE MATERIAL OF 21ST CENTURY

García Gómez proposed the following hypotheses on GR as the material of 21st century.[31]

H1. (Sánchez de Merás, 2014). H_2 *adsorption over* GR: *Coronene as a case study?*[32]

H2. The applications of GR catalysis are: Solar cells, Li^+ batteries, fuel cells, and supercapacitors.

H3. Pyrolized chitosan/alginate are more exfoliable than GR because interlayer distances 6Å *vs.* 3Å.

He provided the following conclusion (C).

C1. GRs are photocatalysts for solar fuels production.

Q1. (Bernabeu). How much does the preparation of GR cost?

Q2. (Bernabeu). Why not instead of preparing GR do you prepare other converter of solar energy?

Q3. (Bernabeu). What is the most efficient system humans can prepare to convert solar energy?

Q4. (Bernabeu). How close are we to the most efficient system to convert solar energy?

7.4 PRESENT AND FUTURE OF QUANTUM TECHNOLOGIES AND CHEMISTRY

Dénia moderated a round table on present and future of quantum technologies and chemistry.[33]

Q1.   What is quantum mechanics?

Q2.   What is it going to change?

Q3.   Which business is going to be affected?

Q4.   Projects of quantum computing?

Q5.   Is photonics going to be supported?

Q6.   Could people speak about terms?

Q7.   In which measure will chemistry contribute?

Q8.   Which role does chemistry play in quantum computing?

Q9.   In AI, persons will need a *computational thinking*, will they need a quantum thinking?

Q10. (Tomás). What is quantum computing?

Q11. Gender gap: Otilia, how will your gender perspective be applied in this theme?

Q12. In technology, space exists for people, will not people have to give incentive to girls?

Q13. Spain occupies the fourth place in EU Flagship, what would you say to young persons?

Q14. (Yáñez). Water is neutral, how to transmit this to students?

Q15. (Cardona). AI and quantum computing, are they the same?

Q16. (Cardona). Parallel?

Q17. (Cardona). Competing?

Q18. (Coronado). Is Flagship a scientists' invention to do lobbies to distribute the game, for example, GR?

7.5 THE REVOLUTION OF Li⁺: THE START OF A NEW ENERGY WORLD

Muelas raised the following questions on Li^+ revolution and the start of a new energy world.[34]

Q1.   Is it either a technological change or a revolution?

Q2.   And if it is a revolution, is there enough Li in the planet?

Q3.   The economy of scale decreases prices, does over demand increase them?

Q4.   Consumer electronics, electric vehicles (EVs), and renewables: the three main applications?

Q5.   Do you self-consume? Do you?

Q6.   Multimegawatt parks. Keep something for later?

Q7.   The anxiety of reach.

Q8.   How are the nets of transport prepared?

Q9.   Thirty million EVs that work with Pb since 70 years?

7.6 SCIENTIFIC INTEGRITY/ETHICS

Fasce interviewed Aluja Schuneman Hofer proposing Q/A on scientific integrity/ethics.[35–38]

Q1.   Where does it come in your interest in the ethics of science?

Q2.   Was it aroused by any particularly relevant incident or did it go with you always?

A2.   It was a gradual process.

Q3.   Which would the difference be between a moralistic science and an ethical science?

A3.   (Ribero Weber, 2004). Moral is an imposed theme; ethics, whereas, does not vary.[39]

Q4.   Is science a neutral tool to obtain knowledge?

A4.   No, it is a delicate theme because one is creating tools that will be used by other persons.

Q5.   One speaks about scientist's individual acts but, what about scientific production system?

Q6.   Do ultraquantification/competitiveness, precariousness, and so on push scientists to ethical faults?

A6.   The process became aggressive, competitive, and this obviously also causes high risks.

Q7.   Till which point do ethical faults among authors of low impact go unnoticed?

A7.   It is more pernicious/harmful to science system the accumulation of small faults than scandals.

Q8.   A problem could be the indefinition of many terms, for example, what is plagiarism exactly?

A8.   Plagiarism is the appropriation of ideas of other person without giving the corresponding credit.

Q9.   Which should the author of an article be?

A9.   The universal definition to justify an authorship is the intellectual contribution.

Q10. When one observes favors traffic/editors behavior, do not you find filters are hacked?

A10. Such problems could be avoided generating scientific-integrity culture rooting in referees.

Q11. Traffic of influence occurs in all ambits: Why should not it also happen in the scientific ambit?

Q12. Soccer referees have training academies, but who does it teach scientists to be good referees?

A12. People should institutionalize workshops to train the new teams of scientific referees.

Q13. Who do you think that should ethically control scientists?

A13. Scientists should regulate themselves from laboratory and root a scientific-integrity culture.

Q14. Has meaning to leave ethics on hands of a community so much heterogeneous as scientific?

A14. The problem is that many are not captured or it occurs much later when evil is already done.

Q15. How does science work?

7.7 HOW TO WRITE GREAT REPORTS/GET PUBLISHED: UNDERSTANDING PUBLISHING

Newman and Bearzot raised questions on how to write great reports and get published.[40]

Q1. How to write great reports and get published?

Q2. How to write a great research report and get it accepted by a good journal?

Q3. How do editors and publishers think?

Q4. What do they expect?

Q5. How does the peer review process work?

Q6. What aspects of authors' reports do editors, reviewers, and publishers look at critically?

Q7. What are people responsibilities?

Q8. What is allowed?

Q9. What is not permitted?

They provided the following conclusion.

C1. The insights above into the publishing process will enable people to be more confident as an author in the world of science publishing and so should help them get their reports published more easily.

7.8 FINAL REMARKS

From the present results, the following final remark can be drawn.

1. Things are because rationalization/theoretical-representation production gives satisfaction.

2. Theoretician's triangular home consists of theory, computer simulation, and understanding.

3. It is needed an intensive dialogue between methodologists, experimentalists, and society.
4. It is necessary to realize and notice untrue hypotheses.
5. In the computation of GR, models are important as case studies.
6. GR catalysis applications are solar cells; Li^+ batteries; fuel cells; supercapacitors.
7. Pyrolized chitosan/alginate are more exfoliable than GR because of interlayer distances.
8. GRs are photocatalysts for solar fuels production.
9. Moral is an imposed theme; ethics, whereas, does not vary.
10. Science is delicate theme because one is creating tools that will be used by other persons.
11. The process became aggressive, competitive, and this obviously also causes high risks.
12. Accumulation of small faults is more pernicious/harmful to science system than scandals.
13. The universal definition to justify an authorship is the intellectual contribution.
14. Editors/referees' problems could be avoided generating scientific-integrity culture.
15. People should institutionalize workshops to train the new teams of scientific referees.
16. Scientists should regulate themselves from laboratory rooting scientific-integrity culture.
17. The insights above into the publishing process will enable people to be more confident as an author in the world of science publishing and so should help them get their reports published more easily.

ACKNOWLEDGMENTS

The authors acknowledge support from Generalitat Valenciana (Project No. PROMETEO/2016/094) and Universidad Católica de Valencia *San Vicente Mártir* (Project No. 2019-217-001).

KEYWORDS

- quantum chemistry
- graphene
- material
- lithium ion
- new energy world
- scientific integrity
- scientific ethics

REFERENCES

1. Bañó-Polo, M.; Baeza-Delgado, C.; Tamborero, S.; Hazel, A.; Grau, B.; Nilsson, I. M.; Whitley, P.; Gumbart, J. C.; von Heijne, G.; Mingarro, I. Transmembrane but Not Soluble Helices Fold Inside the Ribosome Tunnel. *Nat. Commun.* **2018,** *9,* 5246-1-9.
2. Torrens, F.; Castellano, G. Reflections on the Nature of the Periodic Table of the Elements: Implications in Chemical Education. In *Synthetic Organic Chemistry*; Seijas, J. A., Vázquez Tato, M. P., Lin, S. K., Eds.; MDPI: Basel, Switzerland, 2015; Vol. 18; pp 1–15.
3. Torrens, F.; Castellano, G. Nanoscience: From a Two-Dimensional to a Three-Dimensional Periodic Table of the Elements. In *Methodologies and Applications for Analytical and Physical Chemistry*; Haghi, A. K., Thomas, S., Palit, S., Main, P., Eds.; Apple Academic–CRC: Waretown, NJ, 2018; pp 3–26.
4. Torrens, F.; Castellano, G. Periodic Table. In *New Frontiers in Nanochemistry: Concepts, Theories, and Trends*; Putz, M. V., Ed.; Apple Academic–CRC: Waretown, NJ, in press.
5. Torrens, F.; Castellano, G. Ideas in the History of Nano/Miniaturization and (Quantum) Simulators: Feynman, Education and Research Reorientation in Translational Science. In *Synthetic Organic Chemistry*; Seijas, J. A., Vázquez Tato, M. P., Lin, S. K., Eds.; MDPI: Basel, Switzerland, 2015; Vol. 19; pp 1–16.
6. Torrens, F.; Castellano, G. Reflections on the Cultural History of Nanominiaturization and Quantum Simulators (Computers). In *Sensors and Molecular Recognition*; Laguarda Miró, N., Masot Peris, R., Brun Sánchez, E., Eds.; Universidad Politécnica de Valencia: València, Spain, 2015; Vol. 9; pp 1–7.
7. Torrens, F.; Castellano, G. Nanominiaturization and Quantum Computing. In *Sensors and Molecular Recognition*; Costero Nieto, A. M., Parra Álvarez, M., Gaviña Costero, P., Gil Grau, S., Eds.; Universitat de València: València, Spain, 2016; Vol. 10; pp 31–1-5.
8. Torrens, F.; Castellano, G. Nanominiaturization, Classical/Quantum Computers/Simulators, Superconductivity, and Universe. In *Methodologies and Applications for Analytical and Physical Chemistry*; Haghi, A. K., Thomas, S., Palit, S., Main, P., Eds.; Apple Academic–CRC: Waretown, NJ, 2018; pp 27–44.

9. Torrens, F.; Castellano, G. Superconductors, Superconductivity, BCS Theory and Entangled Photons for Quantum Computing. In *Physical Chemistry for Engineering and Applied Sciences: Theoretical and Methodological Implication*; Haghi, A. K., Aguilar, C. N., Thomas, S., Praveen, K. M., Eds.; Apple Academic–CRC: Waretown, NJ, 2018; pp 379–387.

10. Torrens, F.; Castellano, G. EPR Paradox, Quantum Decoherence, Qubits, Goals and Opportunities in Quantum Simulation. In *Theoretical Models and Experimental Approaches in Physical Chemistry: Research Methodology and Practical Methods*; Haghi, A. K., Ed.; Apple Academic–CRC: Waretown, NJ, 2018; Vol. 5; pp 317–334.

11. Torrens, F.; Castellano, G. Nanomaterials, Molecular Ion Magnets, Ultrastrong and Spin–Orbit Couplings in Quantum Materials. In *Physical Chemistry for Chemists and Chemical Engineers: Multidisciplinary Research Perspectives*; Vakhrushev, A. V., Haghi, R., de Julián-Ortiz, J. V., Allahyari, E., Eds.; Apple Academic–CRC: Waretown, NJ, in press.

12. Torrens, F.; Castellano, G. Nanodevices and Organization of Single Ion Magnets and Spin Qubits. In *Chemical Science and Engineering Technology: Perspectives on Interdisciplinary Research*; Balköse, D., Ribeiro, A. C. F., Haghi, A. K., Ameta, S. C., Chakraborty, T., Eds.; Apple Academic–CRC: Waretown, NJ, in press.

13. Torrens, F.; Castellano, G. *Superconductivity and Quantum Computing* via *Magnetic Molecules*. In *New Insights in Chemical Engineering and Computational Chemistry*; Haghi, A.K., Ed.; Apple Academic–CRC: Waretown, NJ, in press.

14. Torrens, F.; Castellano, G. Developing Sustainability via Nanosystems and Devices: Science–Ethics. In *Chemical Science and Engineering Technology: Perspectives on Interdisciplinary Research*; Balköse, D., Ribeiro, A. C. F., Haghi, A. K., Ameta, S. C., Chakraborty, T., Eds.; Apple Academic–CRC: Waretown, NJ, in press.

15. Torrens, F.; Castellano, G. Green Nanotechnology: An Approach towards Environment Safety. In *Advances in Nanotechnology and the Environmental Sciences: Applications, Innovations, and Visions for the Future*; Vakhrushev, A. V.; Ameta, S. C.; Susanto, H., Haghi, A. K., Eds.; Apple Academic–CRC: Waretown, NJ, in press.

16. Torrens, F.; Castellano, G. Molecular Devices/Machines: Hybrid Organic–Inorganic Structures. In *Research Methods and Applications in Chemical and Biological Engineering*; Pourhashemi, A., Deka, S. C., Haghi, A. K., Eds.; Apple Academic–CRC: Waretown, NJ, in press.

17. Torrens, F.; Castellano, G. The Periodic Table, Quantum Biting its Tail, and Sustainable Chemistry. In *Chemical Nanoscience and Nanotechnology: New Materials and Modern Techniques*; Torrens, F., Haghi, A. K., Chakraborty, T., Eds.; Apple Academic–CRC: Waretown, NJ, in press.

18. Torrens, F.; Castellano, G. Quantum Molecular Spintronics, Nanoscience and Graphenes. In *Molecular Physical Chemistry*; Haghi, A. K., Ed.; Apple Academic–CRC: Waretown, NJ, in press.

19. Torrens, F.; Castellano, G. Cancer and Hypotheses on Cancer. In *Molecular Chemistry and Biomolecular Engineering: Integrating Theory and Research with Practice*; Pogliani, L., Torrens, F., Haghi, A. K., Eds.; Apple Academic–CRC: Waretown, NJ, in press.

20. Torrens, F.; Castellano, G. Precision Personalized Medicine from Theory to Practice: Cancer. In *Molecular Physical Chemistry*; Haghi, A. K., Ed.; Apple Academic–CRC: Waretown, NJ, in press.

21. Torrens, F.; Castellano, G. AIDS Destroys Immune Defences: Hypothesis. *New Front. Chem.* **2014**, *23*, 11–20.

22. Torrens-Zaragozá, F.; Castellano-Estornell, G. Emergence, Spread and Uncontrolled Ebola Outbreak. *Basic Clin. Pharmacol. Toxicol.* **2015**, *117* (Suppl. 2) 38–38.

23. Torrens, F.; Castellano, G. 2014 Spread/Uncontrolled Ebola Outbreak. *New Front. Chem.* **2015**, *24*, 81–91.

24. Torrens, F.; Castellano, G. Ebola Virus Disease: Questions, Ideas, Hypotheses and Models. *Pharmaceuticals* **2016**, *9*, 14-6-6.

25. Torrens, F.; Castellano, G. Metaphors That Made History: Reflections on Philosophy/Science/DNA. In *Molecular Physical Chemistry*; Haghi, A. K., Ed.; Apple Academic–CRC: Waretown, NJ, in press.

26. Torrens, F.; Castellano, G. Scientific Integrity Ethics: Science Communication and Psychology. In *Molecular Physical Chemistry*; Haghi, A. K., Ed.; Apple Academic–CRC: Waretown, NJ, in press.

27. Coronado, E., Ed. Book of Abstracts, XVIII Jornada Científica del ICMol, València, Spain, December 14, 2018, Universitat de València: València, Spain, 2018.

28. Malrieu, J. P. Book of Abstracts, XVIII Jornada Científica del ICMol, València, Spain, December 14, 2018, Universitat de València: València, Spain, 2018; O-2.

29. Malrieu, J. P. *Dans le Poing du Marché: Sortir de l'Emprise Libérale*; Rue des Gestes: Toulouse, France, 2009.

30. Malrieu, J. P. *La Science Gouvernée: Essay sur le Triangle Sciences/Techniques/Pouvoir*; Rue des Gestes: Toulouse, France, 2011.

31. García Gómez, H. Book of Abstracts, XVIII Jornada Científica del ICMol, València, Spain, December 14, 2018, Universitat de València: València, Spain, 2018; O-3.

32. Yeamin, B.; Faginas-Lago, N.; Albertí, M.; Cuesta, I.; Sánchez-Marín, J.; Sánchez de Merás, A. M. J. Multi-Scale Theoretical Investigation of Molecular Hydrogen Adsorption Over Graphene: Coronene As a Case Study. *RSC Adv.* **2014**, *4*, 54447–54453.

33. Dénia, O. Book of Abstracts, XVIII Jornada Científica del ICMol, València, Spain, December 14, 2018, Universitat de València: València, Spain, 2018; RT-1.

34. Muelas, A. Personal Communication.

35. Fasce, A. Entrevista a Martín Aluja: Investigador de l'Institut d'Ecologia (Mèxic). *Mètode* **2018**, *2018* (99), 10–16.

36. Aluja, M.; Birke, A., Eds. *El Papel de la Ética en la Investigación Científica y la Educación Superior*; Academia Mexicana de Ciencia: México, México, 2003.

37. Aluja, M.; Birke, A., Eds. *El Papel de la Ética en la Investigación Científica y la Educación Superior*; Fondo de Cultura Económica: México, México, 2004.

38. Aluja Schuneman Hofer, M. R. Curso/Taller sobre Integridad/Ética Científica, València, Spain, May 17–18, 2018, Universitat de València: València, Spain, 2018.

39. Rivero Weber, P. Apología de la inmoralidad. *Este País (México)* **2004**, *2004* (8), 46–50.

40. Newman, A.; Bearzot, M. Personal Communication.

CHAPTER 8

COMPREHENSIVE HIGHLIGHTS OF SOME NOVEL SMALL-MOLECULE INHIBITORS OF CHECKPOINT KINASE FOR CANCER THERAPY

AHMED A. EL-RASHEDY*

*Department of Natural and Microbial Product,
Research Division of Pharmaceutical and Drug Industries,
National Research Centre, Dokki, Cairo 12622, Egypt*

E-mail: ahmedelrashedy45@gmail.com

ABSTRACT

One of the most important part in the cellular response to DNA damage is the activation of Chk, Checkpoint kinase (Chk1 and Chk2) phosphorylation are a key enzyme to obtain cell-cycle arrests. Chks inhibition is believed to sensitize the tumor cells to cancer drugs that damage the DNA, because of the absence of both efficient DNA repair and checkpoints, the cell death or senescence will occur. There are several rationales for the development of Chk inhibitors. First, a wide range of anticancer drugs and ionizing radiation (IR) caused activation of Chk in tumor cells which seriously limited their effectiveness in these cancer cells. These shortcomings of current chemotherapeutic approaches can be addressed by selective inhibition of Chk. Second, inhibition of Chk in normal cells leads to protection of the normal tissues during chemotherapy or radiation therapy that increase the therapeutic index of DNA-targeted and IR agents in these cells. Therefore, Chk inhibitors would protect healthy tissues as well as sensitize the tumor to chemotherapy and IR. Hence, the Chks have been identified as promising targets for anticancer drug design. This chapter will describe and discuss in more detail the most recent inhibitors of Chk1 and Chk2, as reported in the literature including an evaluation of chemical structure and biological activity.

8.1 INTRODUCTION

One of the major causes of pathogenic disorder is intracellular or intercellular communication disorders. Protein phosphorylation is one of the most important single transduction mechanisms through which intercellular or intracellular processes such as cell proliferation and differentiation, ion transport and hormone response are performed. The modern drug design has focused on single transduction therapy such as kinases. Protein kinases (PTKs) are enzymes that control the activity of the protein by phosphorylation of particular amino acids with ATP as a source of phosphate, because of that, it is induced the conformational change from an inactive form to an active form of the protein (Fig. 8.1).

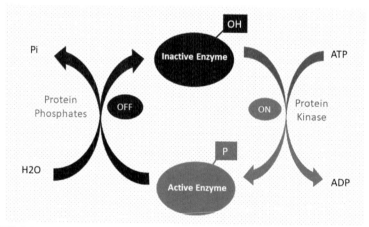

FIGURE 8.1   Protein kinase phosphorylation.

The PTKs are classified according to the amino acid side chain that they can phosphorylate:

- Tyrosine kinases (TKs) phosphorylate the tyrosine phenolic hydroxyl group.

- Histidine kinases phosphorylate the nitrogen group of histidine residues.
- Serine-Threonine (Ser/Thr) kinases that phosphorylate the two-hydroxyl group of the serine and threonine amino acids.

Cell-cycle checkpoint act as a restriction point between each phase of the cell cycle where the entire process can be delayed or stopped to ensure the exact duplication and transmission of the genetic material to progeny cells or to allow the time for DNA repairing.[1–3] Chk 1 (ChK1), is a Ser/Thr kinase type which activated the phosphorylation of both ATR (Ataxia-telengiectasia and Rad3-related) and ATM (Ataxia-telengiectasia, mutated) in response to DNA damage, followed by phosphorylation of a number of substrates and beginning signal cascades that result in cell-cycle arrest. Activation of ATM and ATR lead to phosphorylation/activation of the checkpoint effectors (CDC25A and CDC25C, p53, BRCA1) via phosphorylation/activation of the Chk1 and Chk2 kinases.[4] This pathway is illustrated in Figure 8.2.

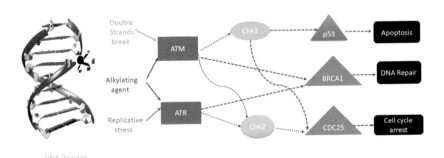

FIGURE 8.2   Summary of DNA response stress.

Phosphorylation of multiple serine residues on the protein phosphatase Cdc25 (cell division cycle 25) is a result on recognition by ubiquitin ligases which result in proteolysis and control the progression through the S phase.[5–8] In addition, Chk1 results in cell-cycle arrest in the G2 phase, this occurs through phosphorylation of Cdc25, preventing the activation and dephosphorylation of Cdk1 (cyclin-dependent kinase inhibitory protein) (Fig. 8.3).[9–11]

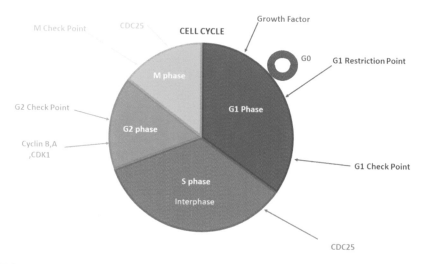

FIGURE 8.3   Detailed function of the mammalian cell cycle.

siRNA studies have demonstrated the importance of Chk1 in control-ling the S, intra S, and the G2-M checkpoints phase; inhibition of Chk1 resulting to abolish the S and G2 checkpoints and impairing DNA repair and increasing the tumor cell death.[5,12–14] Similar to Chk1, the effect of Chk2 activation on the effector protein on Cdc25a, Cdc25c, and p53 are similar. Stimulating of Chk2 is induced by the factor that causes DNA breaks such as ionizing radiation (IR) or chemotherapeutic agents.[6,15–17] Although their effects (Chk1, Chk2) are similar on the downstream substrate, but their outcomes are similar. For instance, in the knock out animal studies on both Chk1, Chk2 have striking outcomes. Chk1 leads in developing lethality, whereas Chk2(-/-) mice are viable and appear to be normal. Even though tissues from Chk2(-/-) mice have shown significant defects in both IR-induced apoptosis and G_1/S checkpoint.[18] there are many studies that have been published to study the relationship between both Chk1 and Chk2 and their crosstalk between the down-stream pathway.[19,20] However, there are many studies that confirmed that the inhibition of both Chk1 and Chk2 has no beneficial over the inhibi-tion of Chk1 alone (Fig. 8.4).[21,22]

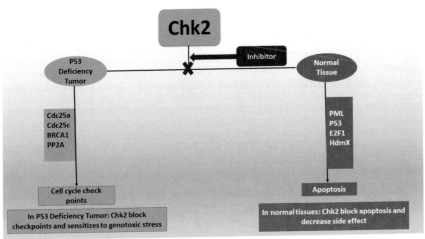

FIGURE 8.4 Chk inhibitors as chemotherapeutic agents. (A) In a p53-deficient tumor, Chk act as cell-cycle checkpoint inducer. Chk inhibition would induce the tumor to DNA-damaging agents used in chemotherapy. (B) In contrast, in normal tissues, Chk act as pro-apoptotic effectors. Chk inhibitors would protect healthy tissues but sensitize the tumor to chemotherapy.

Because a lot of cancer has missed the G_1 checkpoint so that the repairing the damage can occur at the G2/M checkpoint which is mainly regulated by Chk. In a cancer cell, when the DNA damage occurs, an inhibition of Chk1 would allow the cancer cell to get rid of the checkpoint and proceed into mitosis. In a cancer cell, when DNA damage occurs, inhibition of Chk1 would allow the cancer cell to get rid of the checkpoint and proceed with mitosis. When DNA damage occurred, a mitotic disaster would result and cell death would occur. Therefore, the Chk inhibitor would potentiate the effects of DNA damage and sensitize the cancer cell to chemotherapy or radiation therapy without any side effect associated with these therapies.

8.2 CHK INHIBITORS

There have been many recent advances in the design and development of Chk inhibitors. Three of the most advanced inhibitors as XL-844, AZD7762, and PF-473336 are now in Phase-II clinical trials. A fourth agent from Lilly/ICOS (IC83) has recently been disclosed as entering Phase-I trials in combination with pemetrexed. AZD7762 is a thiophene carboxamide urea,[23,24] XL844 an aminopyrazine carboxamide, and PF00477736 and PF-473336 are the diazapinoindolone compounds. All three are selective kinase inhibitors that show activity against both Chk1 and Chk2, but with different degrees. The structure of PF00477736 has not been published. It has a 100-fold selectivity for Chk1 (IC_{50} = 0.49 nM) over Chk2.[25] It is interesting that each inhibitor contains a different hinge-binding region; urea for AZD7762, and a cyclic hydrazine amide in the case of PF477736. Interestingly, in vivo studies had shown that PF477736 should be delayed at least 24 h after administration of DNA damaging agent (gemcitabine) in Colo205 colon cancer xenografts.[25] This is to allow more accumulation of PF477736 in S and G2/M arrested cells in response to the initial genotoxic insult. PF00477736 was less than 100-fold selectivity against VEGF2R, Aurora-A, FGFR3, Flt3, Fms, Ret, and Yes.[25] In preclinical studies, the cellular potency of PF00477736 was measured by assessing cells entering mitosis (histone H3 phosphorylation by spectral dot-blot analysis). The cellular EC_{50} by this method was 45 nM.[25]

XL9844 is a potent oral aminopyrazine inhibitor for both Chk1 and Chk2 (IC_{50} = 2.2 nM and 0.07 nM, respectively).[26] There is no structure published. The inhibition is correlated with ATP concentration. In addition, XL9844 inhibited VEGFR2 (IC_{50} = 12 nM) and Flt-4 (IC_{50} = 6 nM). CEP-3891 (Cephalon) was developed as a more specific small molecular inhibitor of Chk1.[6] The cellular IC_{50} of CEP-3891 is 4 nM. Other kinases inhibited by CEP-3891 (determined by the reduction in Cdc25A phosphorylation) included TrkA (9 nM), MLK1 (42 nM), and VEGFR2 (164 nM). No structure of CEP-3891 has been published.

V158411 is a potent inhibitor for both Chk1 and Chk2 with IC_{50} 3.5 nM and 2.5 nM for both Chk1 and Chk2, respectively.[27] The structure of V158411 has not been published yet. The majority of Chk1 inhibitors are ATP competitive inhibitors, which bind directly to the hinge peptide region that is found between the N and C terminal lobes of the kinase domain, while there are other allosteric binding inhibitors.[28,29] The crystal structure of ATP competitive inhibitors has shown that these inhibitors are usually anchored by hydrogen bonds of one or more Glu85, Tyr86, or Cys87 amino acids in the hinge region, and the polar substituents toward the ribose pocket and lipophilic groups to the selectivity surface. Outside this surface, the cleft opens up to the solvent and the hydrophilic groups are often added to balance the physiochemical properties of the compound.

Chk1 has been proven to be highly amenable to crystallography since Apo-structure has been determined.[30] This helps in the discovery of a number of inhibitors series using structure-based drug design (SBDD).

8.2.1 BISARYLUREAS TEMPLATE-BASED INHIBITOR

Bisarylureas were the earliest reported Chk inhibitors, and one of the most abundant with regard to Chks inhibitor applications.[22,31–36] Following optimization of Chk1 potency and selectivity, this series and analogs generally had good physicochemical properties and enzyme potency. (S)-5-(3-fluorophenyl)-N-(piperidin-3-yl)-3-ureidothiophene-2-carboxa mide (AstraZeneca: AZD7762) as shown in Figure 8.5 was developed and derived from a high-throughput screen that revealed the thiophene urea carboxamides as potent inhibitors of Chk1. AZD7762 is a relatively selective inhibitor of Chk and potently inhibits both Chk1 (IC_{50} = 5 nM) and Chk2 (IC_{50} <10 nM). Overall, AZD7762 has been shown to potentiate the effects of a number of different DNA-damaging agents across a number of different cell lines, with the precise degree of potentiating depending upon both the cell line and the DNA-damaging agent used. Early biomarker work with AZD7762 has focused on the measurement of the changes in levels of both p-Chk1 (at the activation site, Ser345) and p-H2AX. Significant increases in these markers have been observed in both in vitro study (using western blotting) and in vivo study (by immunohistochemistry staining of both xenografts and hair follicles within skin biopsies).[23,24] At present, AZD7762 is in Phase-I clinical trials.

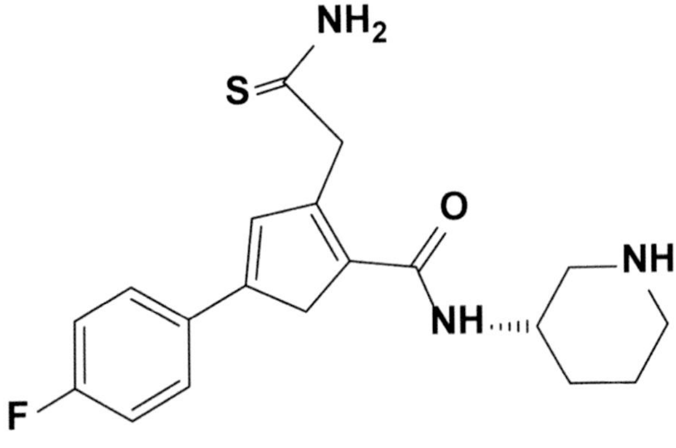

FIGURE 8.5 Astrazeneca; AZD7762, a prototype molecule.

Bisarylurea-based Chk1 inhibitors have six different formulae (Fig. 8.6). For bisarylureas of the general formula **1**, there are six preferred subseries of compounds with variations at W, although all variants are pyrazine derived. Within each subseries, additional points of variation are at R_6 and R_{10} (compound **7**).[33] The compounds tested have IC_{50} values for Chk1 ranging from 8 to 500 nM and show at least 100× selectivity for Chk1 over Chk2.

For Bisarylureas of the general formula **2** (Fig. 8.6), having H as the preferred R_5 substituent (compound **8**). All examples are reported to have IC_{50} potency ranging between 0.1 and 200 nM against Chk1.[37] The X-ray crystallography of lead compound 1-(5-chloro-2,4-dimethoxyphenyl)-3-(5-cyanopyrazin-2-yl) urea (compound **19**) in the Chk 1 (Chk1) enzyme showed R_2 toward the ribose pocket of the Chk1 enzyme, while R_4 points toward the solvent front. Based on this, modification R_4 led to the improvement of physical properties such as polarity and solubility while keeping similar potency. Compound **9** provided the best overall results in the cellular assays as it abrogated doxorubicin-induced cell cycle arrest (IC_{50} = 1.7 µM) and enhanced doxorubicin cytotoxicity (IC_{50} = 0.44 µM) while displaying no single agent activity.

For bisarylureas of the general formula **3** (Fig. 8.6), there were seven preferred heterocyclic groups described for W, wherein in each case R_6 is preferably a basic amino group. The compounds tested had IC_{50} values for Chk1 from 8 to 500 nM and showed at least 100-folds selectivity for Chk1 over Chk2.

For bisarylureas of the general formula **4**, they have a number of quinoline and quinoxaline-N-oxides (Fig. 8.6) as dual DNA-damaging agents/Chk1 inhibitors.[34] These Chk1 inhibitors can enhance the efficacy of DNA-damaging therapeutics. It was envisaged that di-N-oxides such as compound **10** would undergo selective reduction to the corresponding mono-N-oxide in hypoxic tumor cells[38] and that this process would be accompanied by DNA damage and provide some antitumor activity. Chk1 inhibitory activity of these compounds leads to abrogation of the DNA damage-induced checkpoints, prevent normal repair processes from taking place, and further increase cell death (Fig. 8.6).

In diaryl urea derivatives of the general formula **5**, based on the finding that N-oxide formation maintains Chk1 inhibitory activity, the N-oxide **11** has a Chk1 IC_{50} of 71 nM and hERG IC_{50} (functional assay) of 26.7 µM, in marked contrast to the corresponding tertiary amine **12**, which has a Chk1 IC_{50} of 41 nM but is also very potent with an IC_{50} of 108 nM (Fig. 8.6) .[35]

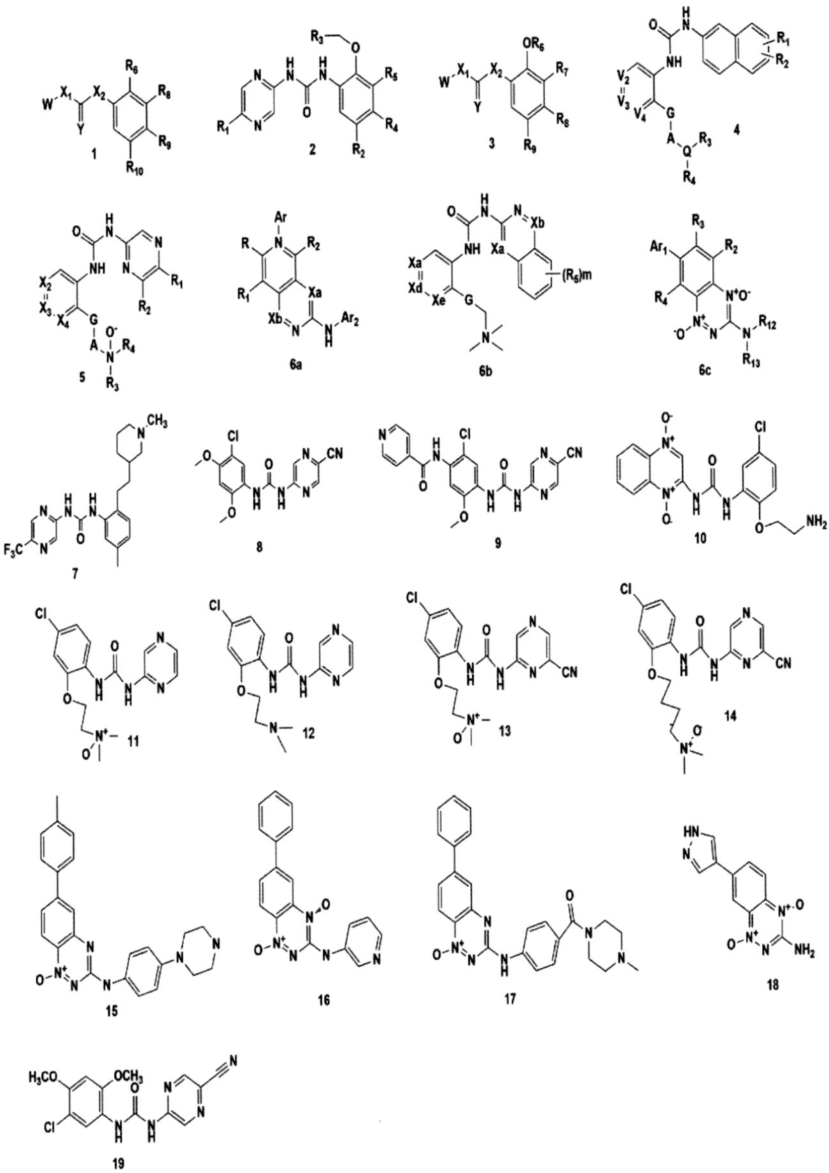

FIGURE 8.6 General formula and specific bisarylurea inhibitors of Chk1.

Building on the N-oxide theme, compounds of three general formulae **6a-c** were formed. All specific examples are fused triazines.[34] For example, N-oxides such as compound **15** of formula **6a**, (Chk1 IC_{50} = 41 nM). The ureas of general formula **6b** are similar to those in formula b but contain fused triazine N-oxides or di-N-oxides instead of quinoxaline N-oxides, the corresponding di-N-oxides such as **16** is potent Chk-1 inhibitor with IC_{50} = 75 nM.[34] Finally, all examples of formula **6c** have all R groups only as H, with variations in the aryl or the heteroaryl substitution at Ar_1. It is interesting to note that there is a very specific claim for a limited generic structure where Ar_1 is a pyrazole, as in compound **18**. Interestingly, the position of the aryl substituent on the fused ring in compounds of formula **6c** is changed relative to that of formula **6a**. Presumably, the lack of substitution on the aniline results in a different binding mode to Chk1 (Fig. 8.6).[36] Compound **19** is a potent ATP competitive inhibitor with IC_{50} = 1.7 µM which synergistically improve the doxorubicin cytotoxicity (IC_{50} = 0.44 µM) while displaying no single activity (Fig. 8.6).[39]

8.2.2   3-DIBENZOAZEPINONES TEMPLATE-BASED INHIBITORS

Dibenzoazepinones template-based inhibitors; PF-394691 (**20a**) and PF477736 (**20b**) are highly selective Chk 1 inhibitors. PF-394691 (Pfizer) is a potent, selective Chk1 inhibitor (300-fold selective over Chk2), with IC_{50} ranging from 40 to 50 nM. In vivo study had shown that PF-394691 has the capability to dissolve the DNA damage induced by cell-cycle arrest,[40] adding to that, PF-394691 has shown to be a dose-dependent antagonism and potentiating the effect of gemcitabine, irinotecan, and cisplatin in human tumor xenograft models.

PF-477736 is a potent Chk1 inhibitor with IC_{50} = 0.49 nM and moderate selectivity of Chk 1 over Chk2. In vitro study has shown that PF-477736 has the capacity to abolish the cell-cycle arrest induced by cell-cycle arrest. This response has been shown in several cell lines and several DNA damaging agents such as gemcitabine, SN-38, carboplatin, doxorubicin, and mitomycin-C. PF-477736 is in Phase-I clinical trials.[41] Compound **21** was stated to have IC_{50} ranging from 0.2 nM to 280 µM, with the most preferred inhibitor having IC_{50} ranging from 0.2 to 30 nM.[42] R_6 is mainly aryl or heteroaryl, being commonly azaindole (pyrrolopyridine) following the general formula **22**. R is usually benzylic, whereas R_6 is most commonly—CH_2CH_2O—substituted with phenyl-4-morpholino or 2-methyl-3-pyridyl, although some examples contain R_2 as a two-carbon linker to an amine. Conversely, in a large number of examples, R_6 is a 3-methoxyphenyl further substituted exclusively on the 4-position.[42–44] N-substituted-2-amino-$5H,7H$-benzopyrimido[4,5,d]azepin-6-one (compound **23**) are not only Chk1, Chk2 inhibitors but also Aurora-A kinase, and polio-like kinase-1 inhibitors. The relative potency and selectivity of Compound **23** is dependent on the specific example chosen, for example, Aurora A kinase ($IC_{50} < 0.5$ μM), Chk1 with $IC_{50} < 0.5$ μM, and polio-like kinase-1 (PLK1) with $IC_{50} < 0.5$ μM (Fig. 8.7).[45,46]

A novel series of 5,10-dihydro-dibenzo[b,e][1,4]diazepin-11-ones have been synthesized as potent and selective Chk 1 (Chk1) inhibitors via structure-based design. Compound **24** exhibited a potent Chk1 with low cytotoxicity, arrested G2 arrest and elevated the cytotoxicity of camptothecin by 19-fold against SW620 cells. Pharmacokinetic studies have revealed that the compound **24** has moderate bioavailability in 20% of mice.[44]

PF 477736 is a selective ATP competitive inhibitor with IC_{50} 0.49 and 47 nM for Chk1 and Chk2, respectively. It causes cell-cycle arrest at S and G2-M checkpoints and sensitizes cells to DNA damage. PF-00477736 sensitized docetaxel-induced suppression of tumor survival.[47] Recently, PF-00477736 has synergistically improved the activity of bosutinib (SKI-606) in highly imatinib-resistant BCR/ABL+ leukemia cells.[48]

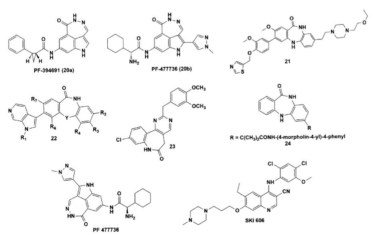

FIGURE 8.7 Specific examples of some dibenzoazepinone based Chk1 inhibitors.

8.2.3 4-SQUARIC ACID DERIVATIVES TEMPLATE-BASED INHIBITORS

Squaric acid inhibitors[49–52] are considered as a novel inhibitors for Chk1, Chk2, and SGK (serum and glucocorticoid-induced kinase). Mainly, the individual applications are varying by having different aryl system attached to the squaric acid scaffold (general formula structure **25-30**). The preferred position for squaric acid derivatives is at positions 3-hydroxy or 3-methoxybenzyl, and sometimes containing a chiral alpha-methyl group. In compound **31-32**, the prominent aryl ring is the biaryl 3-(2-pyridyl)-4-hydroxyphenyl group. Other examples, such as compounds **33** and **34** contain alternative phenolic groups. Compounds **35** and **36** have benzimidazoles ring systems and act as Chk1 inhibitors with $IC_{50} < 100$ nM. There are several other examples of indazolone containing squaric acid (**37-40**) having IC_{50} of about 10 nM[53,54] (Fig. 8.8).

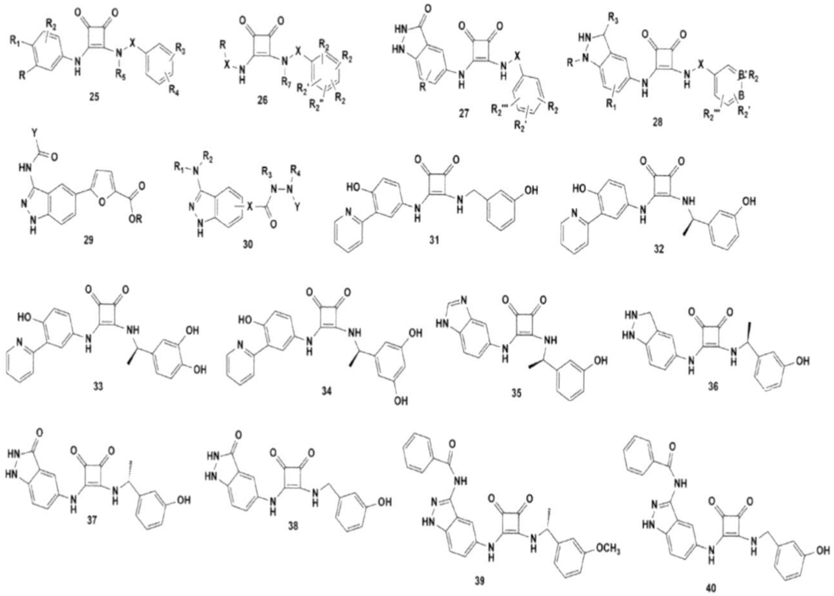

FIGURE 8.8   Squaric acid molecules as Chk1 inhibitors.

8.2.4 INDOLES, INDAZOLES, AND BENZIMIDAZOLES TEMPLATE-BASED INHIBITORS

Several biaryl aromatic ring systems such as indoles, indazoles, and benzimidazoles of the general formulae **41-44** act as scaffolds for Chk1 inhibitors.[55-58] CHIR-124 (Chiron) [(S)-3-(1H-benzo[d]imidazol-2-yl)-6-chloro-4-(quinuclidin-3-ylamino)-quinolin-2(1H)-one] is a novel quinolone-based small molecular inhibitor of Chk2 with $IC_{50} = 697$ nM[59] and Chk1 with an $IC_{50} = 0.3$ nM[60] (2000-fold lower than that against Chk2) (Fig. 8.9). This was determined in a cell-free kinase assay examining the ability of Chk1 to inhibit Cdc25C phosphorylation. CHIR-124 also has some limited activity against PDGFR, FLT3 (FMS-like tyrosine kinase-3) and GSK3 (glycogen synthase kinase 3), but with 10 to 100-fold higher IC_{50} values. It has synergistic effect on topoisomerase-I in both in vivo and in vitro study.[59]

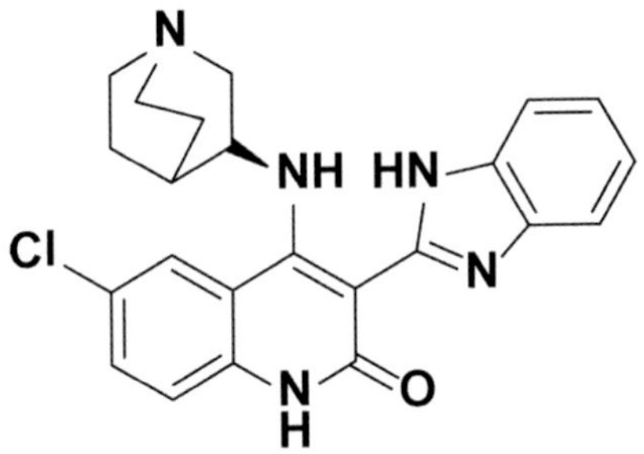

FIGURE 8.9 Chiron; CHIR-124, a prototype molecule.

Derivatives of indolylquinolinone[56] act as Chk1 inhibitors **41** and are very similar to the previously disclosed benzimidazole series from Chiron (e.g., CHIR-124).[59,60] Represented examples are shown in Figure 8.10 (**45a-d**). All these compounds suffered from lower biological activity with $IC_{50} < 50$ μM against the substrate in a homogeneous time-resolved fluorescence (HTRF) assay system.

A series of indolylindazoles of general formula **42** are revealed as Chk1 inhibitors. There are subsets of compounds as defined by the substituent at R_2 as **46** and **47** are shown in Figure 8.10. Pyrazolo benzimidazoles with the general formula **43** act inhibitor for kinase enzyme, but mostly Chk1 inhibitor. R_2 is always basic amide wherein only two examples: R_1

as H; the rest having R_1 as methyl were found to be active. For Instance, piperidine amide 69 shows Chk1 inhibition with $IC_{50} = 0.25$ µM, at the same time, adding another methyl group in the 5-position (R_1) of pyrazole 44 leads to increase in the activity against Chk1 with $IC_{50} = 98$ nM. The addition of another R_4 amid group leads to increase both activity and potency against Chk1 with $IC_{50} = 2$ nM, simple exchange in the amide and N-methylation of the piperidine in compound 51 had shown no change in both selectivity and potency, but, 1-cyclopropyl-3-[3-(5-morphplin-4-methyl-1H-benzoimidazol-2-yl)1H-pyrazol-4-yl]urea 52 had shown high potency and selectivity against different kinds of kinases.[61–64]

3,3'-diindolylmethane (DIM) 53 declined the growth of SKOV-3, TOV-21G, and OVCAR-3 ovarian cancer cells in both a dose- and time-dependent manner with effective concentrations ranging from 40 to 100 µM. Growth-inhibitory effects of DIM were mediated by cell-cycle arrest in G2/M phase in all the three cell lines. G2/M arrest was associated with DNA damage as indicated by phosphorylation of H(2)A.X at Ser139 and activation of Chk 2 (Chk2) in all the three cell lines.[65]

2-aryl benzimidazoles were the first selective ATP competitive Chk2 inhibitors which were identified from HTS.[66] The 4-chloro analog 54 (BML-277) had improved the overall potency, and it was suggested that the chlorine atom was partially solvent exposed. Adding to that, the replacement of the terminal aryl ring with alkyl-linked alcohol has improved the solubility (Fig. 8.10).[67]

Recently, Galal et al. had synthesized compound 55 which is potent Chk2 inhibitors. This compound was evaluated alone and in combination with doxorubicin on cell-cycle phases of MCF-7 cells using flow cytometry analysis. The results revealed their potencies as Chk2 inhibitors with IC_{50} ranges from 9.95 to 65.07 nM.[68] PD0407824 (9-hydroxy-4-phenyl-6 H-pyrrolo[3,4-c]carbazole-1,3-dione) 56 also known as PD407824, is a potent selective, small molecular Chk1 inhibitor with potential anticancer activity ($IC_{50} = 47$ nM).[69,70]

4,4-diacetyldiphenylurea-bis(guanylhydrazone) (NSC 109555) was reported as a novel Chk2 inhibitor (Fig. 8.11). NSC 109555 and PV1019 (NSC 744039) [7-nitro-1H-indole-2-carboxylic acid {4-[1-(guanidinohyd razone)-ethyl]-phenyl}-amide] had shown high selectivity as Chk2 inhibitor with submicromolar activity in various in vitro studies. PV1019 is ATP competitive Chk2 inhibitor which inhibits autophosphorylation process, Cdc25C phosphorylation, and HDMX degradation in response to DNA damage. PV1019 has been founded to protect normal mouse thymocytes against ionizing radiation-induced apoptosis. In addition, it synergizes the antiproliferative activity with topotecan, camptothecin, and radiation in human tumor cell lines. PV1019 and Chk2 showed small interfering with RNAs that can increase the antiproliferative activity against cancer cell lines with high Chk2 expression in the NCI-60 screen. These data indicate that PV1019 is a potent and selective inhibitor of Chk2 with chemotherapeutic and radiosensitization potential. The cocrystal structure of PV1019 bound in the ATP binding pocket of Chk2.[71]

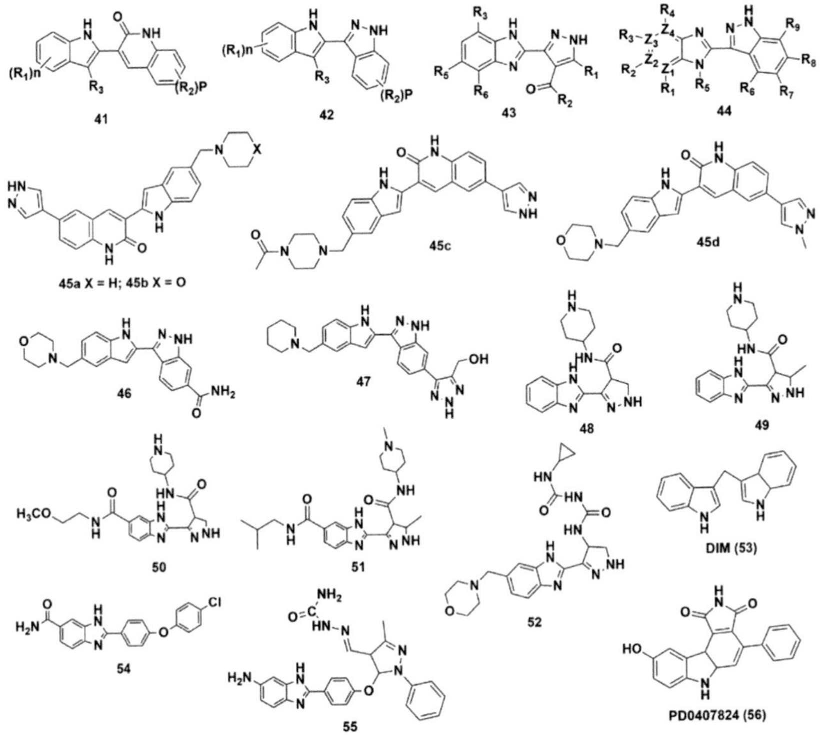

FIGURE 8.10 Generic structures and examples of indole, indazole, indolylindazoles, pyrazolo benzimidazoles, and benzimidazole Chk1 inhibitors.

NSC109555 belongs to a family of compounds known as the bis(guanylhydrazones), including the aliphatic derivative methylglyoxal-bis(guanylhydrazone) (MGBG). NSC109555 is a potent, selective, revisable ATP competitive inhibitor with $IC_{50} = 0.2$ μM. It inhibits histone H_1 phosphorylation ($IC_{50} = 0.24$ μM), in addition it declined the mitochondrial ATP synthesis. NSC109555 has shown in vivo anticancer activity in the number of leukemia cell study.[71,72]

PD 407824 is a potent selective Chk1 inhibitor with IC_{50} 47 nM (Fig. 8.11). Recently, Feng et al. found that PD 407824 increases the sensitivity of cells to sub-threshold amounts of BMP4. In addition, PD 407824 had depleted p21 levels, so that, activating CDK8/9, which then phosphorylates the SMAD2/3 linker region, leading to declining the levels of SMAD2/3 protein and improved the levels of nuclear SMAD1.[74]

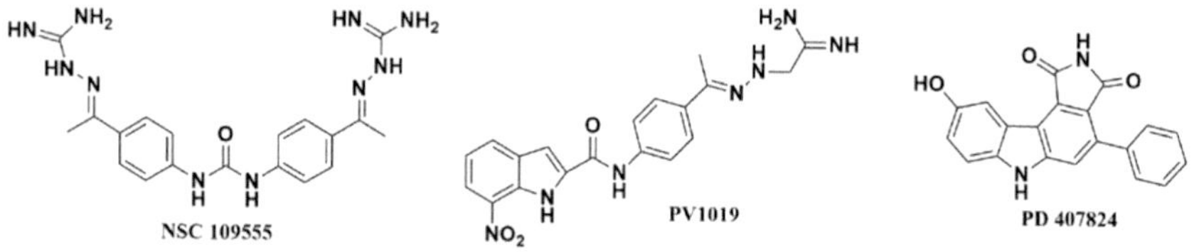

FIGURE 8.11   Drugs at clinical trials; NSC 744039, NSC 109555, and PD 407824.

8.2.5 THIENOPYRIDINE, IMIDAZOPYRAZINE, AND OTHER FUSED HETEROCYCLES TEMPLATE-BASED INHIBITORS

Five or six fused aromatic ring systems of general formula **57-64** were considered as the largest structurally related series of recently disclosed Chk inhibitor scaffold.[74-80] Varieties of fused 5- or 6-heteroaromatic ring system containing a carboxamide moiety fitting general formula **57** acts as Chk1, PDK1, and PAK inhibitors. A series pyrrolo[3,4-c]carbazoles of the general formula **57** not only inhibit Chks but also broader to be used as Ser/Thr kinases inhibitors kinases (CDKs and CHKs), receptor tyrosine kinases (e.g., HER subfamily), and non-receptor tyrosine kinases (e.g., Src family).

Most of the examples are thienopyridine carboxamides, in which the preferred L contains a basic amine, most commonly 3*S*-aminopiperidine, and R_1 can be substituted phenyl, such as in compounds **65** or aromatic heterocycles such as pyrazole such as in compounds **66**. Adding to the piperidine ring, the addition of basic amine, for example, pyrrolidine **67**, and homopiperidine **68**, and change the linkers to the amine, such as ether

69, all act as Chk1 inhibitors. Some of the alternate ring system revealed in the application are thiazolopyridines, thienopyridazines exemplified by **70**, and indoles like **70** from the above-mentioned example, it is clear that stereochemical orientation of the amide plays an important role in increasing the selectivity and potency against Chk1, PDK, or PAK. The cyclic amine having *S* stereochemistry are more likely to be preferred than the R stereochemistry, like indole **71**, non-chiral amines but still being used as Chk1 inhibitors but with low biological activity. This series of ChK inhibitors have been designed by scaffold morphing from the AZD7762 class of thiophene carboxamide ureas. Recently, Isono et al. had founded that AZD7762 strongly sensitizes urothelial carcinoma cells to gemcitabine.[84]

5-substituted pyrrolo[3,4-c]carbazole-1,3(2*H*,6*H*)-dione derivatives **73** had high potent anticancer activity (Chk1 inhibitor) with $IC_{50} = 2.8$ nM with higher activity than UNC-01.[88] 3,5-Diaryl-2-aminopyridines such as compound **74** was identified by the Institute of Cancer Research, London as Chk2 inhibitors following HTS of a 7000 member kinase-focused library.[89] In WO2009/044162, the aryl group in the general formula **64** was exemplified by 2-cyano-pyrazin-5-yl. The second aryl group is usually coupled with pyrazine via an amine linker with either pyridine or pyrimidine, and R covers a wide range of chemical space. Compound **75** was shown to be a potent anticancer activity with IC_{50} value of 600 nM against Chk1 (Fig. 8.12).[90]

UCN-01 (7-hydroxystaurosporine) is an indolocarbazole natural product, it has been founded to enhance the therapeutic activity of DNA damaging agent in animal models.[82] UCN-01 has been founded to be an extremely long half-life 25.9 days (range 6–161 days) (because it avoids binding with the human plasma protein).[83] UCN-01 is in the Phase-II clinical trial at present.[84] Although staurosporine is a chemical analog to UCN-01 and isogranulatimide, but these compounds do not suffer from an extremely long half-life, and all are known to have Chk1 inhibitor activity. Therefore, the pyrrolo[3,4-c]carbazole is considered as a good scaffold to develop novel Chk1 inhibitors (Fig. 8.12).[85–87]

MK-8776 (SCH 900776) is a selective Chk1 inhibitor with IC_{50} of 3 nM with minimal intrinsic antagonistic properties. It is highly selective (500-fold selectivity against Chk2 compared to Chk1) with IC_{50} of 1.5 μmol/L and it is a weak CDK2 ($IC_{50} = 160$ nM) inhibitor.[91] SCH900776 enhances the γ-H2AX response of hydroxyurea, 5-fluoruracil, and cytarabine. In combination with an anti-metabolite, SCH900776 induces accumulation of γ-H2AX within 2 h, indicative of replication fork collapse and double-stranded DNA breaks. Finally, SCH900776 decline the accumulation of the Chk1 pS296 autophosphorylation in a dose-dependent manner.[92] Herůdková et al. reported that SCH900776 significantly increased the cytotoxic response produced by platinum-based drugs in colon cancer cells.[93] Recently, SCH900776 has been found to synergistically increase the anticancer activity of MLN4924[94] and also improved radiosensitizing effect compared to UCN-01 by exacerbating radiation-induced aberrant mitosis. MK-8776 is in Phase-II clinical trials in combination with chemotherapy.[95–97]

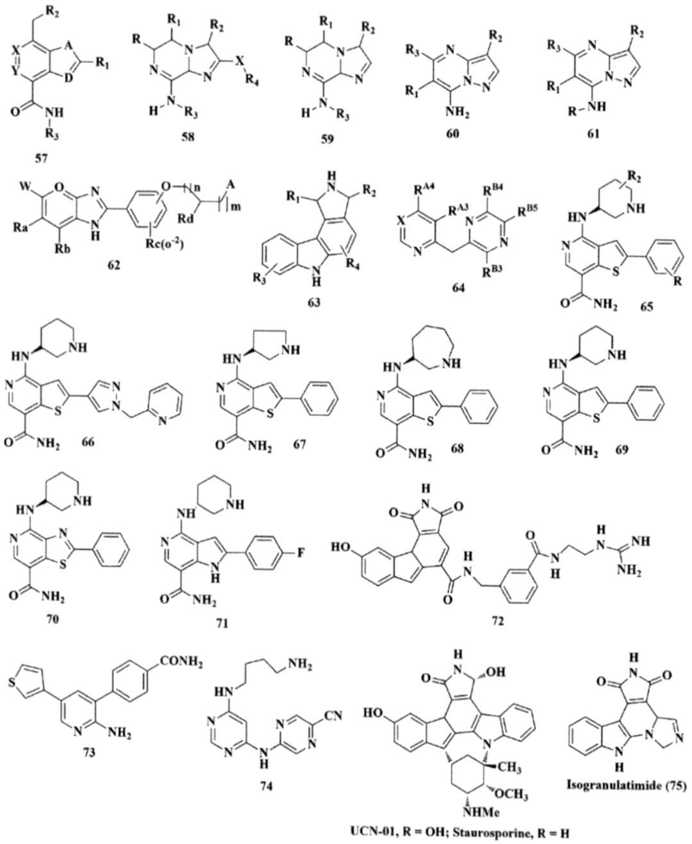

FIGURE 8.12 Thienopyridine, imidazopyrazine, and other fused heterocycles as Chk inhibitors.

Recently, Samadder et al. had synthesized MU380, an analogue of SCH900776, having N-trifluoromethylpyrazole motif which interferes with metabolic oxidative dealkylation; this provides greater robustness to MU380. Comparing to SCH900776, MU380 in combination with GEM causes higher accumulation of DNA damage in tumor cells and subsequent enhanced cell death.[98] CCT241533 is a potent Chk2 ATP competitive inhibitor (IC_{50} = 3 nM), it stopped Chk2 activity in human tumor cell lines in response to DNA damage, as exhibited by inhibition of Chk2 autophosphorylation at S516, HDMX degradation and band-shift mobility changes. It synergistically improves the cytotoxicity of PARP inhibitors.[99] SB 218078 is a potent ATP competitive Chk1 inhibitor with IC_{50} of 15 nM. It is important for G_2/M arrest in response to DNA damage. In cellular assay, SB 218078 was able to abrogate G_2 arrest in response to DNA damage and improve the cytotoxicity of DNA-damaging drug.[100]

TCS 2312 is a potent selective Chk1 inhibitor (Ki = 0.38 nM, EC_{50} = 60 nM). TCS 2312 synergistically improve the activity of gemcitabine against breast and prostate cancer cell lines and display antiproliferative effects in vitro.[101]

SAR-020106 is a pyrazolo[1,5-a]pyrimidine potent, selective for Chk2 (IC_{50} = 13 nM) and CDK1 (IC_{50} = 13 nM). In addition, in vitro studies had shown that SAR-020106 synergistically inhibit the cancer cell growth when used in combination with SN38 in HT-29, SW620, and Colo205 colon cell lines. It has an IC_{50} for CHK2 and CDK1 of >10 µM. Other kinases that were modestly inhibited included FLT3, IRAK4, Met, MST2, p70S6K, Ret, RSK1, and TrkA.[102] Adding to that, it potentiates the anticancer activity of irinotecan and gemcitabine in an SW620 colon cancer xenograft model.[103]

Eli Lilly and Company (Indianapolis, US) had synthesis LY2606368 which act as Chk1 (IC_{50}<50 nM) and Chk2 (IC_{50} < 4.7nM) inhibitors (Fig. 8.13). This compound had shown to reduce the tumor growth by 6-fold in both HT-29 colon cancer and Calu-6 lung cancer tumor xenografts when used with gemcitabine.[104] Furthermore, LY2606368 showed a strong cytotoxic activity on B-/T-All cell lines as a single agent and in combination with imatinib and dasatinib or with the purine nucleoside anti-metabolite clofarabine.[105] LY2606368 is in Phase-I clinical testing. Recently, prexasertib showed clinical activity and was tolerable in patients with BRCA wild-type high-grade serous ovarian carcinoma.[106–108]

PD-321852 is a potent Chk1 inhibitor which synergist the effect of gemcitabine-induced clonogenic death in a panel of pancreatic cancer cell lines (Fig. 8.13). PD-321852 inhibited Chk1 in all cell lines as evidenced by stabilization of Cdc25A.[109] Its IC_{50} in a cell-free inhibition assay for Chk1 is 5 nM.[110] CCT244747 is a novel oral Chk1 inhibitor developed by the Institute for Cancer Research in London and Sareum Pharmaceuticals.[111] It has been developed from the compound SAR-020106. Its IC_{50} Chk1 inhibitor is 8 nM. It shows >75 times selectivity against FLT3 and >1000-fold selectivity against Chk2 and CDK1. Mouse xenograft models of human tumors have confirmed that clinically relevant concentrations of CCT244747 are detectable following oral administration with an oral bioavailability of 62%.

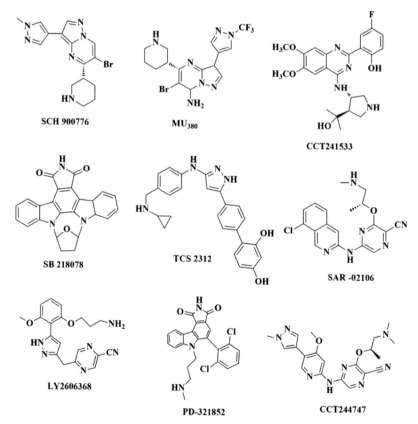

FIGURE 8.13   Some potent Chk1/2 inhibitors in the clinical trial.

8.2.6 FUSED QUINOLINONE AND OTHER MULTI-RING DERIVATIVES TEMPLATE-BASED INHIBITOR

Merck & Co. has filed a great number of patent applications using the tri- and tetracyclic scaffold Chk1 inhibitors of general formulae **76-80** (Fig. 8.14).[112–116] Many of the applications cover tricyclic ring cores very similar to those reported by AstraZeneca in 2005.[117] A series of fused pyrazoles of the general formula **76** (e.g., **81**) act as Chk1 inhibitors. The R_1 substitution is usually alkylamino with a benzyl group as in **82** or sometimes amid and urea 83. A series of triazolo-quinazolinones of general formula **78** (e.g., **84**) are maintained to act as Chk1 inhibitor. Compounds **81-87** had been founded to be a potent Chk inhibitory activity with IC_{50} <50 µM. Another series of fused imidazoles with general formula **79** (e.g., compounds **88-92**), benzoisoquinolinones of general formula **80** (e.g., compounds **93-96**) had shown to act as potent Chk inhibitor represented in Figure 8.14. A series of triazolones of general formula **78** (e.g., compound **97**) had been identified as a potent, selective Chk1 inhibitor with good pharmacokinetic properties and high water solubility.[122] Compound **98** is a thioquinazolinone derivative with potent Chk1 inhibitor that bound allosterically to the active site.[29] The carbonyl from the quinazolinone ring formed a water-mediated hydrogen bond to Glu134, while the piperidine amine and amide carbonyl interacted directly with Glu205 and the backbone of Leu206, respectively. The 3-chlorophenyl group fitted securely into a narrow hydrophobic cleft.[28]

GNE-900 (**99**) ((9*H*-Pyrrole[2,3-b:5,4-c']-dipyridine-6-carbonitrile-3-[4-(1-piperidinylmethyl)phenyl]) is a potent oral bioavailable inhibitor of Chk 1 with IC_{50} = 1.1 nM, developed by Genentech by high-throughput screening of their small molecule library.[119] GNE-900 inhibited an SN-38-induced G2/M checkpoint in HT-29 colon cancer cells with an EC_{50} of 29.3 nM. GNE-900 (Fig. 8.15) is an orally bioavailable ATP-competitive small molecular inhibitor, with high selectivity (1000-fold selective for Chk1 over Chk2). It inhibits Chk1 with a notably high IC_{50} value of 1.1 nM. It synergistically improves the activity, when combined with gemcitabine in an HT-29 colon cancer xenograft. Optimal efficacy was observed in vivo when S-phase arrest was induced first using gemcitabine, followed by checkpoint abrogation by subsequent dosing of the CHK1 inhibitor.[120] GDC-0425 (Fig. 8.15) is an orally bioavailable, ATP-competitive Chk1 inhibitors known to synergize the activity of gemcitabine by abolishing the S and G2 checkpoints, thereby resulting in a premature entry into mitosis and mitotic catastrophe. At present, the molecule is in the Phase-I clinical trial.[121]

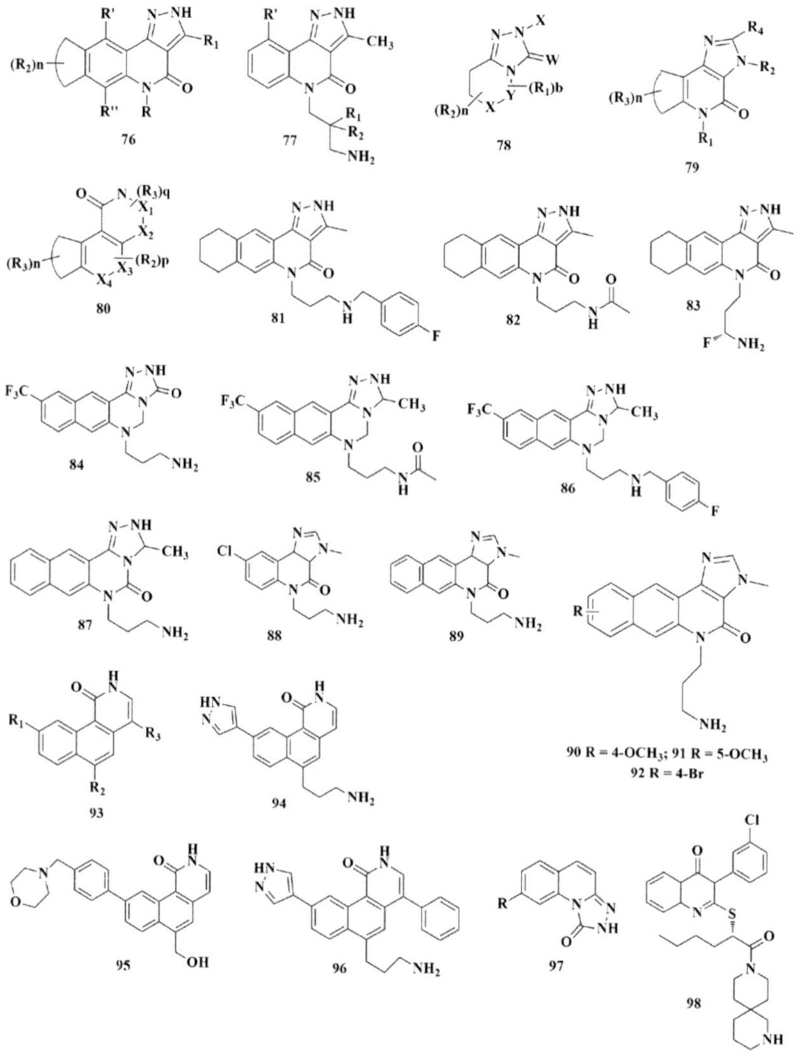

FIGURE 8.14 Generic formula and compounds of fused quinolinone and other fused-ring as Chk1 inhibitors.

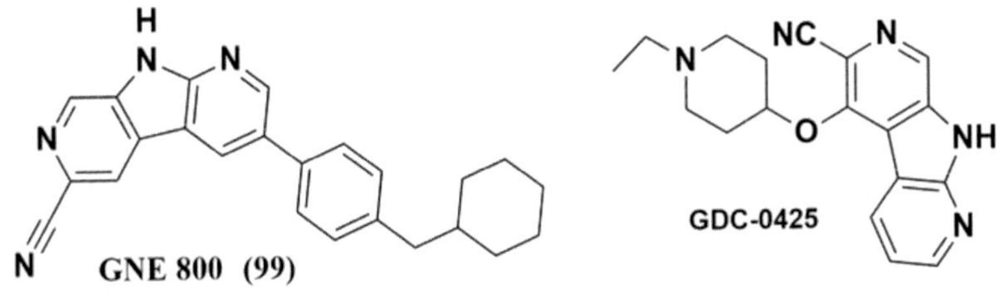

FIGURE 8.15   GNE 800 (G2/M checkpoint inhibitor) and GDC-0425 (S and G2 checkpoints inhibitor) as emerging leads.

8.2.7 AMINOTHIAZOLE TEMPLATE-BASED INHIBITOR

Series of aminothiazole derivatives of the general formula **100-113** are claimed as Chk1 ,[122] they are also used for the treatment of inflammation, proliferation disorder, central nervous system disorders, and cardiovascular disorder.[123,1249] The 2-pyridylaminothiazoles of the general formula **99**, having a more specific substructure 104, is shown in Figure 8.16. Different positions of attachment for R_1 were studied, but mostly 4-position substitution (absent in the 3-position) and morpholino-piperazines were the most common, as in compound **105**. Examples of R_2 variation covered mainly amides, but also included heteroaryls and amino alkylamino substitution compounds such as **106**. It is interesting that a third generic structure 103 is mentioned in the text but not in the claims although examples such as **108** are disclosed (Fig. 8.17).[123] In anilinopiperazinyl aminothiazole derivatives with general formula 101,[123] there are 161 examples with 18 example having the generic formula **108**, R_1 is usually heteroaryl or aryl (mostly pyrazole and indazole), and R_3 are usually H or CH_3. Also, there are 16 examples with the general formula **108** when Q3 is mostly H, whereas Q1 is usually COOH; $n = 1$; w is usually CH linker or an amine. Finally, there are four examples with general formula **110**, where $R_1 = CH_3$. The most specific compound claim is for general formula **111** where R_2 is either H or alkyl (Fig. 8.16). In the final, there are 323 examples of aminothiazole with general formula **102**.[124] Compounds **112** and **113** are examples illustrated in this series.

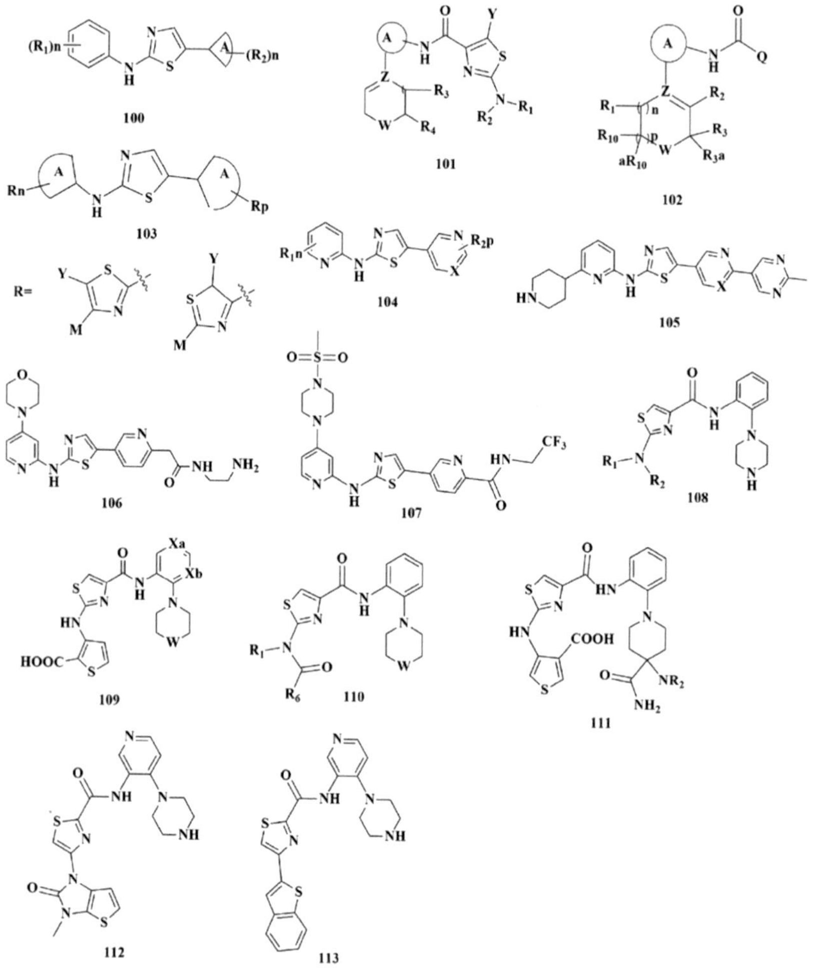

FIGURE 8.16   Aminothiazole compounds as Chk1 inhibitors.

8.2.8   3-HYDROXYISOTHIAZOLE-4-CARBOXYMIDINES TEMPLATE-BASED INHIBITOR

A series of 3-hydroxyisothiazole-4-carboxymidines with general formula **114-116** act as ATP competitive inhibitor,[125] and selectively inhibit Chk2.[126–128] Ar_1 and Ar_2 are usually phenylderivatives, or pyridyl derivatives while R_1 is usually OH, halo, alkoxy alkyl, and finally,

R_2 are hydrogen or halogen. One of the most important isothiazoles derivatives is VRX0466617 **117**, which selectivity inhibit Chk2 enzyme through blocking the enzymatic activity of recombinant Chk2. VRX0466617 at dose 5–10 μmol/L activate the phosphorylation of Chk2 Thr68 even in the absence of DNA damage, because of blocking of Chk2 enzymatic activity. Although VRX0466617 increased the multinucleated cells, it did not mutate the cell-cycle distribution. It did not affect the cytotoxicity of anticancer drugs such as doxorubicin, taxol, and cisplatin as it attenuated the IR-induced apoptosis in a short-term assay. These results underscore the specificity of VRX0466617 for Chk2 inhibitor for both in vitro and in vivo studies (Fig. 8.17) and support the use of this compound as a biological probe to study the Chk2-dependent pathways.

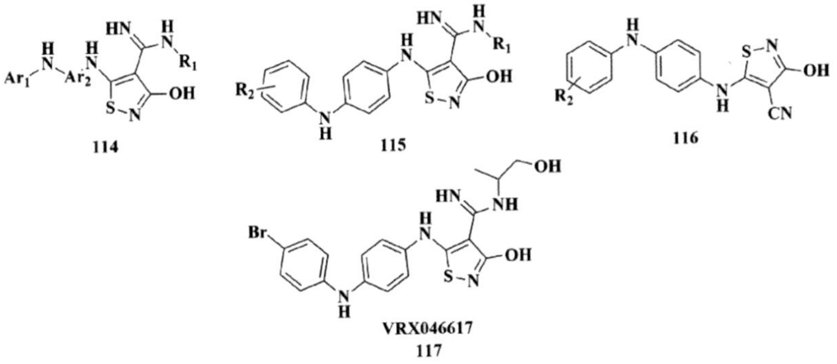

FIGURE 8.17   3-Hydroxyisothiazole-4-carboxymidines as Chk2 inhibitor.

8.2.9   2-(QUINAZOLIN-2-YL)PHENOLS TEMPLATE-BASED INHIBITOR

2-(quinazolin-2-yl)phenols are considered as a new series of Chk2 inhibitor [General formula **118**], for example, **119-121**.[129] Structure–activity relationship for multiple substitution positions were optimized separately, and in combination leading to compound 4-fluoro-2-(4-((3S,4R)-4-(2-hydroxypropan-2-yl)pyrrolidin-3-ylamino)-6,7-dimethoxyquinazolin-2-yl)phenol **121** with IC$_{50}$ 3 nM, with high selectivity against Chk2 in comparison to Chk1 and a wider panel of kinases (Fig. 8.18).

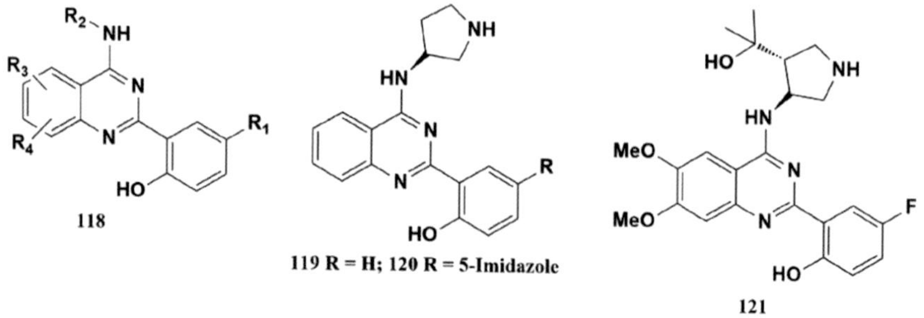

FIGURE 8.18   2-(quinazolin-2-yl)phenols-based Chk2 inhibitors.

8.3   CONCLUSION

Tremendous advances in the inhibition of Chks (ChKs) by small molecules have occurred over the past 12 years. These inhibitors can be organized into seven closely related scaffolds: bisaryl ureas, dibenzoazepinones, squaric acid derivatives, bi-heteroaryl rings, bicyclic fused heteroaromatic rings, tricyclic fused rings, and aminothiazoles. These inhibitors have different adenine (Hing-binding) functional group that interacts with both Chk1 and Chk2 in the kinase active site. From the screening of the preferred substitution of these inhibitors, it becomes evident that these inhibitors interact with certain key residues in, or surrounding the ATP-binding pocket in either the "buried" hydrophobic pocket or near the adjacent ribose sugar-binding pocket. The biological importance of the Ser/Thr Chks; Chk1 and Chk2 are to inhibit the damaging DNA cells from replications. Preclinical data suggested that the combination therapy between Chk inhibitors and DNA-damaging agent are a promising anticancer treatment. Furthermore, recent developments in Chk biology have the potential to impact future development of Chk inhibitors and clinical trials. In addition to Chk1 and Chk2, other emerging therapeutic targets for potentiating the effects of DNA damage are PARP, ATM, ATR, CDC25, DNA-PK, Wee1 kinase, and hsp90. Judging from the intense efforts being made in the field of sensitization approaches, we can expect additional clinical candidates to be brought forward for evaluation in the near future.

KEYWORDS

- checkpoint kinase
- anticancer
- clinical trials
- inhibitors
- PF477736
- V158411

REFERENCES

1. Harper, J. W.; Elledge, S. J. The DNA Damage Response: Ten Years After. *Mol. Cell* **2007,** *28,* 739–745.
2. O'Connor, M. J.; Martin, N. M. B.; Smith, G. C. M. Targeted Cancer Therapies Based on the Inhibition of DNA Strand Break Repair. *Oncogene* **2007,** *26,* 7816–7824.
3. Brosh, R. M., Jr. DNA Repair as a Target for Anti-Cancer Therapy. *Anticancer Agents Med. Chem.* **2008,** *8* (4), 350
4. Pommier, Y.; Sordet, O.; Rao, V. A.; Zhang, H.; Kohn, K. W. Targeting Chk2 Kinase: Molecular Interaction Maps and Therapeutic Rationale. *Curr. Pharm. Des.* **2005,** *11,* 2855–2872.
5. Zhao, H.; Watkins, J. L.; Piwnica-Worms, H. Disruption of the Chk 1/Cell Division Cycle 25A Pathway Abrogates Ionizing Radiation-Induced S and G2 Checkpoints. *Proc. Natl. Acad. Sci. U. S. A.* **2002,** *99,* 14795–14800.
6. Sørensen, C. S.; Syljuåsen, R. G.; Falck, J.; Schroeder, T.; Rönnstrand, L.; Khanna, K. K.; Zhou, B. -B.; Bartek, J.; Lukas, J. Chk1 Regulates the S Phase Checkpoint by Coupling the Physiological Turnover and Ionizing Radiation-Induced Accelerated Proteolysis of Cdc25A. *Cancer Cell* **2003,** *3,* 247–258.
7. Mailand, N.; Falck, J.; Lukas, C.; Syljuåsen, R. G.; Welcker, M.; Bartek, J.; Lukas, J. Rapid Destruction of Human Cdc25A in Response to DNA Damage. *Science* **2000,** *288,* 1425–1429.
8. Mailand, N.; Podtelejnikov, A. V.; Groth, A.; Mann, M.; Bartek, J.; Lukas, J. Regulation of G(2)/M Events by Cdc25A Through Phosphorylation-Dependent Modulation of its Stability. *EMBO J.* **2002,** *21,* 5911–5920.
9. Cunat, S.; Anahory, T.; Berthenet, C.; Hedon, B.; Franckhauser, C.; Fernandez, A.; Hamamah, S.; Lamb, N. J. C. The Cell Cycle Control Protein cdc25C is Present, and Phosphorylated on Serine 214 in the Transition From Germinal Vesicle to Metaphase II in Human Oocyte Meiosis. *Mol. Reprod. Dev.* **2008,** *75,* 1176–1184.
10. Zhang, Y.; Zhang, Z.; Xu, X. -Y.; Li, X. -S.; Yu, M.; Yu, A. -M.; Zong, Z. -H.; Yu, B. -Z. Protein Kinase A Modulates Cdc25B Activity During Meiotic Resumption of Mouse Oocytes. *Dev. Dyn.* **2008,** *237,* 3777–3786.

11. Perry, J. A.; Kornbluth, S. Cdc25 and Wee1: Analogous Opposites? *Cell Div.* **2007,** *2*, 12.

12. Zachos, G.; Rainey, M. D.; Gillespie, D. A. F. Chk1-Deficient Tumour Cells are Viable But Exhibit Multiple Checkpoint and Survival Defects. *EMBO J.* **2003,** *22*, 713–723.

13. Gatei, M.; Sloper, K.; Sörensen, C.; Syljuäsen, R.; Falck, J.; Hobson, K.; Savage, K.; Lukas, J.; Zhou, B. -B.; Bartek, J.; Khanna, K. K. Ataxia-Telangiectasia-Mutated (ATM) and NBS1-Dependent Phosphorylation of Chk1 on Ser-317 in Response to Ionizing Radiation. *J. Biol. Chem.* **2003,** *278*, 14806–14811.

14. Xiao, Z.; Chen, Z.; Gunasekera, A. H.; Sowin, T. J.; Rosenberg, S. H.; Fesik, S.; Zhang, H. Chk1 Mediates S and G2 Arrests Through Cdc25A Degradation in Response to DNA-Damaging Agents. *J. Biol. Chem.* **2003,** *278*, 21767–21773.

15. Bartek, J.; Lukas, J. Chk1 and Chk2 Kinases in Checkpoint Control and Cancer. *Cancer Cell* **2003,** *3*, 421–429.

16. Ahn, J.; Urist, M.; Prives, C. The Chk2 Protein Kinase. *DNA Repair (Amst).* **2004,** *3*, 1039–1047.

17. Falck, J.; Mailand, N.; Syljuåsen, R. G.; Bartek, J.; Lukas, J. The ATM–Chk2–Cdc25A Checkpoint Pathway Guards Against Radioresistant DNA Synthesis. *Nature* **2001,** *410*, 842–847.

18. Takai, H.; Naka, K.; Okada, Y.; Watanabe, M.; Harada, N.; Saito, S.; Anderson, C. W.; Appella, E.; Nakanishi, M.; Suzuki, H.; Nagashima, K.; Sawa, H.; Ikeda, K.; Motoyama, N. Chk2-Deficient Mice Exhibit Radioresistance and Defective p53-Mediated Transcription. *EMBO J.* **2002,** *21*, 5195–5205.

19. Zaugg, K.; Su, Y. -W.; Reilly, P. T.; Moolani, Y.; Cheung, C. C.; Hakem, R.; Hirao, A.; Liu, Q.; Elledge, S. J.; Mak, T. W. Cross-Talk Between Chk1 and Chk2 in Double-Mutant Thymocytes. *Proc. Natl. Acad. Sci. U. S. A.* **2007,** *104*, 3805–3810.

20. Niida, H.; Katsuno, Y.; Banerjee, B.; Hande, M. P.; Nakanishi, M. Specific Role of Chk1 Phosphorylations in Cell Survival and Checkpoint Activation. *Mol. Cell. Biol.* **2007,** *27*, 2572–2581.

21. Chen, Z.; Xiao, Z.; Gu, W. -Z.; Xue, J.; Bui, M. H.; Kovar, P.; Li, G.; Wang, G.; Tao, Z. -F.; Tong, Y.; Lin, N. -H.; Sham, H. L.; Wang, J. Y. J.; Sowin, T. J.; Rosenberg, S. H.; Zhang, H. Selective Chk1 Inhibitors Differentially Sensitize p53-Deficient Cancer Cells to Cancer Therapeutics. *Int. J. Can.* **2006,** *119*, 2784–2794.

22. Li, G.; Hasvold, L. A.; Tao, Z. -F.; Wang, G. T.; Gwaltney, S. L.; Patel, J.; Kovar, P.; Credo, R. B.; Chen, Z.; Zhang, H.; Park, C.; Sham, H. L.; Sowin, T.; Rosenberg, S. H.; Lin, N. -H. Synthesis and Biological Evaluation of 1-(2,4,5-trisubstituted phenyl)-3-(5-cyanopyrazin-2-yl)ureas as Potent Chk1 Kinase Inhibitors. *Bioorg. Med. Chem. Lett.* **2006,** *16*, 2293–2298.

23. Mitchell, J. B.; Choudhuri, R.; Fabre, K.; Sowers, A. L.; Citrin, D.; Zabludoff, S. D.; Cook, J. A. In Vitro and In Vivo Radiation Sensitization of Human Tumor Cells by a Novel Chk Inhibitor, AZD7762. *Clin. Cancer Res.* **2010,** *16*, 2076–2084.

24. McNeely, S.; Conti, C.; Sheikh, T.; Patel, H.; Zabludoff, S.; Pommier, Y.; Schwartz, G.; Tse, A. Chk1 Inhibition After Replicative Stress Activates a Double Strand Break Response Mediated by ATM and DNA-Dependent Protein Kinase. *Cell Cycle* **2010,** *9*, 995–1004.

25. Blasina, A.; Hallin, J.; Chen, E.; Arango, M. E.; Kraynov, E.; Register, J.; Grant, S.; Ninkovic, S.; Chen, P.; Nichols, T.; O'Connor, P.; Anderes, K. Breaching the DNA Damage Checkpoint via PF-00477736, a Novel Small-Molecule Inhibitor of Chk 1. *Mol. Cancer Ther.* **2008**, *7*, 2394–2404.

26. Matthews, D. J.; Yakes, F. M.; Chen, J.; Tadano, M.; Bornheim, L.; Clary, D. O.; Tai, A.; Wagner, J. M.; Miller, N.; Kim, Y. D.; Robertson, S.; Murray, L.; Karnitz, L. M. Pharmacological Abrogation of S-Phase Checkpoint Enhances the Anti-Tumor Activity of Gemcitabine In Vivo. *Cell Cycle* **2007**, *6*, 104–110.

27. Bryant, C.; Scriven, K.; Massey, A. J. Inhibition of the Chk Chk1 Induces DNA Damage and Cell Death in Human Leukemia and Lymphoma Cells. *Mol. Cancer* **2014**, *13*, 147.

28. Converso, A.; Hartingh, T.; Garbaccio, R. M.; Tasber, E.; Rickert, K.; Fraley, M. E.; Yan, Y.; Kreatsoulas, C.; Stirdivant, S.; Drakas, B.; Walsh, E. S.; Hamilton, K.; Buser, C. A.; Mao, X.; Abrams, M. T.; Beck, S. C.; Tao, W.; Lobell, R.; Sepp-Lorenzino, L.; Zugay-Murphy, J.; Sardana, V.; Munshi, S. K.; Jezequel-Sur, S. M.; Zuck, P. D.; Hartman, G. D. Development of Thioquinazolinones, Allosteric Chk1 Kinase Inhibitors. *Bioorg. Med. Chem. Lett.* **2009**, *19*, 1240–1244.

29. Vanderpool, D.; Johnson, T. O.; Ping, C.; Bergqvist, S.; Alton, G.; Phonephaly, S.; Rui, E.; Luo, C.; Deng, Y. -L.; Grant, S.; Quenzer, T.; Margosiak, S.; Register, J.; Brown, E.; Ermolieff, J. Characterization of the Chk1 Allosteric Inhibitor Binding Site. *Biochemistry* **2009**, *48*, 9823–9830.

30. Chen, P.; Luo, C.; Deng, Y.; Ryan, K.; Register, J.; Margosiak, S.; Tempczyk-Russell, A.; Nguyen, B.; Myers, P.; Lundgren, K.; Kan, C. C.; O'Connor, P. M. The 1.7 Å Crystal Structure of Human Cell Cycle Chk Chk1: Implications for Chk1 Regulation. *Cell* **2000**, *100*, 681–692.

31. Diaz FA, Holcomb R, Farouz F, Thorsett G. *Development of highly selective Chk-1 inhibitors with low nanomolar cellular activity.* In: Abstracts of Papers of the American Chemical Society 2007;233:518-518.

32. Kesicki EA, Gaudino JJ, Cook AW, Kaufman RJ, Brandhuber BJ, Vigers GP, Howard ML, Weidner MF, Dickinson E, Keegan KS. *Discovery of Pyrazinyl Ureas as Inhibitors of the Cell Cycle Checkpoint Kinase Chk1.* J. Med. Chem. 2001;44:4615.

33. Diaz, F.; Farouz, F. S.; Holcomb, R.; Kesicki, E. A.; Ooi, H. C.; Rudolph, A.; Stappenbeck, F.; Thorsett, E.; Gaudino, J. J.; Fischer, K. L.; Cook, A. W. Heteroaryl Urea Derivatives Useful for Inhibiting Chkl, US2006/011584; 2006.

34. Limited., S. O. Preparation of Quinoline and Quinoxaline N-oxides as Chk-1 Inhibitors. WO2008015423, **2008**.

35. Limited, S. O. *Preparation of Diarylurea N-oxides as CHK1 Inhibitors for Treatment of Cancer,* WO2007144579; **2007**.

36. Limited, S. O. *Preparation of 3-substituted-1,2,4-benzotriazine Derivatives as Kinase Inhibitors,* WO2008059259; **2008**.

37. Corporation, I. *Preparation of Bisarylurea Derivatives Useful for Inhibiting Chk1,* WO2006012308; **2006**.

38. McKeown, S. R.; Cowen, R. L.; Williams, K. J. Bioreductive Drugs: from Concept to Clinic. *Clin. Oncol.* **2007**, *19*, 427–442.

39. Li, G.; Hasvold, L. A.; Tao, Z. -F.; Wang, G. T.; Gwaltney, S. L.; Patel, J.; Kovar, P.; Credo, R. B.; Chen, Z.; Zhang, H.; Park, C.; Sham, H. L.; Sowin, T.; Rosenberg,

S. H.; Lin, N. -H. Synthesis and Biological Evaluation of 1-(2,4,5-trisubstituted phenyl)-3-(5-cyanopyrazin-2-yl)ureas as Potent Chk1 Kinase Inhibitors. *Bioorg. Med. Chem. Lett.* **2006**, *16*, 2293–2298.

40. Alessandra, B.; Jill, K.; Enhong, C.; Anderes, K. A Novel Inhibitor of the Protein Kinase Chk1: Studies on the Mechanism of Action. *Cell. Mol. Biol.* **2005**, *65*, 1045.

41. McArthur, G. A. Imaging with FLT-PET Demonstrates that PF-477736, an Inhibitor of CHK1 Kinase, Overcomes a Cell Cycle Checkpoint Induced by Gemcitabine in PC-3 Xenografts. *Proc. Am. Soc. Clin. Oncol.* **2006**, *25*, 3045.

42. Abbott Laboratories. Preparation of dibenzo[b,e][1,4]diazepin-11-ones as kinase inhibitors for treatment of cancer. US2007254867; **2007**, Cont.-in-part of US Ser. No. 785,120.

43. Hasvold, L. A.; Wang, L.; Przytulinska, M.; Xiao, Z.; Chen, Z.; Gu, W. -Z.; Merta, P. J.; Xue, J.; Kovar, P.; Zhang, H.; Park, C.; Sowin, T. J.; Rosenberg, S. H.; Lin, N. -H. Investigation of Novel 7,8-disubstituted-5,10-dihydro-dibenzo[b,e][1,4] diazepin-11-ones as Potent Chk1 Inhibitors. *Bioorg. Med. Chem. Lett.* **2008**, *18*, 2311–2315.

44. Wang, L.; Sullivan, G. M.; Hexamer, L. A.; Hasvold, L. A.; Thalji, R.; Przytulinska, M.; Tao, Z. -F.; Li, G.; Chen, Z.; Xiao, Z.; Gu, W. -Z.; Xue, J.; Bui, M. -H.; Merta, P.; Kovar, P.; Bouska, J. J.; Zhang, H.; Park, C.; Stewart, K. D.; Sham, H. L.; Sowin, T. J.; Rosenberg, S. H.; Lin, N. -H. Design, Synthesis, and Biological Activity of 5,10-dihydro-dibenzo[b,e][1,4]diazepin-11-one-based potent and Selective Chk-1 Inhibitors. *J. Med. Chem.* **2007**, *50*, 4162–4176.

45. Millennium Pharmaceuticals, Inc. Preparation of diarylureas as Chk1 kinase inhibitors for treating cancer. WO2005072733; **2005**.

46. Millennium Pharmaceuticals, Inc. Preparation of 2,5-dihydro-pyrazolo[4,3-c] quinolin-4-ones as Chk-1 inhibitors for treating cancer. WO2005118583; **2005**.

47. Zhang, C.; Yan, Z.; Painter, C. L.; Zhang, Q.; Chen, E.; Arango, M. E.; Kuszpit, K.; Zasadny, K.; Hallin, M.; Hallin, J.; Wong, A.; Buckman, D.; Sun, G.; Qiu, M.; Anderes, K.; Christensen, J. G. PF-00477736 Mediates Chk 1 Signaling Pathway and Potentiates Docetaxel-Induced Efficacy in Xenografts. *Clin. Cancer Res.* **2009**, *15*, 4630–4640.

48. Nguyen, T.; Hawkins, E.; Kolluri, A.; Kmieciak, M.; Park, H.; Lin, H.; Grant, S. Synergism Between Bosutinib (SKI-606) and the Chk1 Inhibitor (PF-00477736) in Highly Imatinib-Resistant BCR/ABL+ Leukemia Cells. *Leuk. Res.* **2015**, *39*, 65–71.

49. Patent, M. *Preparation of Squaramides as Serine Threonine Kinase Inhibitors*, DE102005035742 WO2007014608; **2007**.

50. GmbH, M. P. *Preparation of N-pyridinylphenyl-3-4-diaminocyclobut-3-ene-1, 2-diones as CHK1, CHK2, and/or SGK Kinase Inhibitors for Treating Cancer*, WO2007014607; **2007**.

51. GmbH, M. P. *Preparation of 3-oxoindazolyl-substituted Squaric Acid Derivatives as CHK1, CHK2 and/or SGK Kinase Inhibitors*, WO2007022858; **2007**.

52. Merck Patent GmbH. Preparation of 3-amino-4-[(phenylmethyl)amino]-3-cyclobutene-1,2-diones as CHK1, CHK2 and SGK kinase inhibitors. WO2006105865; **2006**.

53. Patent, M. *Preparation of 5-(2-furanyl)-1H-indazoles as CHK1/CHK2 Kinase Inhibitors*, DE102006005180 [WO2007090493]; **2007**.

54. Patent, M. *Preparation of 3-aminoindazoles as CHK1/CHK2 Kinase Inhibitors*, DE102006005179 [WO2007090494]; **2007**.

55. Merck & Co, Inc,. Quinolinone inhibitors of Checkpoint Kinase CHK1 for Treatment of Cancer. WO2007084135; **2007**.

56. Merck & Co, I. *Preparation of Indolylindazole Derivatives as Inhibitors of Chks*, 2003.

57. Corporation., C. *Preparation of (indazolyl)benzimidazoles and Analogs for Inhibiting c-ABL*, US2006079564; **2006**, Cont.-in-part of US Ser. No. 187, 967.

58. Vernalis R & D Limited. Preparation of Pyrazolylbenzimidazoles as PDK1 and CHK1 Kinase Inhibitors for the Treatment of Cancer and Autoimmune Disorders. WO2006134318; **2006**.

59. Tse, A. N.; Rendahl, K. G.; Sheikh, T.; Cheema, H.; Aardalen, K.; Embry, M.; Ma, S.; Moler, E. J.; Ni, Z. J.; Lopes de Menezes, D. E.; Hibner, B.; Gesner, T. G.; Schwartz, G. K. CHIR-124, a Novel Potent Inhibitor of Chk1, Potentiates the Cytotoxicity of Topoisomerase I Poisons In Vitro and In Vivo. *Clin. Cancer Res.* **2007**, *13*, 591–602.

60. Ni, Z. -J.; Barsanti, P.; Brammeier, N.; Diebes, A.; Poon, D. J.; Ng, S.; Pecchi, S.; Pfister, K.; Renhowe, P. A.; Ramurthy, S.; Wagman, A. S.; Bussiere, D. E.; Le, V.; Zhou, Y.; Jansen, J. M.; Ma, S.; Gesner, T. G. 4-(Aminoalkylamino)-3-benzimidazole-quinolinones as Potent CHK-1 Inhibitors. *Bioorg. Med. Chem. Lett.* **2006**, *16*, 3121–3124.

61. Tong, Y.; Claiborne, A.; Stewart, K. D.; Park, C.; Kovar, P.; Chen, Z.; Credo, R. B.; Gu, W. -Z.; Gwaltney, S. L.; Judge, R. A.; Zhang, H.; Rosenberg, S. H.; Sham, H. L.; Sowin, T. J.; Lin, N. -H. Discovery of 1,4-dihydroindeno[1,2-c]Pyrazoles as a Novel Class of Potent And Selective Chk 1 Inhibitors. *Bioorg. Med. Chem.* **2007**, *15*, 2759–2767.

62. Tong, Y.; Claiborne, A.; Pyzytulinska, M.; Tao, Z. -F.; Stewart, K. D.; Kovar, P.; Chen, Z.; Credo, R. B.; Guan, R.; Merta, P. J.; Zhang, H.; Bouska, J.; Everitt, E. A.; Murry, B. P.; Hickman, D.; Stratton, T. J.; Wu, J.; Rosenberg, S. H.; Sham, H. L.; Sowin, T. J.; Lin, N. 1,4-Dihydroindeno[1,2-c]pyrazoles as Potent Chk 1 Inhibitors: Extended Exploration on Phenyl Ring Substitutions and Preliminary ADME/PK Studies. *Bioorg. Med. Chem. Lett.* **2007**, *17*, 3618–3623.

63. Tong, Y.; Przytulinska, M.; Tao, Z. -F.; Bouska, J.; Stewart, K. D.; Park, C.; Li, G.; Claiborne, A.; Kovar, P.; Chen, Z.; Merta, P. J.; Bui, M. -H.; Olson, A.; Osterling, D.; Zhang, H.; Sham, H. L.; Rosenberg, S. H.; Sowin, T. J.; Lin, N. -H. Cyanopyridyl Containing 1,4-dihydroindeno[1,2-c]pyrazoles as Potent Chk 1 Inhibitors: Improving Oral Biovailability. *Bioorg. Med. Chem. Lett.* **2007**, *17*, 5665–5670.

64. Tao, Z. -F.; Li, G.; Tong, Y.; Stewart, K. D.; Chen, Z.; Bui, M. -H.; Merta, P.; Park, C.; Kovar, P.; Zhang, H.; Sham, H. L.; Rosenberg, S. H.; Sowin, T. J.; Lin, N. -H. Discovery of 4'-(1,4-dihydro-indeno[1,2-c]pyrazol-3-yl)-benzonitriles and 4'-(1,4-dihydro-indeno[1,2-c]pyrazol-3-yl)-pyridine-2'-Carbonitriles as Potent Chk 1 (Chk1) Inhibitors. *Bioorg. Med. Chem. Lett.* **2007**, *17*, 5944–5951.

65. Kandala, P. K.; Srivastava, S. K. Activation of Chk 2 by 3,3'-Diindolylmethane Is Required for Causing G2/M Cell Cycle Arrest in Human Ovarian Cancer Cells. *Mol. Pharmacol.* **2010**, *78*, 297–309.

66. Arienti, K. L.; Brunmark, A.; Axe, F. U.; McClure, K.; Lee, A.; Blevitt, J.; Neff, D. K.; Huang, L.; Crawford, S.; Pandit, C. R.; Karlsson, L.; Breitenbucher, J. G. Chk

Inhibitors: SAR and Radioprotective Properties of a Series of 2-Arylbenzimidazoles. *J. Med. Chem.* **2005,** *48* (6), 1873–1885

67. Neff, D. K.; Lee-Dutra, A.; Blevitt, J. M.; Axe, F. U.; Hack, M. D.; Buma, J. C.; Rynberg, R.; Brunmark, A.; Karlsson, L.; Breitenbucher, J. G. 2-Aryl benzimidazoles Featuring Alkyl-Linked Pendant Alcohols and Amines as Inhibitors of Chk Chk2. *Bioorg. Med. Chem. Lett.* **2007,** *17,* 6467–6471.

68. Galal, S. A.; Khairat, S. H. M.; Ali, H. I.; Shouman, S. A.; Attia, Y. M.; Ali, M. M.; Mahmoud, A. E.; Abdel-Halim, A. H.; Fyiad, A. A.; Tabll, A.; El-Shenawy, R.; El Abd, Y. S.; Ramdan, R.; El Diwani, H. I. Part II: New Candidates of Pyrazole–Benzimidazole Conjugates as Chk 2 (Chk2) Inhibitors. *Eur. J. Med. Chem.* **2018,** *144,* 859–873.

69. Squire, C. J.; Dickson, J. M.; Ivanovic, I.; Baker, E. N. Structure and Inhibition of the Human Cell Cycle Chk, Wee1A Kinase. *Structure* **2005,** *13,* 541–550.

70. Palmer, B. D.; Thompson, A. M.; Booth, R. J.; Dobrusin, E.M.; Kraker, A. J.; Lee, H. H.; Lunney, E. A.; Mitchell, L. H.; Ortwine, D. F.; Smaill, J. B.; Swan, L. M.; Denny, W. A. 4--Phenylpyrrolo[3,4-c]carbazole-1,3(2H,6H)-dione Inhibitors of the Chk Wee1. Structure−Activity Relationships for Chromophore Modification and Phenyl Ring Substitution. *J. Med. Chem.* **2006,** *49* (16), 4896–4991.

71. Jobson, A. G.; Lountos, G. T.; Lorenzi, P. L.; Llamas, J.; Connelly, J.; Cerna, D.; Tropea, J. E.; Onda, A.; Zoppoli, G.; Kondapaka, S.; Zhang, G.; Caplen, N. J.; Cardellina, J. H.; Yoo, S. S.; Monks, A.; Self, C.; Waugh, D. S.; Shoemaker, R. H.; Pommier, Y. Cellular Inhibition of Chk 2 (Chk2) and Potentiation of Camptothecins and Radiation by the Novel Chk2 Inhibitor PV1019 [7-nitro-1H-indole-2-carboxylic acid {4-[1-(guanidinohydrazone)-ethyl]-phenyl}-amide]. *J. Pharmacol. Exp. Ther.* **2009,** *331,* 816–826.

72. Jobson, A. G.; Cardellina, J. H.; Scudiero, D.; Kondapaka, S.; Zhang, H.; Kim, H.; Shoemaker, R.; Pommier, Y. Identification of a Bis-guanylhydrazone [4,4'-Diacetyldiphenylurea-bis(guanylhydrazone); NSC 109555] as a Novel Chemotype for Inhibition of Chk2 kinase. *Mol. Pharmacol.* **2007,** *72,* 876–884.

73. Feng, L.; Cook, B.; Tsai, S. -Y.; Zhou, T.; LaFlamme, B.; Evans, T.; Chen, S. Discovery of a Small-Molecule BMP Sensitizer for Human Embryonic Stem Cell Differentiation. *Cell Rep.* **2016,** *15,* 2063–2075.

74. AstraZeneca UK Limited. *Substituted Thienopyridines and Related Compounds and their Preparation, Pharmaceutical Compositions, and Use as CHK1, PDK1 and PAK Inhibitors in the Treatment Of Cancer,* WO2006106326; **2006.**

75. Schering Corporation. *Imidazopyrazines as Protein Kinase Inhibitors and Their Preparation, Pharmaceutical Compositions and Use in the Treatment of Kinase-Mediated Diseases,* WO2007145921; **2007.**

76. Schering Corporation. *Preparation of Imidazopyrazines as Protein Kinase Inhibitors,* WO2007058942; **2007.**

77. Schering Corporation. *Preparation of Pyrazolopyrimidines as Protein Kinase Inhibitors,* WO2007041712; **2007.**

78. Schering Corporation. *Pyrazolo[1,5-a]pyrimidine Compounds as Protein Kinase Inhibitors and their Preparation, Pharmaceutical Compositions and their Use in the Treatment of Protein Kinase-Mediated Diseases,* US2007082900 [WO2007044441]; **2007.**

79. Janssen Pharmaceutica, N. *Preparation of Aryl-Substituted Benzimidazole and Imidazopyridine Ether Check Point Kinase Inhibitors for Treating Cancer*, US2006004039 [WO2006004791]; **2006**.

80. Cancer Research Technology Limited. *Morpholino-bicyclo-heteroaryl Compounds as CHK1 Kinase Inhibitors And Their Preparation, Pharmaceutical Compositions and Use in the Treatment of Cancer*, WO2008075007; **2008**.

81. Isono, M.; Hoffmann, M. J.; Pinkerneil, M.; Sato, A.; Michaelis, M.; Cinatl, J.; Niegisch, G.; Schulz, W. A. Chk Inhibitor AZD7762 Strongly Sensitises Urothelial Carcinoma Cells To Gemcitabine. *J. Exp. Clin. Cancer Res.* **2017**, *36*, 1.

82. Akinaga, S.; Nomura, K.; Gomi, K.; Okabe, M. Enhancement of Antitumor Activity of Mitomycin C In Vitro and In Vivo by Ucn-01, A Selective Inhibitor of Protein Kinase C. *Cancer Chemother. Pharmacol.* **1993**, *32*, 183–189.

83. Fuse, E.; Tanii, H.; Kurata, N.; Kobayashi, H.; Shimada, Y.; Tamura, T.; Sasaki, Y.; Tanigawara, Y.; Lush, R. D.; Headlee, D.; Figg, W. D.; Arbuck, S. G.; Senderowicz, A. M.; Sausville, E. A.; Akinaga, S.; Kuwabara, T.; Kobayashi, S. Unpredicted Clinical Pharmacology of UCN-01 Caused by Specific Binding to Human Alpha1-acid glycoprotein. *Cancer Res.* **1998**, *58*, 3248–3253.

84. Sausville, E. A.; Arbuck, S. G.; Messmann, R.; Headlee, D.; Bauer, K. S.; Lush, R. M.; Murgo, A.; Figg, W. D.; Lahusen, T.; Jaken, S.; Jing, X.; Roberge, M.; Fuse, E.; Kuwabara, T.; Senderowicz, A. M. Phase I Trial of 72-hour Continuous Infusion UCN-01 in Patients with Refractory Neoplasms. *J. Clin. Oncol.* **2001**, *19*, 2319–2333.

85. Hugon, B.; Anizon, F.; Bailly, C.; Golsteyn, R. M.; Pierré, A.; Léonce, S.; Hickman, J.; Pfeiffer, B.; Prudhomme, M. Synthesis and Biological Activities of Isogranulatimide Analogues. *Bioorg. Med. Chem.* **2007**, *15*, 5965–5980.

86. Jiang, X.; Zhao, B.; Britton, R.; Lim, L. Y.; Leong, D.; Sanghera, J. S.; Zhou, B.-B. S.; Piers, E.; Andersen, R. J.; Roberge, M. Inhibition of Chk1 by the G2 DNA Damage Checkpoint Inhibitor Isogranulatimide. *Mol. Cancer Ther.* **2004**, *3*, 1221–1227.

87. BerlinckR. G. S.; Britton, R., Piers, E.; Lim, L.; Roberge, M.; da Rocha, R. M.; Andersen, R. J. Granulatimide and Isogranulatimide, Aromatic Alkaloids with G2 Checkpoint Inhibition Activity Isolated from the Brazilian Ascidian Didemnum granulatum: Structure Elucidation and Synthesis. *J. Org. Chem.* **1998**, *63* (26), 9850–9856

88. Sako, Y.; Ichikawa, S.; Osada, A.; Matsuda, A. Synthesis and Evaluation of 5-substituted 9-hydroxypyrrolo[3,4-c]carbazole-1,3(2H,6H)-diones as Checkpoint 1 Kinase Inhibitors. *Bioorg. Med. Chem.* **2010**, *18*, 7878–7889.

89. Hilton, S.; Naud, S.; Caldwell, J. J.; Boxall, K.; Burns, S.; Anderson, V. E.; Antoni, L.; Allen, C. E.; Pearl, L. H.; Oliver, A. W.; Wynne Aherne, G., Garrett, M. D.; Collins, I. Identification and Characterisation of 2-aminopyridine Inhibitors of Chk 2. *Bioorg. Med. Chem.* **2010**, *18*, 707–718.

90. Cancer Research Technology Ltd. Pyrazin-2-yl-pyridin-2-yl-amine and pyrazin-2-yl-pyrimidin-4-yl-amine Compounds and Their Use, US8058045B2.

91. Guzi, T. J.; Paruch, K.; Dwyer, M. P.; Labroli, M.; Shanahan, F.; Davis, N.; Taricani, L.; Wiswell, D.; Seghezzi, W.; Penaflor, E.; Bhagwat, B.; Wang, W.; Gu, D.; Hsieh, Y.; Lee, S.; Liu, M.; Parry, D. Targeting the Replication Checkpoint Using SCH 900776, a Potent and Functionally Selective CHK1 Inhibitor Identified via High Content Screening. *Mol. Cancer Ther.* **2011**, *10*, 591–602.

92. Guzi, T. J.; Paruch, K.; Dwyer, M. P.; Labroli, M.; Shanahan, F.; Davis, N.; Taricani, L.; Wiswell, D.; Seghezzi, W.; Penaflor, E.; Bhagwat, B.; Wang, W.; Gu, D.; Hsieh, Y.; Lee, S.; Liu, M.; Parry, D. Targeting the replication Checkpoint Using SCH 900776, a Potent and Functionally Selective CHK1 Inhibitor Identified Via High Content Screening. *Mol. Cancer Ther.* **2011**, *10*, 591–602.

93. Herůdková, J.; Paruch, K.; Khirsariya, P.; Souček, K.; Krkoška, M.; Vondálová Blanářová, O.; Sova, P.; Kozubík, A. Hyršlová Vaculová, A. Chk1 Inhibitor SCH900776 Effectively Potentiates the Cytotoxic Effects of Platinum-Based Chemotherapeutic Drugs in Human Colon Cancer Cells. *Neoplasia* **2017**, *19*, 830–841.

94. Li, J.; Song, C.; Rong, Y.; Kuang, T.; Wang, D.; Xu, X.; Yuan, J.; Luo, K.; Qin, B.; Nowsheen, S.; Lou, Z.; Lou, W. Chk1 Inhibitor SCH 900776 Enhances the Antitumor Activity of MLN4924 on Pancreatic Cancer. *Cell Cycle* **2018**, 1–9.

95. Engelke, C. G.; Parsels, L. A.; Qian, Y.; Zhang, Q.; Karnak, D.; Robertson, J. R.; Tanska, D. M.; Wei, D.; Davis, M. A.; Parsels, J. D.; Zhao, L.; Greenson, J. K.; Lawrence, T. S.; Maybaum, J.; Morgan, M. A. Sensitization of Pancreatic Cancer to Chemoradiation by the Chk1 Inhibitor MK8776. *Clin. Cancer Res.* **2013**, *19*, 4412–4421.

96. Grabauskiene, S.; Bergeron, E. J.; Chen, G.; Chang, A. C.; Lin, J.; Thomas, D. G.; Giordano, T. J.; Beer, D. G.; Morgan, M. A.; Reddy, R. M. Chk1 Levels Correlate with Sensitization to Pemetrexed by CHK1 Inhibitors in Non-Small Cell Lung Cancer Cells. *Lung Cancer* **2013**, *82*, 477–484.

97. Dai, Y.; Chen, S.; Kmieciak, M.; Zhou, L.; Lin, H.; Pei, X. -Y.; Grant, S. The Novel Chk1 Inhibitor MK-8776 Sensitizes Human Leukemia Cells to HDAC Inhibitors by Targeting the Intra-S Checkpoint and DNA Replication and Repair. *Mol. Cancer Ther.* **2013**, *12*, 878–889.

98. Samadder, P.; Suchánková, T.; Hylse, O.; Khirsariya, P.; Nikulenkov, F.; Drápela, S.; Straková, N.; Vaňhara, P.; Vašíčková, K.; Kolářová, H.; Binó, L.; Bittová, M.; Ovesná, P.; Kollár, P.; Fedr, R.; Ešner, M.; Jaroš, J.; Hampl, A.; Krejčí, L.; Paruch, K.; Souček, K. Synthesis and Profiling of a Novel Potent Selective Inhibitor of CHK1 Kinase Possessing Unusual N-trifluoromethylpyrazole Pharmacophore Resistant to Metabolic N-dealkylation. *Mol. Cancer Ther.* **2017**, *16*, 1831–1842.

99. Anderson, V. E.; Walton, M. I.; Eve, P. D.; Boxall, K. J.; Antoni, L.; Caldwell, J. J.; Aherne, W.; Pearl, L. H.; Oliver, A. W.; Collins, I.; Garrett, M. D. CCT241533 is a Potent and Selective Inhibitor of CHK2 that Potentiates the Cytotoxicity of PARP Inhibitors. *Cancer Res.* **2011**, *71*, 463–472.

100. Wang, X. -M.; Li, J.; Feng, X. -C.; Wang, Q.; Guan, D. -Y.; Shen, Z. -H. Involvement of the Role of Chk1 in Lithium-Induced G2/M Phase Cell Cycle Arrest in Hepatocellular Carcinoma Cells. *J. Cell. Biochem.* **2008**, *104*, 1181–1191.

101. Teng, M.; Zhu, J.; Johnson, M. D.; Chen, P.; Kornmann, J.; Chen, E.; Blasina, A.; Register, J.; Anderes, K.; Rogers, C.; Deng, Y.; Ninkovic, S.; Grant, S.; Hu, Q.; Lundgren, K.; Peng, Z.; Kania, R. S. Structure-Based Design of (5-Arylamino-2 *H*-pyrazol-3-yl)-biphenyl-2',4'-diols as Novel and Potent Human CHK1 Inhibitors. *J. Med. Chem.* **2007**, *50*, 5253–5256.

102. Matthews, T. P.; Klair, S.; Burns, S.; Boxall, K.; Cherry, M.; Fisher, M.; Westwood, I. M.; Walton, M. I.; McHardy, T.; Cheung, K. -M. J.; Van Montfort, R.; Williams, D.;

Aherne, G. W.; Garrett, M. D.; Reader, J.; Collins, I. Identification of Inhibitors of Chk 1 Through Template Screening. *J. Med. Chem.* **2009**, *52*, 4810–4819.

103. Pfizer, I. *Substitued 2-heterocyclylamino Pyrazine Compounds as CHK-1 Inhibitors*, US8518952.

104. Eli Lilly and Co. *Compounds Useful for Inhibiting CHK1*, WO2010077758A1.

105. Luserna Di Rora, A. G.; Iacobucci, I.; Imbrogno, E.; Derenzini, E.; Ferrari, A.; Guadagnuolo, V.; Robustelli, V.; Soverini, S.; Papayannidis, C.; Abbenante, M. C.; Cavo, M.; Martinelli, G. (2015) The Inhibition of Chk 1 As a Promising Strategy to Increase the Effectiveness of Different Treatments in Acute Lymphoblastic Leukemia. *Blood* **2015**, *126*.

106. Lee, J. -M.; Karzai, F. H.; Zimmer, A.; Annunziata, C. M.; Lipkowitz, S.; Parker, B.; Houston, N.; Ekwede, I.; Kohn, E. C. A Phase II Study of the Cell Cycle Chks 1 and 2 Inhibitor (LY2606368; Prexasertib monomesylate monohydrate) in Sporadic High-Grade Serous Ovarian Cancer (HGSOC) and Germline BRCA Mutation-Associated Ovarian Cancer (gBRCAm+ OvCa). *Ann. Oncol.* **2016**, *27*.

107. Hong, D.; Infante, J.; Janku, F.; Jones, S.; Nguyen, L. M.; Burris, H.; Naing, A.; Bauer, T. M.; Piha-Paul, S.; Johnson, F. M.; Kurzrock, R.; Golden, L.; Hynes, S.; Lin, J.; Lin, A. B.; Bendell, J. Phase I Study of LY2606368, a Chk 1 Inhibitor, in Patients With Advanced Cancer. *J. Clin. Oncol.* **2016**, *34*, 1764–1771.

108. Lee, J. -M.; Nair, J.; Zimmer, A.; Lipkowitz, S.; Annunziata, C. M.; Merino, M. J.; Swisher, E. M.; Harrell, M. I.; Trepel, J. B.; Lee, M. -J.; Bagheri, M. H.; Botesteanu, D. -A.; Steinberg, S. M.; Minasian, L.; Ekwede, I.; Kohn, E. C. Prexasertib, a Cell Cycle Chk 1 and 2 Inhibitor, in BRCA Wild-Type Recurrent High-Grade Serous Ovarian Cancer: A First-In-Class Proof-Of-Concept Phase 2 Study. *Lancet Oncol.* **2018**, *19*, 207–215.

109. Leslie, A.; Joshua, D.; William, H. R. J.; Denny, W. A.; Kraker, A. J.; Maybaum, J. Cancer Research : The Official Organ of the American Association for Cancer Research, Inc. *Cancer Res.* Waverly Press.

110. Parsels, L. A.; Morgan, M. A.; Tanska, D. M.; Parsels, J. D.; Palmer, B. D.; Booth, R. J.; Denny, W. A.; Canman, C. E.; Kraker, A. J.; Lawrence, T. S.; Maybaum, J. Gemcitabine Sensitization by Chk 1 Inhibition Correlates with Inhibition of a Rad51 DNA Damage Response in Pancreatic Cancer Cells. *Mol. Cancer Ther.* **2009**, *8*, 45–54.

111. Walton, M. I.; Eve, P. D.; Hayes, A.; Valenti, M. R.; De Haven Brandon, A. K.; Box, G.; Hallsworth, A.; Smith, E. L.; Boxall, K. J.; Lainchbury, M.; Matthews, T. P.; Jamin, Y.; Robinson, S. P.; Aherne, G. W.; Reader, J. C.; Chesler, L.; Raynaud, F. I.; Eccles, S. A.; Collins, I.; Garrett, M. D. CCT244747 is a Novel Potent and Selective CHK1 Inhibitor with Oral Efficacy Alone and in Combination with Genotoxic Anticancer Drugs. *Clin. Cancer Res.* **2012**, *18*, 5650–5661.

112. Merck & Co. *Substituted Triazoloquinazolinones as Inhibitors of Chk CHK1 in the Treatment of Cancer*, US2007254879 [WO2007127138]; **2007**.

113. Merck & Co. *Pyrazoloquinolinone Inhibitors of Chk CHK1 for Use in Cancer Treatment*, WO2006074281; **2006**.

114. Merck & Co. *Inhibitors of Chk CHK1 for Use as Antitumor Agents*, WO2007081572; **2007**.

115. Merck & Co. *Imidazole Derivatives as Antitumor Inhibitors of Human Chk CHK1*, WO2007015837; **2007**.

116. Merck & Co. *Benzoisoquinolines and Aza Derivatives as Antitumor Inhibitors of Human Chk CHK1*, WO2007008502; **2007**.

117. AstraZeneca UK Limited. *Preparation of Novel Fused Triazolones as Antitumor Agents*, WO2004081008; **2004**.

118. Oza, V.; Ashwell, S.; Brassil, P.; Breed, J.; Deng, C.; Ezhuthachan, J.; Haye, H.; Horn, C.; Janetka, J.; Lyne, P.; Newcombe, N.; Otterbien, L.; Pass, M.; Read, J.; Roswell, S.; Su, M.; Toader, D.; Yu, D.; Yu, Y.; Valentine, A.; Webborn, P.; White, A.; Zabludoff, S.; Zheng, X. Discovery of a Novel Class of Triazolones as Chk Inhibitors—Hit to Lead Exploration. *Bioorg. Med. Chem. Lett.* **2010**, *20*, 5133–5138.

119. Blackwood, E.; Epler, J.; Yen, I.; Flagella, M.; O'Brien, T.; Evangelista, M.; Schmidt, S.; Xiao, Y.; Choi, J.; Kowanetz, K.; Ramiscal, J.; Wong, K.; Jakubiak, D.; Yee, S.; Cain, G.; Gazzard, L.; Williams, K.; Halladay, J.; Jackson, P. K.; Malek, S. Combination Drug Scheduling Defines a "Window of Opportunity" for Chemopotentiation of Gemcitabine by an Orally Bioavailable, Selective ChK1 Inhibitor, GNE-900. *Mol. Cancer Ther.* **2013**, *12*, 1968–1980.

120. Blackwood, E.; Epler, J.; Yen, I.; Flagella, M.; O'brien, T.; Evangelista, M.; Schmidt, S.; Xiao, Y.; Choi, J.; Kowanetz, K.; Ramiscal, J.; Wong, K.; Jakubiak, D.; Yee, S.; Cain, G.; Gazzard, L.; Williams, K.; Halladay, J.; Jackson, P. K.; Malek, S. Combination Drug Scheduling Defines a;Window of Opportunity for Chemopotentiation of Gemcitabine by an Orally Bioavailable, Selective ChK1 Inhibitor, GNE-900. *Mol. Cancer Ther.* **2013**, *12*, 1968–1980.

121. Infante, J. R.; Hollebecque, A.; Postel-Vinay, S.; Bauer, T. M.; Blackwood, E. M.; Evangelista, M.; Mahrus, S.; Peale, F. V.; Lu, X.; Sahasranaman, S.; Zhu, R.; Chen, Y.; Ding, X.; Murray, E. R.; Schutzman, J. L.; Lauchle, J. O.; Soria, J. -C.; LoRusso, P. M. Phase I Study of GDC-0425, a Chk 1 Inhibitor, in Combination with Gemcitabine in Patients with Refractory Solid Tumors. *Clin. Cancer Res.* **2017**, *23*, 2423–2432.

122. Garbaccio, R. M.; Huang, S.; Tasber, E. S.; Fraley, M. E.; Yan, Y.; Munshi, S.; Ikuta, M.; Kuo, L.; Kreatsoulas, C.; Stirdivant, S.; Drakas, B.; Rickert, K.; Walsh, E. S.; Hamilton, K. A.; Buser, C. A.; Hardwick, J.; Mao, X.; Beck, S. C.; Abrams, M. T.; Tao, W.; Lobell, R.; Sepp-Lorenzino, L.; Hartman, G. D. Synthesis and Evaluation of Substituted Benzoisoquinolinones as Potent Inhibitors of Chk1 Kinase. *Bioorg. Med. Chem. Lett.* **2007**, *17*, 6280–6285.

123. Schering Corporation. *2-Aminothiazole-4-carboxylic Acid Amides as Protein Kinase Inhibitors and Their Preparation, Pharmaceutical Compositions and Use in the Treatment of Diseases*, WO2008054701; **2008**.

124. Reddy, P. A. P.; Wong, T. T.; Zhao, L.; Tang, S.; Labroli, M. A.; Guzi, T. J.; M. A. S. *Thiazole Derivatives as Protein Kinase Inhibitors*, US 2010/0331313.

125. Garbaccio, R. M.; Huang, S.; Tasber, E. S; Fraley, M. E.; Yan, Y.; Munshi, S.; Ikuta, M.; Kuo, L.; Kreatsoulas, C.; Stirdivant, S.; Drakas, B.; Rickert, K.; Walsh, E. S.; Hamilton, K. A.; Buser, C. A.; Hardwick, J.; Mao, X.; Beck, S. C.; Abrams, M. T.; Tao, W.; Lobell, R.; Sepp-Lorenzino, L.; Hartman, G. D. Synthesis and Evaluation of Substituted Benzoisoquinolinones as Potent Inhibitors of Chk1 Kinase. *Bioorg. Med. Chem. Lett.* **2007**, *17*, 6280–6285.

126. J. Z., W.; Chen, H. 3-Hydroxyisothiazole-4-carboxymidines as Chk2 Inhibitors, US20090137041.
127. Carlessi, L.; Buscemi, G.; Larson, G.; Hong, Z.; Wu, J. Z.; Delia, D. Biochemical and Cellular Characterization of VRX0466617, A Novel and Selective Inhibitor for the Chk Chk2. *Mol. Cancer Ther.* **2007,** *6,* 935–944.
128. Larson, G.; Yan, S.; Chen, H.; Rong, F.; Hong, Z.; Wu, J. Z. Identification of Novel, Selective and Potent Chk2 Inhibitors. *Bioorg. Med. Chem. Lett.* **2007,** *17,* 172–175.
129. Caldwell, J. J.; Welsh, E. J.; Matijssen, C.; Anderson, V. E.; Antoni, L.; Boxall, K.; Urban, F.; Hayes, A.; Raynaud, F. I.; Rigoreau, L. J. M.; Raynham, T.; Aherne, G. W.; Pearl, L. H.; Oliver, A. W.; Garrett, M. D.; Collins, I. Structure-Based Design of Potent and Selective 2-(quinazolin-2-yl)phenol Inhibitors of Chk 2. *J. Med. Chem.* **2011,** *54,* 580–590.

CHAPTER 9

N-METHYL-D-ASPARTATE RECEPTOR ANTAGONISTS: EMERGING DRUGS TO TREAT NEURODEGENERATIVE DISEASES

VINOD G. UGALE[1*], RAHUL WANI[1], SAURABH KHADSE[1], and SANJAY B. BARI[2]

[1]Department of Pharmaceutical Chemistry,
R. C. Patel Institute of Pharmaceutical Education and Research,
Shirpur, Dist. Dhule, Maharashtra 425405, India

[2]Department of Pharmaceutical Chemistry,
H. R. Patel Institute of Pharmaceutical Education and Research,
Shirpur, Dist. Dhule, Maharashtra 425405, India

*Corresponding author. E-mail: vinod.ugale@rediffmail.com

ABSTRACT

N-methyl-D-aspartate (NMDA) receptor is a subtype of ionotropic glutamate receptor. NMDA receptor plays a decisive role in significant high-level brain processes and has been involved in diverse neuropsychological conditions. NMDA receptor antagonists have exposed their clinical effectiveness in neurodegenerative diseases such as epilepsy, Alzheimer's disease, Parkinson's disease, pain, and depression. Depending on the clinical observations and insights into NMDA receptor pharmacology, novel modulatory approaches are beginning to emerge with potential therapeutic benefits. Hence, NMDA receptor is considered to be a prospective target for the treatment of neurodegenerative diseases. NMDA receptor has diverse sites where ligands can bind to provoke bioactivity in a subunit selective manner; the recent pharmacological data also disclosed molecular determinants for their subunit selectivity. By addressing the role of NMDA receptor modulators in neuropsychological consequences, we would certainly be a step closer to a goal of improving the quality of life of individuals suffered from neurodegenerative diseases. We discussed more recent results and significance of subunit selective NMDA receptor ligands, which have proven to be antagonists that are particularly useful in the management of neurological diseases. A flurry of clinical, functional, and chemical studies summarized in this chapter reinvigorated efforts to identify subunit selective modulators of NMDA receptor as initial proof-of-concept molecules to treat neurodegenerative diseases.

9.1   INTRODUCTION

The most important neurotransmitters released in the central nervous system (CNS) are amino acids. The neurotransmitters involved in high-level brain processes have been classified into two main categories on the basis of their functions: excitatory neurotransmitters (glutamate, aspartate, and cysteate), results in depolarization in the mammalian CNS; and inhibitory neurotransmitters [γ-amino butyric acid (GABA), glycine, taurine and β-alanine], causes hyperpolarization in mammalian neurons.[1] Glutamate is the major excitatory neurotransmitter in the mammalian CNS that acts as an agonist for two types of receptors: second messenger-linked metabotropic glutamate receptors and ionotropic cation-selective ligand-gated channels.[2] Glutamate is considered to be an abundant mediator of excitatory signals in the CNS and involved in functions such as cognition, memory, movement, and learning. The neurotransmitter glutamate has a vital role in brain physiological processes and in the underlying pathophysiology of neurodegenerative disorders.[3] For this reason, ionotropic glutamate receptors (iGluRs) have been extensively focused in recent years.[4] Glutamate is involved in the mammalian brain functions by activation of ionotropic NMDA, α-amino-3-hydroxy-5-methyl-4-isoxazolepropionic acid (AMPA) and kainic acid receptor subtypes.[5] Overstimulation of these exicitatory iGluRs, can cause excitotoxicity through an immense rise in cytoplasmic Ca^{2+} concentration, leads to neuronal death. Excito-toxic processes contribute to a variety of neurological disorders such as epilepsy, ischemic brain damage, Parkinson's and Alzheimer's diseases

(NADs), Huntington's chorea, and amyotrophic lateral sclerosis.[6,7] These findings led to the design and development of selective iGluR antagonists as research tools and potential therapeutic agents against a number of neurological disorders.

9.2 GLUTAMATERGIC SYSTEM

The NMDA receptor is distinctive from other iGluRs in terms of pharmacological properties.[8] NMDA receptor has a decisive role in neurological and psychiatric disorders as well as in vital brain processes.[9] NMDA receptor antagonists have shown clinical benefits in epilepsy, Parkinson's disease, AD, pain, and depression.[10] Depending upon the clinical utility and more insights into NMDA receptor pharmacology, new modulatory approaches have emerged with potential therapeutic benefits.[11] A common feature of NMDA receptor is its construction as tetrameric assemblies of subunits. NMDA tetramers are assembled from two subunits of glycine binding GluN1 (NR1) and two subunits of glutamate binding GluN2 (NR2). The functions of NMDA receptor could be altered by blocking or interacting with one of the following binding sites: (1) glycine agonist site, (2) glutamate agonist site, (3) ion channel pore, and (4) allosteric sites on the amino-terminal domain.[12] NMDA receptors are also considered as heteromeric assemblies containing three different subunits, NR1, NR2, and rarely NR3.[13] Electrophysiological studies confirmed that the NMDA receptor activation requires the occupation of the glycine binding site of NR1 subunit while opening of the gates is triggered through binding of glutamate at NR2 subunit. Conversely, the NR3 subunits seem to inhibit the channel activity.[14]

9.3 NMDA RECEPTOR-BINDING LIGANDS

AD is the most common form of dementia. Cholinergic signaling, which is important in cognition, is slowly lost in AD, so the first-line therapy is to treat symptoms with acetylcholinesterase inhibitors to increase levels of acetylcholine. Out of five available FDA (Food and Drug Administration)-approved AD medications, donepezil, galantamine, and rivastigmine are cholinesterase inhibitors while memantine, NMDA receptor antagonist, blocks the effects of high glutamate levels. The fifth medication consists of a combination of donepezil and memantine. Although these medications can reduce and temporarily slow down the symptoms of AD, they cannot stop the damage to the brain from progressing. For a superior therapeutic effect, multi-target drugs are required. Multitarget-directed ligand strategy has received more attention from scientists who are attempting to develop hybrid molecules that simultaneously modulate multiple biological targets. However, it has been demonstrated, a combination of memantine (an NMDA receptor antagonist), with an acetylcholinesterase inhibitor increases cognitive function when compared to a single AChE (Acetyl-cholinesterase) inhibitor. Biochemical evidence suggests that activity of glutamatergic neurons is also dysfunctional in AD and that their joint dysfunction with the cholinergic system is crucial in AD pathology. Thus, drug combinations that target cholinergic and glutamatergic systems simultaneously are recommended as the current standard of care for AD patients. The new hybrid compounds were designed following a dual-binding approach, by connecting two drug molecules through a variable-length polymethylene linker. Compounds carrying a hexamethylene spacer have the most promising properties of the series.[15]

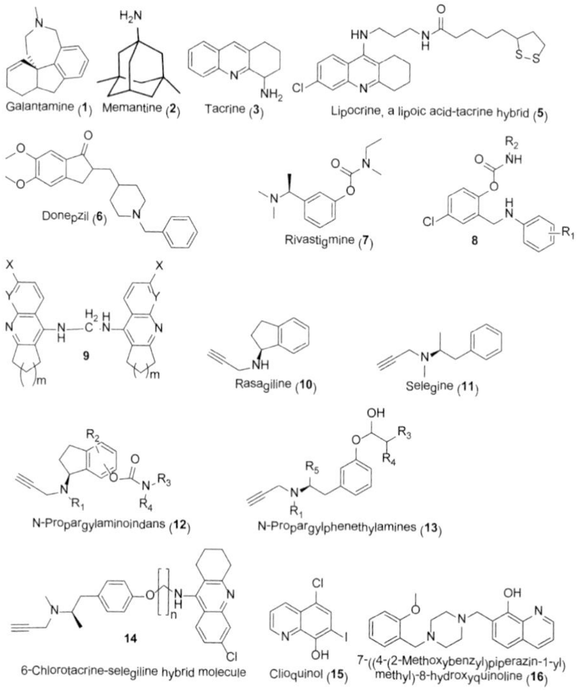

FIGURE 9.1   New hybrid compounds designed by dual-binding approach.

1,4-Dioxane derivative, a potent noncompetitive NMDA receptor antagonist, showed cytotoxic activity in MCF7 breast cancer cell line significantly higher than those of the functionally related compounds (S)-(+)-ketamine and MK-801. Encouraged by this result and considering that copper complexes have been highlighted to be promising anticancer agents, the NMDA receptor ligand **1** was linked to the bifunctionaliz-able species, affording the conjugated derivatives that were used for the preparation of the stable Cu(II) complexes. All the compounds were evaluated against a panel of human cancer cell lines derived from solid tumors. Complex showed the best antitumor activity in all the studied cell lines. This result suggests that might act through synergistic mechanisms of action due to the presence of the NMDA ligand and copper(II) in the same chemical entity. Furthermore, the cellular mechanisms affected by complex were assessed through cytofluorimetric and Western blot analyses. Data suggested the induction of cell death through paraptosis mediated by the endoplasmatic reticulum stress. The in-vitro antitumor activity of the novel copper(II) complexes and the uncoordinated ligands was evaluated against a panel of human cancer cell lines derived from solid tumors.

In summary, the noncompetitive NMDA receptor antagonist shows antitumor activity at MCF-7 breast cancer cell line significantly higher than those of the reference compounds (S)-(+)-ketamine and MK-801. Considering that copper complexes have also been demonstrated to be promising anticancer agents, the ligand was conjugated through an amide function with the bifunctionalizable species to form the conjugated derivatives from which the novel copper(II) complexes were obtained. Among the novel compounds, evaluated by MTT test against a panel of human tumor cell lines, the Cu(II) complex shows the best antitumor activity in all the studied cells, suggesting that it might act through synergistic mechanisms of action due to the presence of the NMDA ligand **1** and Cu(II) in the same chemical entity. Ligands (L^{NMDA}) and (L^{2NMDA}) were prepared according to the procedure reported in Scheme 9.1. The acids LH and L^2H were activated with CDI (Carbonyldiimidazole) and then treated with amine. The ligands are soluble in acetonitrile, chloroform, and DMSO, while **5** is soluble in methanol, acetonitrile, chloroform, and DMSO (dimethyl sulfoxide).[16]

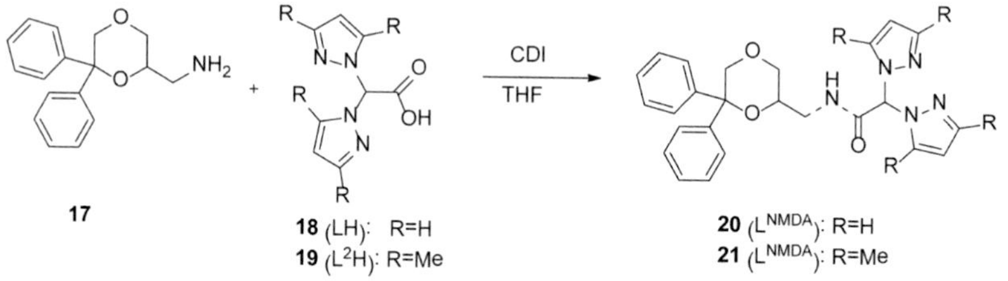

SCHEME 9.1 Reaction scheme for the synthesis of ligands **20** and **21**.[16]

The copper complexes [(LNMDA)CuCl$_2$] and [(L$_2$NMDA)CuCl$_2$·H$_2$O] were prepared from the reaction of CuCl$_2$·2H$_2$O with LNMDA and L$_2$NMDA, respectively, in methanol suspension and in methanol solution, at room temperature (Scheme 9.2). Both compounds are soluble in DMSO, methanol, ethanol, and chloroform.

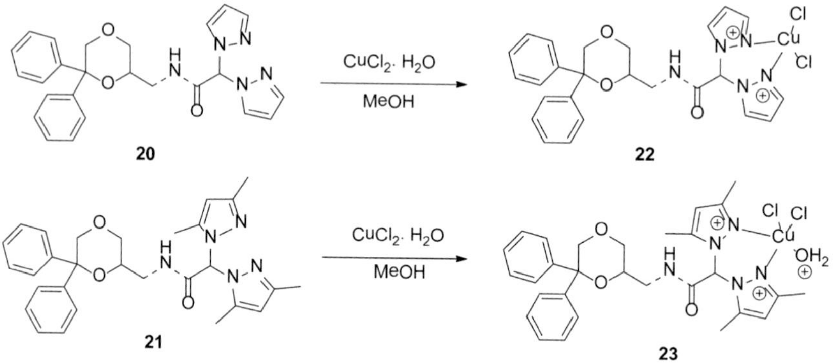

SCHEME 9.2 Reaction scheme for the synthesis of complexes **22** and **23**.[16]

Ketamine is rapidly metabolized in the human body to a variety of metabolites, including the hydroxynorketamines. At least two hydroxynor-ketamines have significant antidepressant action in rodent models, with limited action against the N-methyl-D-aspartate (NMDA) receptor. The synthesis of hydroxynorketamines and their binding affinity to the NMDA receptor is presented.[17]

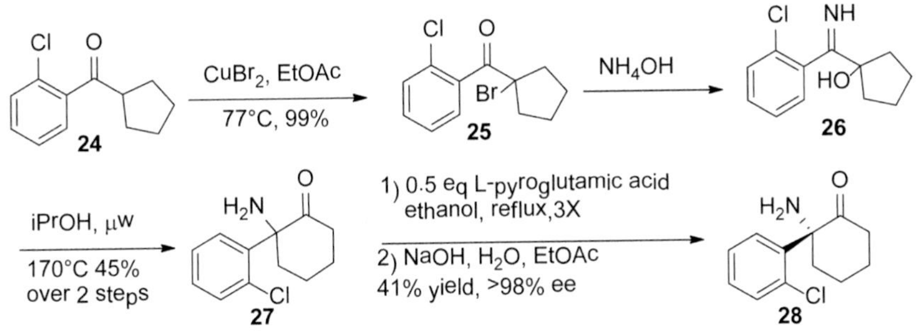

SCHEME 9.3 Synthesis of enantiopure norketamine.[17]

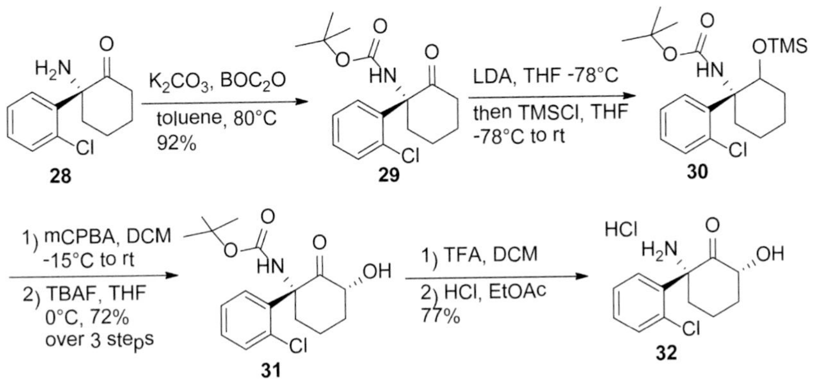

SCHEME 9.4 Synthesis of compound **32**.[17]

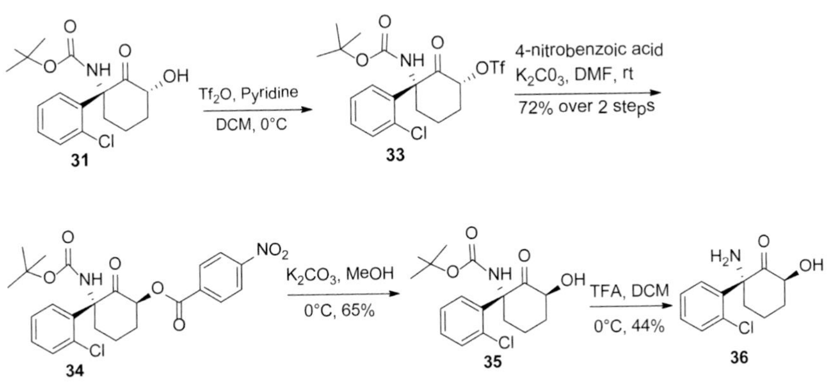

SCHEME 9.5 Synthesis of compound **36**.[17]

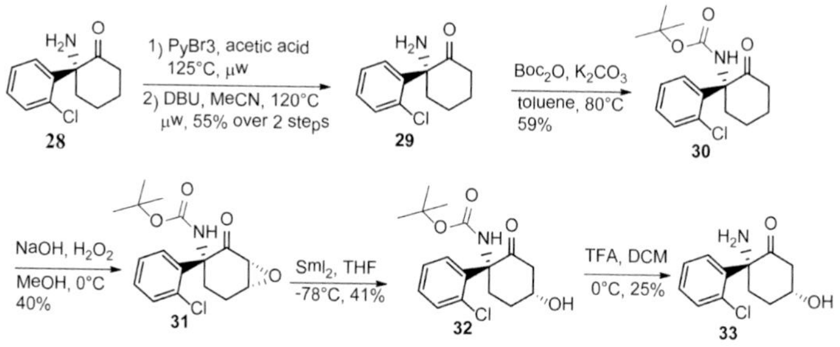

SCHEME 9.6 Synthesis of compound **33**.[17]

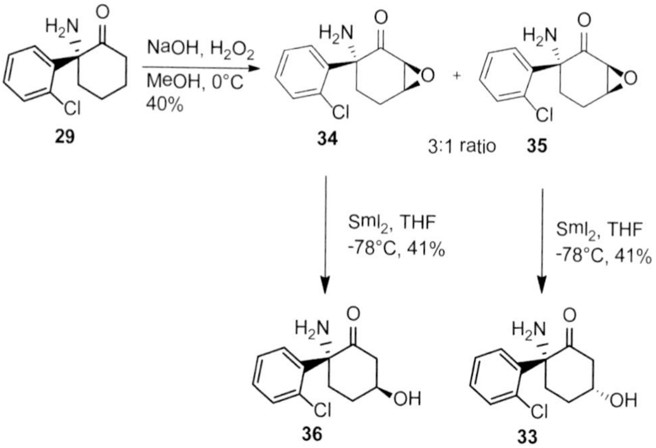

SCHEME 9.7 Synthesis of compound **36**.[17]

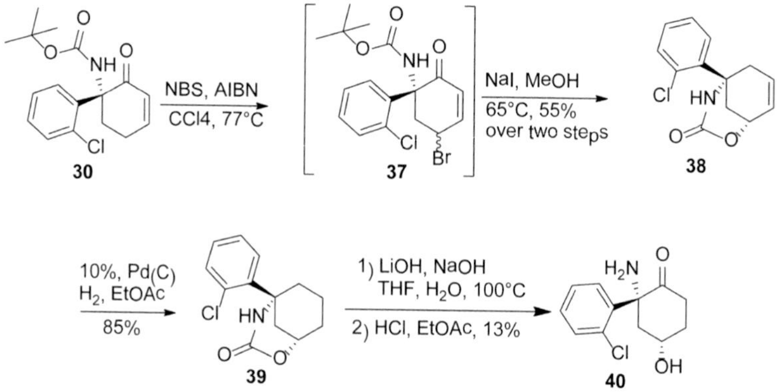

SCHEME 9.8 Synthesis of compound **40**.[17]

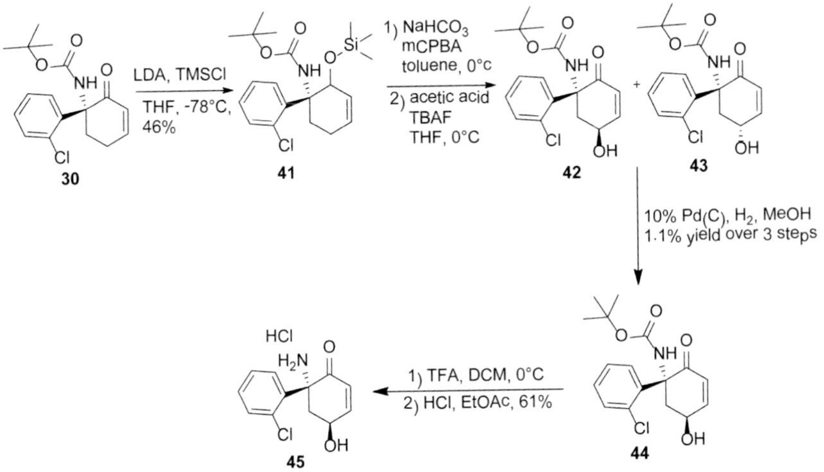

SCHEME 9.9 Synthesis of compound **45**.[17]

Humanin, a 24-amino acid bioactive peptide, has been shown to increase cell survival of neurons after exposure to Aβ and NMDA induced toxicity and thus could be beneficial in the treatment of AD. The neuro-protection by HN is reported to be primarily through its agonist binding properties to the gp130 receptor. However, the peptidic nature of HN presents challenges in its development as a therapeutic for AD. These agents could lead to a new pharmacological class of therapeutic agents for AD.[18] *N*-methyl-D-aspartate receptors (NMDARs) play a central role in epileptogensis and NMDAR antagonists have been shown to have anti-epileptic effects in animals and humans. Despite significant progress in the development of antiepileptic therapies over the previous three decades, a need still exists for novel therapies. An in-house library of small molecules targeting the NMDA receptor was synthesized. A novel indolyl compound, 2-(1,1-dimethyl-1,3-dihydro-benzo[*e*]indol-2-ylidene)-malonaldehyde (DDBM) showed the best binding with the NMDA receptor and compu-tational docking data showed that DDBM antagonized the binding sites of the NMDA receptor at lower docking energies compared to other molecules. Using a rat electroconvulsive shock model of epilepsy showed that DDBM decreased seizure duration and improved the histological outcomes. These indolyls have robust anticonvulsive activity and potential to be developed as novel anticonvulsants.[19]

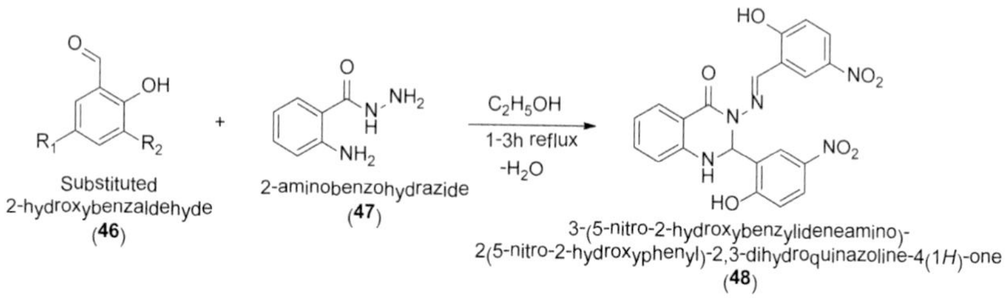

SCHEME 9.10 Syntheis of 3-(5-nitro-2-hydroxybenzylideneamino)-2(5-nitro-2-hydroxyphenyl)-2,3-dihydroquinazoline-4(1*H*)-one (**48**).[19]

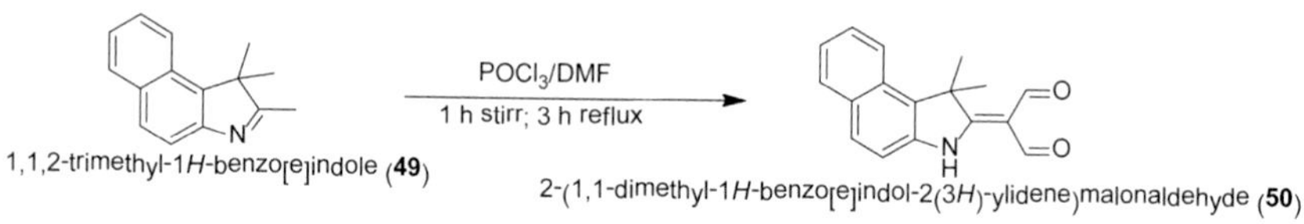

SCHEME 9.11 Synthesis of 2-(1,1-dimethyl-1,3-dihydro-benzo{e}indol-2-ylidene)-malonaldehyde.[19]

These molecules could be a potent lead for more investigations toward finding novel therapeutics against epilepsy and other neurodiseases related to excitotoxic effects of NMDAR. Enantiopure tryptophanol is easily obtained from the reduction of its parent natural amino acid tryptophan and can be used as chiral auxiliary/inductor to control the stereochemical course of a diastereoselective reaction. Furthermore, enantiopure tryptophanol is useful for the syntheses of natural products or biologically active molecules containing the aminoalcohol functionality. In this communication, we report the development of a small library of indolo[2,3-*a*]quinolizidines and evaluation of their activity as NMDA receptor antagonists. The synthesized enantiopure indolo[2,3-*a*] quinolizidines were evaluated as NMDA receptor antagonists and one compound was identified to be 2.9-fold more potent as NMDA receptor blocker than amantadine. This compound represents a hit compound for the development of novel NMDA receptor antagonists with potential applications in neurodegenerative disorders associated with overactivation of NMDA receptors.[20]

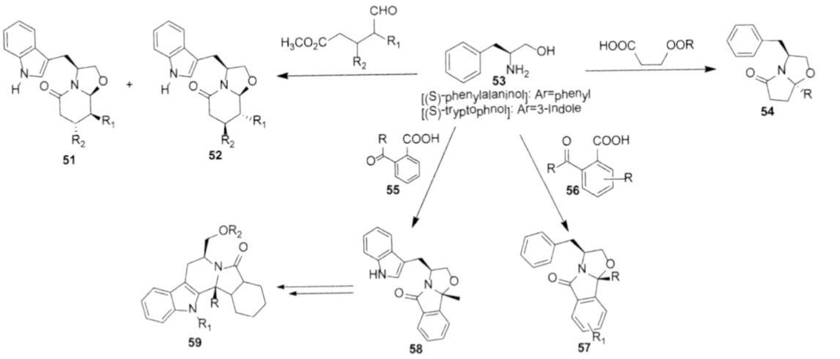

SCHEME 9.12   Synthesis of biologically active small molecules from tryptophanol and phenylalaninol.[20]

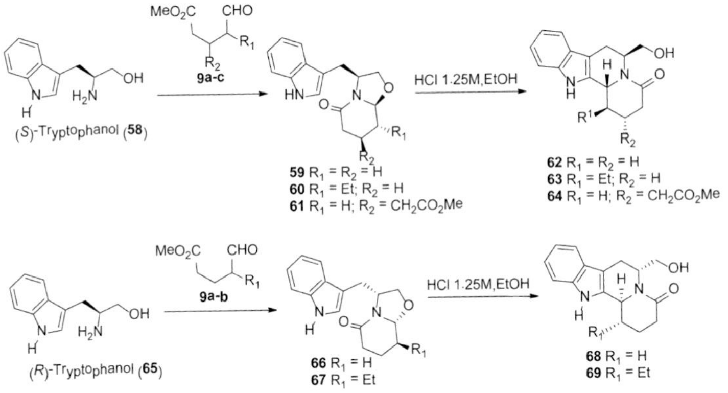

SCHEME 9.13   Synthesis of indolo[2,3-*a*]quinolizidines.[20]

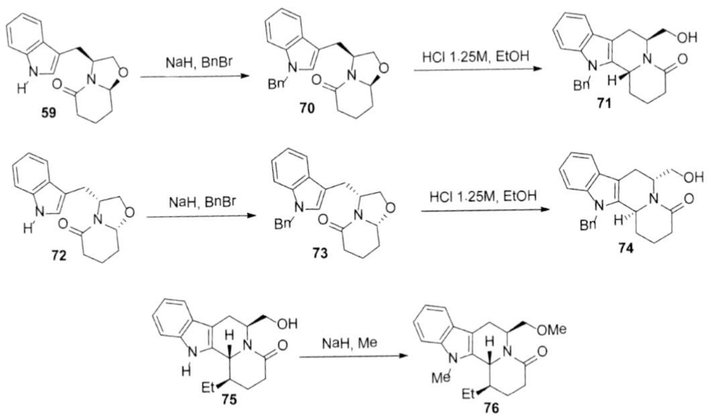

SCHEME 9.14   Synthesis of compounds **71**, **74**, and **76**.[20]

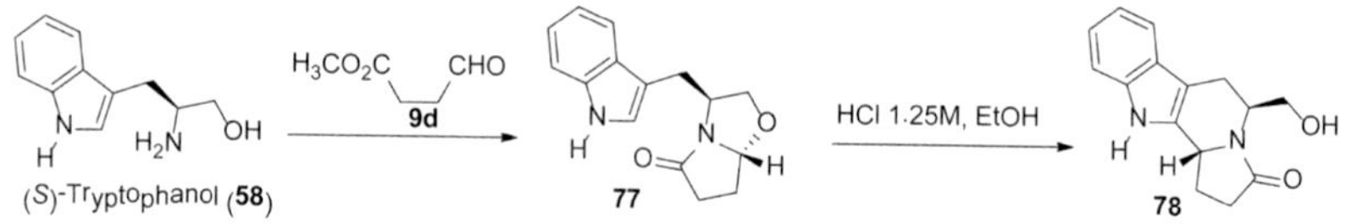

SCHEME 9.15   Synthesis of compound 78.[20]

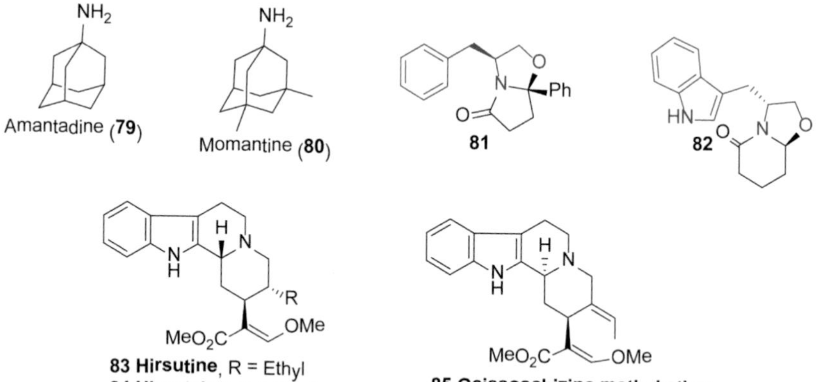

FIGURE 9.2   Some emerging potential NMDA receptor antagonists.[20]

To avoid legislation based on chemical structure, research chemicals, frequently used for recreational purposes, are continually being synthesized. Ephenidine is a diarylethylamine that has recently become popular with recreational users searching for dissociative hallucinogenic effects. The pharmacological basis of its neural actions has been investigated, initially by assessing its profile in CNS receptor binding assays and subsequently in targeted electrophysiological studies. Ephenidine was a potent inhibitor of 3H MK-801 binding (K_i: 66 nM), implying that it acts at the phencyclidine (PCP) site of NMDA receptor. It also showed modest activity at dopamine (379 nM) and noradrenaline (841 nM) transporters and at sigma 1 (629 nM) and sigma 2 (722 nM) binding sites. The new psychoactive substance, ephenidine, is a selective NMDA receptor antagonist with a voltage-dependent profile similar to ketamine. Such properties help explain the dissociative, cognitive, and hallucinogenic effects in man.[21]

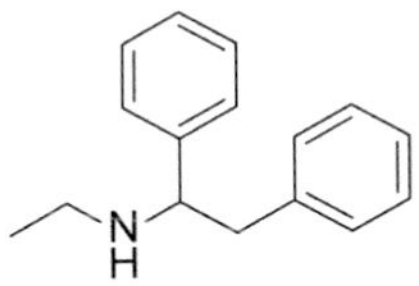

Ephenidine (*N*-ethyl-1,2-diphenylethylamine) (86)

FIGURE 9.3 Ephenidine, the selective diarylethylamine based NMDA antagonist.[21]

Besides the analgesic and neuroprotective properties of ketamine, an exciting novel therapeutic target for ketamine has emerged. Thus, ketamine and some other NMDA receptor antagonists have recently been proposed as rapidly acting antidepressants. During the depressed mood and during stress, memories of unpleasant events may be established through long-term potentiation and long-term depression. The role of NMDA receptors in curcumin-mediated renoprotection against ischemia–reperfusion (I/R)-induced acute kidney injury (AKI) in rats have been reported by the researchers. Rats were subjected to bilateral renal I/R (40 min I, 24 h R) to induce AKI. Kidney injury was assessed by measuring creatinine clearance, blood urea nitrogen, plasma uric acid, potassium level, fractional excretion of sodium, and macroproteinuria. Oxidative stress in renal tissues was assessed by measuring myeloperoxidase activity, thiobarbituric acid reactive substances, superoxide anion generation, and reduced glutathione content. Curcumin (30 and 60 mg/kg) was administered 1 h before subjecting rats to AKI. In separate groups, NMDA receptor agonists, glutamic acid (200 mg/kg), and spermidine (20 mg/kg) were administered prior to curcumin treatment in rats followed by AKI. I/R-induced AKI was demonstrated by a significant change in plasma and urine parameters along with a marked increase in oxidative stress and histological changes in renal tissues that were aggravated with pretreatment of glutamic acid and spermidine in rats. Administration of curcumin resulted in significant protection against AKI. However, glutamic acid and spermidine pretreatments prevented curcumin-mediated renoprotection. It is concluded that NMDA receptor antagonism significantly contributes toward curcumin-mediated protection against I/R-induced AKI. The abolition of curcumin-mediated renoprotection with glutamic acid and spermidine suggests that NMDA receptor antagonism plays an important role in its renoprotective action. However, the exact underlying mechanism of this interaction between curcumin and NMDA receptor still remains to be elucidated.[22]

A new series of benzopolycyclic amines active as NMDA receptor antagonists were synthesized. Most of them exhibited increased activity compared with related analogs previously published. All the tested compounds were more potent than clinically approved amantadine and one of them displayed a lower IC_{50} value than memantine, an anti-Alzheimer's approved drug.[23]

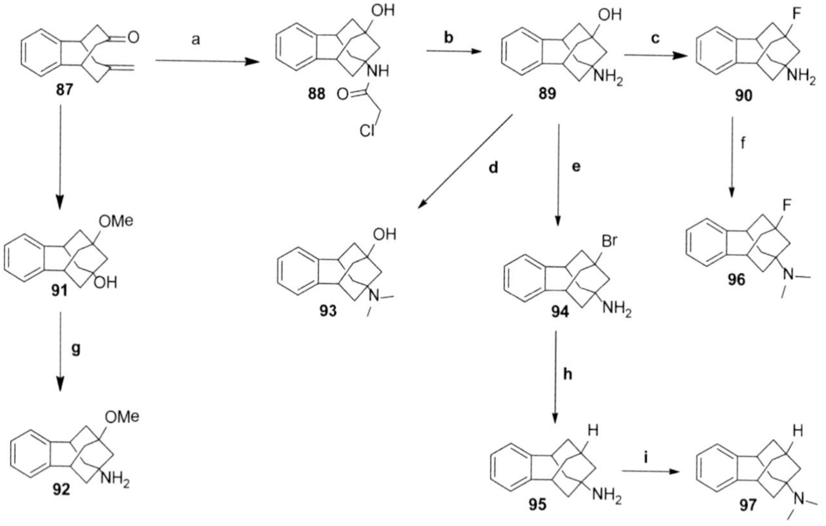

SCHEME 9.16   Synthesis of amines.

Reagents and conditions: (a) Chloroacetonitrile, conc. H_2SO_4, DCM, 0–5°C to RT, 49% yield; (b) thiourea, glacial AcOH, ethanol, reflux; (c) DAST, DCM, 30–5°C, 44% yield; (d) formaldehyde, $NaBH_3CN$, AcOH, methanol, RT, 33% yield; (e) thionyl bromide, toluene, rt, 79% yield; (f) formaldehyde, $NaBH_3CN$, AcOH, methanol, RT, 31% yield; (g) chloroacetonitrile, H_2SO_4, DCM, 0–5°C to RT, 23% yield; thiourea, AcOH, reflux, 59% yield; (h) TBTH, AIBN, toluene, 95°C, 13% yield; (i) formaldehyde, $NaBH_3CN$, glacial AcOH, methanol, RT, 69% yield.[23]

To evaluate if the synthesized compounds were able to antagonize NMDA receptors, we have measured its effect on the increase in intracellular calcium evoked by NMDA on rat cultured cerebellar granule neurons. Seven new polycyclic amines have been synthesized from easily accessible enone. All novel compounds were more potent than amantadine against the NMDA-induced calcium increase in cerebellar granule neurons. Moreover, three derivatives displayed antagonist activities very similar or even higher than that of memantine. While the replacement of the proton of C-9 by a fluorine atom has only a small deleterious effect in the activity, the introduction of polar groups such as a hydroxyl or methoxy group led to much less potent compounds. Also, in going from primary to tertiary amines, the activity diminished. A synthetic method for the preparation of suitably protected 3-carboxy-D$_2$-pyrazolin-5-yl-alanine was developed. This scaffold is amenable to further decoration at the N1 position and was used to generate novel NMDA receptor ligands. Although weaker than the previously reported N1–Ph derivatives, the new ligands retain the ability to selectively bind to NMDA receptor with micromolar to submicromolar affinity. Considering the relevance of the *N*-functionalization for the biological activity, the results presented the full SAR study of this novel class of NMDA receptor antagonists.[24]

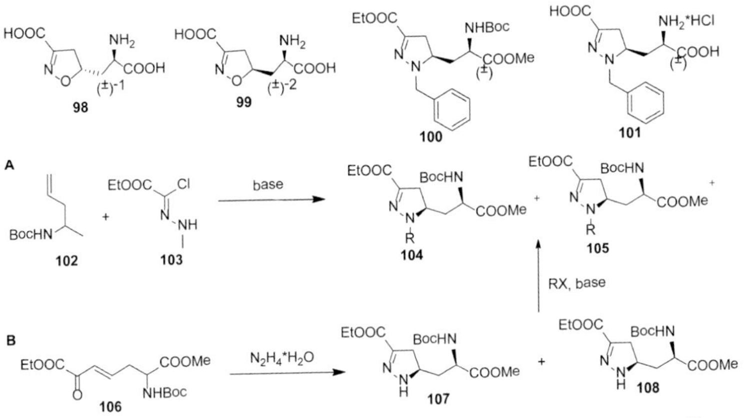

SCHEME 9.17   Two synthetic routes to synthesize N^1-substituted pyrazolines.[24]

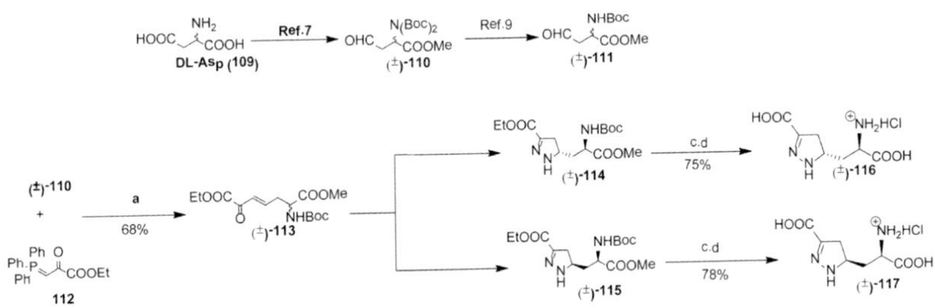

SCHEME 9.18   Synthesis of compounds **116** and **117**.
Reagents and conditions: (a) dioxane, 100°C, MW, 8 h; (b) N$_2$H$_4$·H$_2$O, AcOH, EtOH, 115°C, MW, 10 min; (c) 30% TFA, CH$_2$Cl$_2$, 3 h, 0°C to RT; (d) Ambersep 900-OH, H$_2$O/dioxane, 1 M HCl.[24]

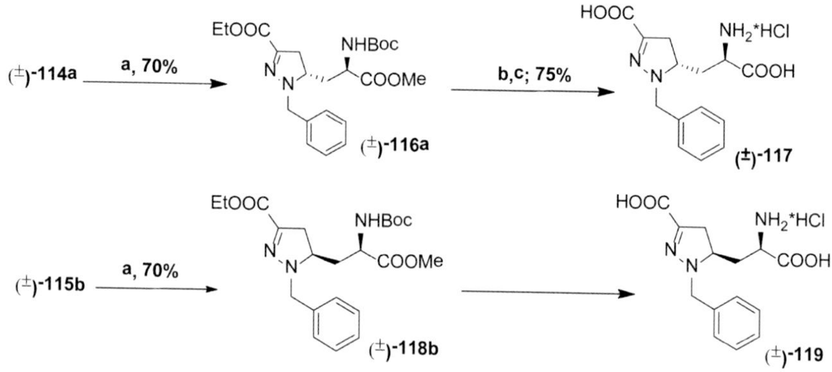

SCHEME 9.19 Synthesis of compound **119**.

Reagents: (a) BnBr, K$_2$CO$_3$, NaI, CH$_3$CN, reflux; (b) 30% TFA, CH$_2$Cl$_2$, 3 h, 0°C to RT; and (c) (i) Ambersep 900-OH, H$_2$O/dioxane and (ii) 1 M HCl.[24]

In the suitable synthetic method, 3-carboxy-D$_2$-pyrazolin-5-yl-alanine scaffold was obtained to generate a series of N-substituted pyrazoline derivatives. Moreover, we have confirmed the bioisosterism between the isoxazoline and the pyrazoline ring and highlighted how the N1 substituent is able to positively or negatively influence the binding affinity. In this light, the synthetic method developed herein will allow us to easily prepare a series of variously functionalized N1 derivatives that will serve to probe the size and electronic properties of the GluN2-binding pocket.

Despite widely reported clinical and preclinical studies of rapid antidepressant actions of glutamate NMDAR antagonists, there has been very little work examining the effects of these drugs in stress models of depression that require chronic administration of antidepressants or the molecular mechanisms that could account for the rapid responses. The results indicate that the structural and functional deficits resulting from long-term stress exposure, which could contribute to the pathophysiology of depression, are rapidly reversed by NMDA receptor antagonists in a mammalian target of rapamycin-dependent manner.[25]

Studies are underway to test additional targets in the glutamate–mTOR signaling pathway that could also be developed as rapid-acting antidepressants. To facilitate the transition from lead compounds in preclinical animal models to drug candidates for human use, it is important to establish whether NMDA receptor ligands have similar properties at rodent and human NMDA receptors. Here, amino acid sequences for human and rat

NMDA receptor subunits and discuss interspecies variation in the context of our current knowledge of the relationship between NMDA receptor structure and function. Studies summarize on the biophysical properties of human NMDA receptors and compare these properties to those of rat orthologs. Finally, we provide a comprehensive pharmacological characterization that allows side-by-side comparison of agonists, uncompetitive antagonists, GluN2B-selective noncompetitive antagonists, and GluN2C/D-selective modulators at recombinant human and rat NMDA receptors. The evaluation of biophysical properties and pharmacological probes acting at different sites on the receptor suggest that the binding sites and conformational changes leading to channel gating in response to agonist binding are highly conserved between human and rat NMDA receptors. In summary, the results of this study suggest that no major detectable differences exist in the pharmacological and functional properties of human and rat NMDA receptors.[26]

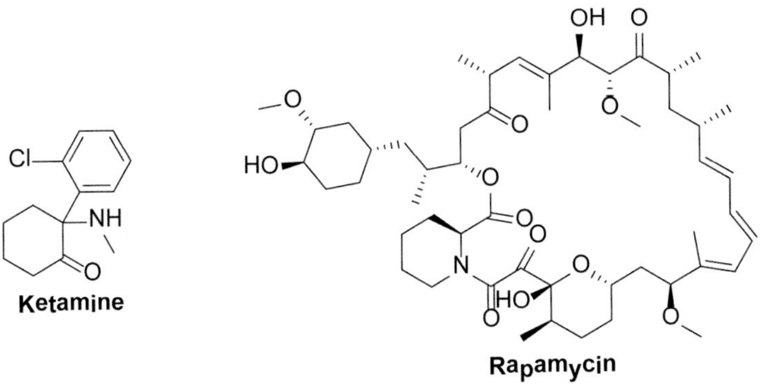

FIGURE 9.4   Structures of ketamine and rapamycin.[26]

Preclinical evaluation of drugs for neurological disorders is usually performed on overfed rodents, without consideration of how metabolic state might affect drug efficacy. Using a widely employed mouse model of focal ischemic stroke, we found that that the NMDA receptor antagonist dizocilpine (MK-801) reduces brain damage and improves functional outcome in mice on the usual ad libitum diet but exhibits little or no therapeutic efficacy in mice maintained on an energy-restricted diet. Thus, NMDA receptor activation plays a central role in the mechanism by which a high dietary energy intake exacerbates ischemic brain injury. These findings suggest that the inclusion of subjects with a wide range of energy intakes in clinical trials for stroke may mask a drug benefit in the overfed/obese subpopulation of subjects. These findings suggest the possibility that NMDAR antagonists might improve stroke outcome in individuals who have an excessive energy intake, but not in those with a healthier low level of energy intake.[27]

The synthesis of several 6,7,8,9,10,11-hexahydro-9-methyl-5,7:9,11-dimethano-5*H*-benzocyclononen-7-amines is reported. Several of them display low micromolar NMDA receptor antagonist and/or trypanocidal activities. Two compounds are endowed with micromolar antivesicular stomatitis virus activity, while only one compound shows micromolar anti-influenza activity. The anti-influenza activity of this compound does not seem to be mediated by blocking of the M2 protein.[28]

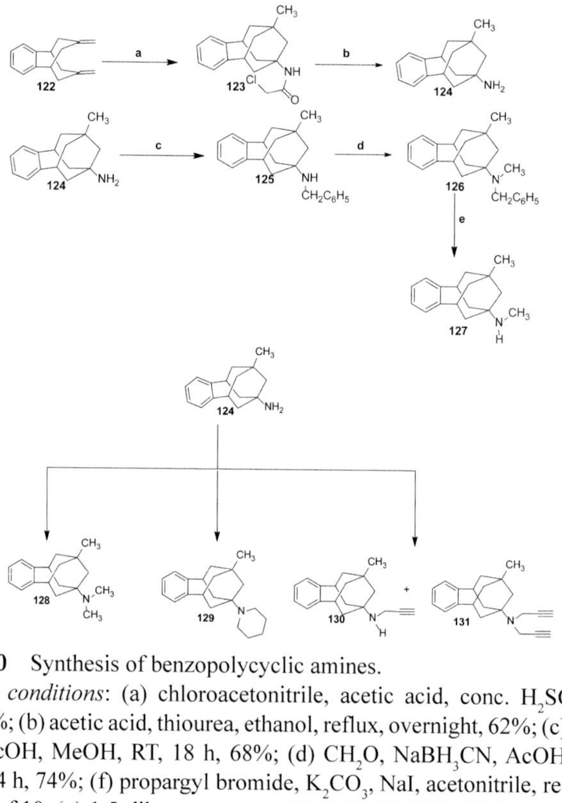

SCHEME 9.20 Synthesis of benzopolycyclic amines.
Reagents and conditions: (a) chloroacetonitrile, acetic acid, conc. H_2SO_4, 0°C to RT, overnight, 71%; (b) acetic acid, thiourea, ethanol, reflux, overnight, 62%; (c) benzaldehyde, $NaBH_3CN$, AcOH, MeOH, RT, 18 h, 68%; (d) CH_2O, $NaBH_3CN$, AcOH; (e) H_2, Pd/C, 1atm, 90°C, 24 h, 74%; (f) propargyl bromide, K_2CO_3, NaI, acetonitrile, reflux, 18 h, 17% of 9 and 48% of 10; (g) 1,5-dibromopentane, Et_3N, DMF, 60°C, 26 h, 35%.[28]

9.4 INHIBITORS AND MODULATORS OF GLUN2A, GLUN2C, AND GLUN2D SUBTYPE RECEPTORS

In screening, the synthesized compounds were able to antagonize NMDA receptors by measuring its effect on the increase in intracellular calcium evoked by glutamate or NMDA on rat cultured cerebellar granule neurons. Inspection of the results reveals that piperidine derivative had a value of IC_{50} (NMDA) very similar to that of amantadine, while the other compounds had values of IC_{50} (NMDA) that were in the micromolar order, that is, lower than amantadine but higher than memantine. Several of the derivatives were more potent than amantadine against NMDA-induced calcium increase in cerebellar granule neurons, although they were less potent than memantine. The functional assay of antagonist activity at NMDA receptors was performed using primary cultures of cerebellar granule neurons that were prepared according to established protocols.[28]

Hallucinations, a hallmark of psychosis, can be induced by the psychotomimetic NMDAR antagonists, ketamine and PCP, and are associated with hypersynchronization in the g-frequency band, but it is unknown how reduced interneuron activation associated with NMDA receptor hypofunction can cause hypersynchronization or distorted perception.[29]

A series of chiral nonracemic dexoxadrol analogs with various substituents in position 4 of the piperidine ring was synthesized and pharmacologically evaluated. Only the enantiomers having (S)-configuration at the 2-position of the piperidine ring and 4-position of the dioxolane ring were considered. Key steps in the synthesis were an imino-Diels–Alder reaction of enantiomerically pure imine (S)-13, which had been obtained from D-mannitol, with Danishefsky's diene 14 and the replacement of the p-methoxybenzyl protective group with a Cbz-group. It was shown that (S,S)-configuration of the ring junction (position 2 of the piperidine ring and position 4 of the dioxolane ring) and axial orientation of the C-4-substituent (($4S$)-configuration) are crucial for high NMDA receptor affinity. 2-(2,2-Diphenyl-1,3-dioxolan-4-yl)piperidines with a hydroxyl moiety ((S,S,S)-5, $K_i = 28$ nM), a fluorine atom ((S,S,S)-6, WMS-2539, $K_i = 7$ nM) and two fluorine atoms ((S,S)-7, $K_i = 48$ nM) in position-4 represent the most potent NMDA antagonists with high selectivity against R1 and R2 receptors and the polyamine-binding site of the NMDA receptor. The NMDA receptor affinities of the new ligands were correlated with their electrostatic potentials, calculated gas-phase proton affinities and dipole moments. According to these calculations decreasing proton affinity and increasing dipole moment are correlated with decreasing NMDA receptor affinity.[30]

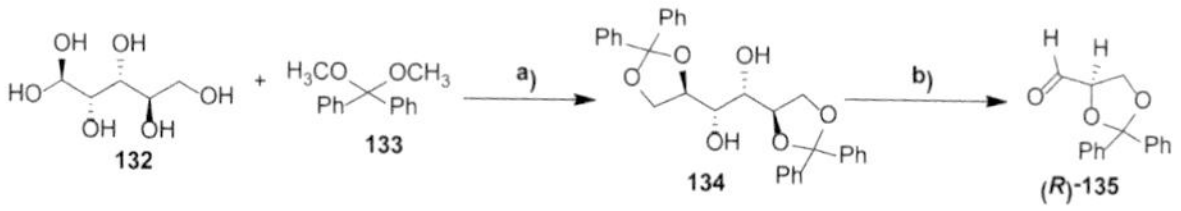

SCHEME 9.21 Synthesis of enantiomerically pure aldehyde **(R)-135**.
Reagents and conditions: (a) SnCl$_2$, dimethoxyethane, 14 h, reflux, 56% and (b) Pb(OAc)$_4$, CH$_2$Cl$_2$, 30 min, 0°C, 95%.[30]

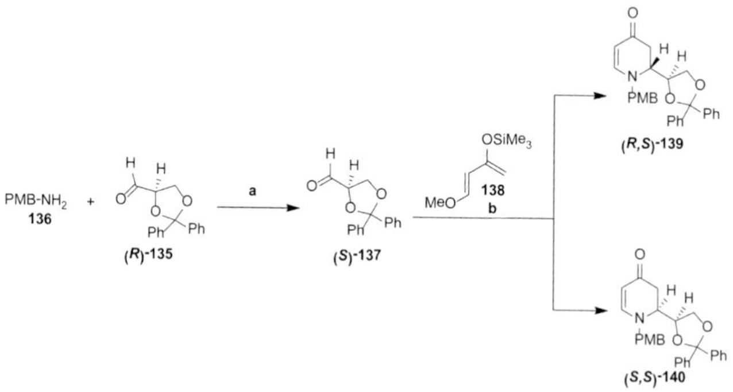

SCHEME 9.22 Synthesis of dihydropyridones.
Reagents and conditions: (a) CH$_3$(OCH$_3$)$_3$, RT, 14 h and (b) reaction conditions.[30]

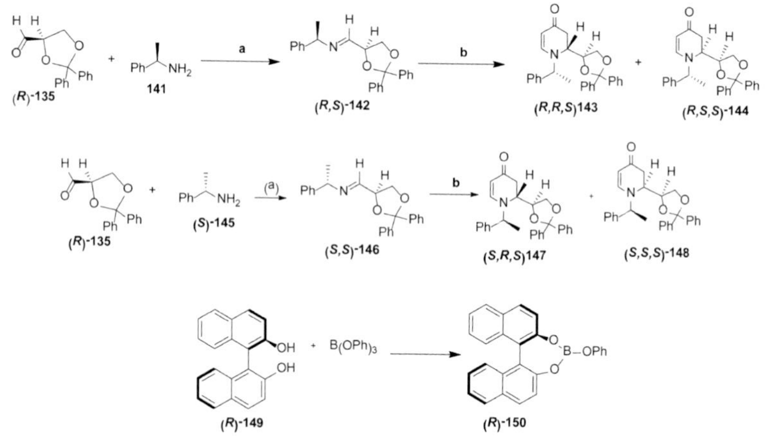

SCHEME 9.23 Diastereoselectivity of the imino-Diels–Alder reaction using chiral 1-phenylethylamine and chiral Lewis acids.
Reagent and conditions: (a) CH$_3$(OCH$_3$)$_3$, RT, 14 h and (b) reaction conditions.[30]

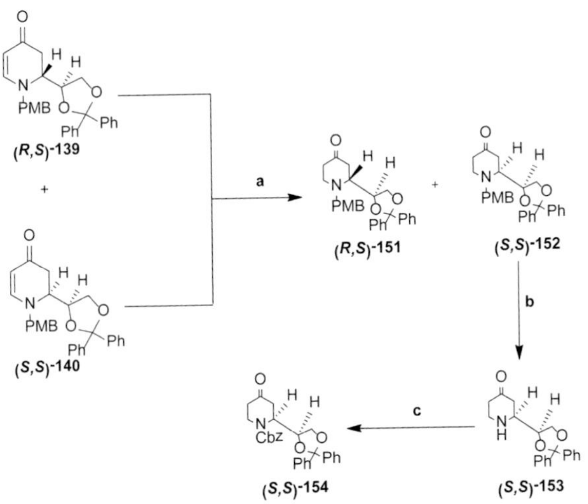

SCHEME 9.24 Identification and separation of diastereomers and replacement of PMB-protective group with the Cbz-protective group.[30]
Reagents and conditions: (a) $BF_3 \cdot OEt_2$, THF, $-78°C$, 30 min, then $LiEt_3BH$, $-78°C$, 2 h, 35% ((R,S)-**22a**), 52% ((S,S)-**22c**); (b) H_2, Pd/C 10%, MeOH, 16 h, RT, 85%; (c) $PhCH_2OCOCl$, NEt_3, THF, 1 h, RT, 90%.

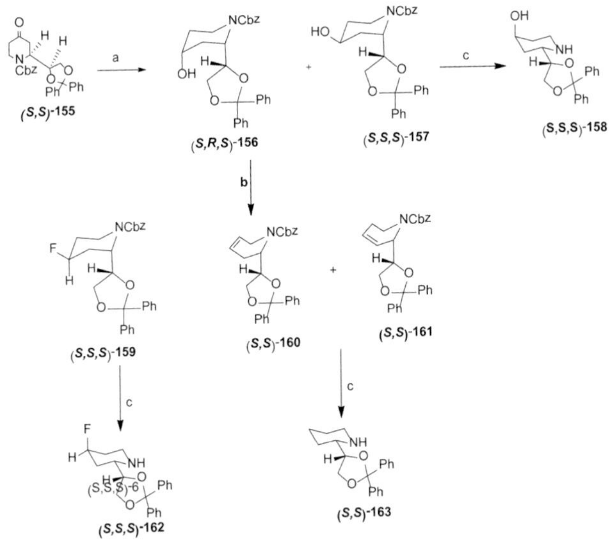

SCHEME 9.25 Synthesis of 4-hydroxydexoxadrol and 4-fluorodexoxadrol.
Reagents and conditions: (a) $NaBH_4$, MeOH, 1 h, 0°C, 45% ((S,R,S)-**24c**), 48% ((S,S,S)-**24d**); (b) DAST, CH_2Cl_2, 3 h, -78°C, 31% ((S,S,S)-**25d**), 55% ((S,S)-**26c**) and ((S,S)-**26d**); (c) H_2, Pd/C 10%, MeOH, 4 h, RT, 90% ((S,R,S)-**5**), 85% ((S,S,S)-**6**), 90% ((S,S)-**3**).[30]

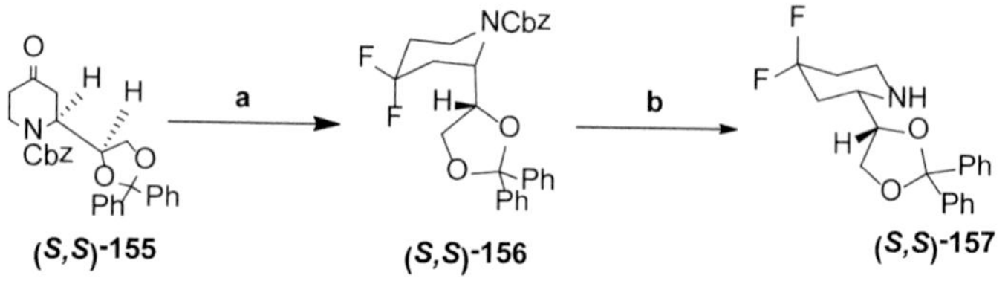

SCHEME 9.26　Synthesis of 4,4-difluorodexoxadrol (*S*,*S*)-**157**.
Reagents and conditions: (a) DAST, CH$_2$Cl$_2$, 16 h, RT, 70% and (b) H$_2$, Pd/C 10%, MeOH, 4 h, RT, 90%.[30]

First stereoselective synthesis of chiral nonracemic dexoxadrol (*S*,*S*)-**3** and analogs with various substituents in 4-position is presented. The enantiomerically enriched ligands display higher NMDA receptor affinities than the racemic mixtures, which prove that the eutomers have been synthesized. The NMDA receptor affinity of the new ligands was correlated with their electrostatic potential, proton affinity, and dipole moment. The calculations showed decreasing NMDA receptor affinity with decreasing proton affinity and increasing dipole moment.[31]

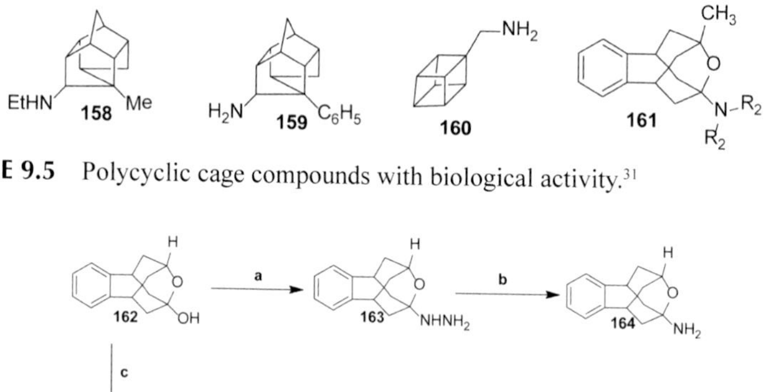

FIGURE 9.5　Polycyclic cage compounds with biological activity.[31]

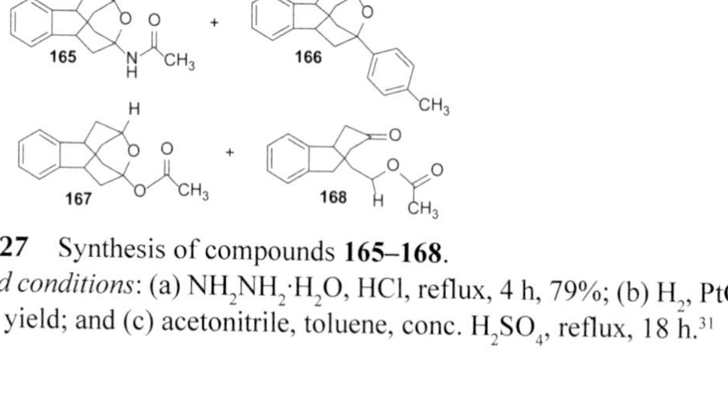

SCHEME 9.27　Synthesis of compounds **165–168**.
Reagents and conditions: (a) NH$_2$NH$_2$·H$_2$O, HCl, reflux, 4 h, 79%; (b) H$_2$, PtO$_2$, 1 atm, RT, 3 days, 82% yield; and (c) acetonitrile, toluene, conc. H$_2$SO$_4$, reflux, 18 h.[31]

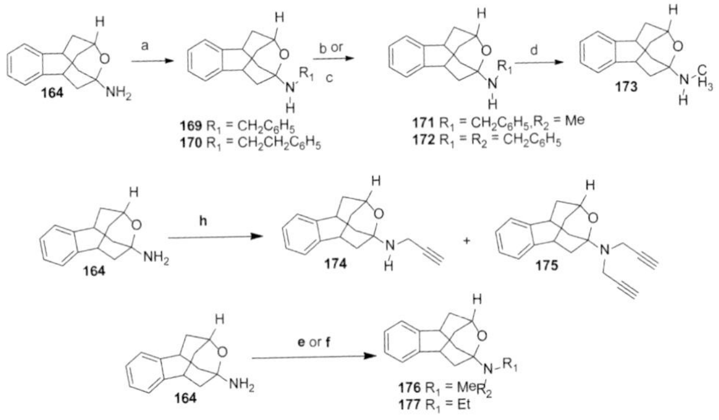

SCHEME 9.28 Synthesis of compounds **165–168** from **164**.
Reagents and conditions: (a) benzaldehyde or phenylacetaldehyde, NaBH$_3$CN, AcOH, MeOH, RT, 18 h; (b) CH$_2$O, NaBH$_3$CN, AcOH, acetonitrile, RT, 2 h; (c) benzyl chloride, K$_2$CO$_3$, NaI, acetonitrile, reflux, 24 h; (d) H$_2$, Pd/C, 38 atm, 100°C, 24 h; (e) HCO$_2$H, 37% aq. CH$_2$O, 80°C, 24 h; (f) acetaldehyde, NaBH$_3$CN, AcOH, acetonitrile, RT, 2 h; (g) 1,5-dibromopentane, Et$_3$N, DMF, 60°C, 26 h, 46%; (h) propargyl bromide, K$_2$CO$_3$, NaI, acetonitrile, reflux, 18 h.[31]

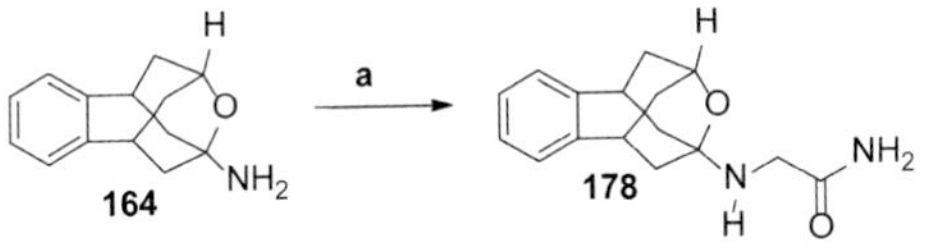

SCHEME 9.29 NMDA receptor antagonists bearing an aminoacetamide group and synthesis of analog **178**.
Reagents: (a) chloroacetamide, K$_2$CO$_3$, NaI, acetonitrile, reflux, 18 h.[31]

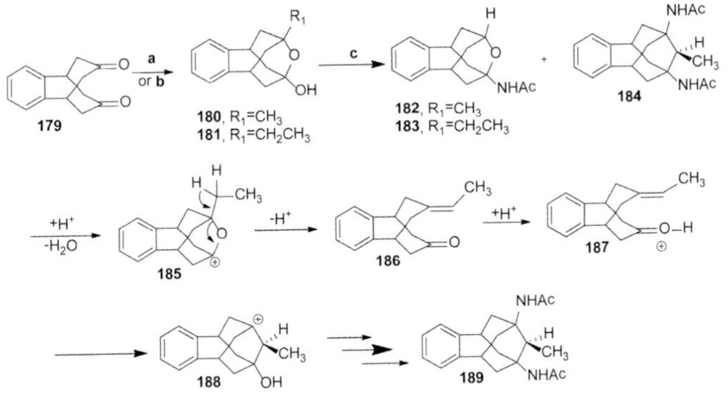

SCHEME 9.30 Synthesis of compound **189**.
Reagents and conditions: (a) Methylmagnesium bromide or ethylmagnesium bromide, toluene, 0°C, overnight; (b) ethylmagnesium bromide, toluene, 0°C, overnight; (c) acetonitrile, H$_2$SO$_4$, reflux, 18 h.[31]

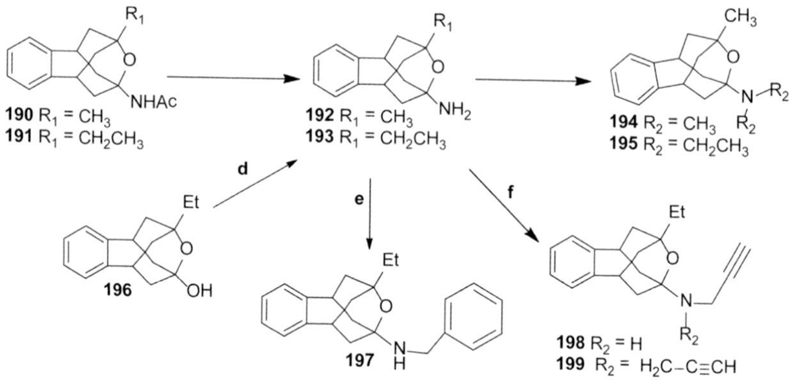

SCHEME 9.31   Synthesis of compounds **197–199**.

Reagents and conditions: (a) HCl, reflux, 18 h; (b) HCOOH, 37% aq. CH_2O, 80°C, 24 h; (c) acetaldehyde, $NaBH_3CN$, AcOH, acetonitrile, RT, 18 h; (d) urea, $CF3CO2H$, 115°C, 18 h; (e) benzaldehyde, $NaBH_3CN$, AcOH, MeOH, RT, 18 h; (f) propargyl bromide, K_2CO_3, NaI, acetonitrile, reflux, 18 h.[31]

   This chapter focuses on the basic biophysical properties and physiological functions of NMDA receptors and how these are modulated by various signaling molecules and biochemical cascades under physiological conditions. The ability of modulators to influence NMDA receptor currents is dependent on their abundance and proximity to the receptor. Proteomic characterization identified synaptic NMDA receptors as part of a remarkably large macromolecular signaling complex called the NMDA receptor complex. NMDA receptors were found linked to receptors, adhesion molecules, scaffolding proteins, signaling molecules, cytoskeletal proteins, and various novel proteins, in complexes lacking non-NMDA receptors. Among the signaling proteins were kinases, phosphatases, GTPases, and GTPase-activating proteins. Physical linkage of these receptors, signaling molecules, and the cytoskeleton to the NMDA receptor is an important way to facilitate rapid modulation of the receptor in response to synaptic activity.[32]

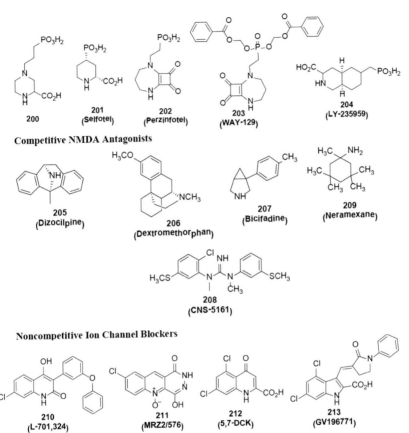

FIGURE 9.6 Structures of competitive NMDA antagonists, noncompetitive ion channel blockers, and glycine antagonists.[32]

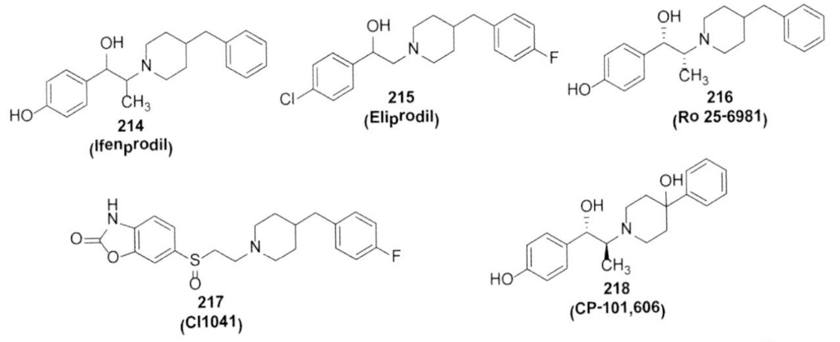

FIGURE 9.7 Structures of NR2B-specific noncompetitive NMDA antagonists.[32]

NMDA receptor antagonists, such as ketamine and phencyclidine, induce perceptual abnormalities, psychosis-like symptoms, and mood changes in healthy humans and patients with schizophrenia. The similarity between NMDA receptor antagonist-induced psychosis and schizophrenia has led to the widespread use of the drugs to provide models to aid the development of novel treatments for the disorder. This chapter investigates the predictive validity of NMDA receptor antagonist models based on a range of novel treatments that have now reached clinical trials. Furthermore, it considers the extent to which the different hypotheses that have been proposed to account for the psychotomimetic effects of NMDA receptor antagonist have been validated by the results of these trials. Finally, the chapter discusses some of the caveats associated with the use of the models and some suggestions as to how greater use of translational markers might ensure progress in understanding the relationship between the models and schizophrenia.[33] In the present study, the effects of intra-cerebroventricular injection of NMDA receptor agonist and antagonist on impairment of memory formation and the state-dependent learning by morphine have been investigated in mice. The results suggest that NMDA receptors are involved in morphine state-dependent learning in mice.[34]

A series of oximes, deriving from 2-arylidene-pyrroline-3,4-diones has been prepared. The presence of tautomers in their solutions has been established by spectroscopic means. The compounds reacted with diazomethane chiefly by N-methylation forming nitrones. The analogously prepared 2-arylidene-4-nitropyrrolin-3-ones, formally derived from nitrotetramic acids, yielded nitronic acid esters upon reaction with diazomethane. The structures were elucidated by spectral evidence and in the case of compounds X-ray diffraction analysis. The binding affinity of some of the new compounds toward the NMDA (glycine site) receptor has been measured thus providing the basis for further structure-activity relationship studies. Oxime showed the highest binding potency ($K_i = 9.2$ µM).

Excitotoxicity, defined as excessive exposure to the neurotransmitter glutamate or overstimulation of its membrane receptors, has been implicated as one of the key factors contributing to neuronal injury and death in a wide range of both acute and chronic neurologic disorders. Excitotoxic cell death is due, at least in part, to excessive activation of NMDA-type glutamate receptors and hence excessive Ca^{2+} influx through the receptor's associated ion channel. Physiological NMDA receptor activity, however, is also essential for normal neuronal function; potential neuroprotective agents that block virtually all NMDA receptor activity will very likely have unacceptable clinical side effects. For this reason, many NMDA receptor antagonists have disappointingly failed advanced clinical trials for a number of diseases including stroke and neurodegenerative disorders such as Huntington's disease. In contrast, studies in my laboratory were the first to show that memantine, an adamantane derivative, preferentially blocks excessive NMDA receptor activity without disrupting normal activity. Memantine does this through its action as an open-channel blocker; it enters the receptor-associated ion channel preferentially when it is excessively open, and, most importantly, its off-rate is relatively fast so that it does not substantially accumulate in the channel to interfere with normal synaptic transmission. Past clinical use for other indications has demonstrated that memantine is well tolerated, and it has recently been approved in both Europe and the USA for the treatment of dementia of the Alzheimer's type. Clinical studies of the safety and efficacy of memantine for other neurological disorders, including glaucoma and other forms of dementia, are currently underway. A series of second-generation memantine derivatives are currently in development and may prove to have even greater neuroprotective properties than does memantine. These second-generation drugs take advantage of the fact that the NMDA receptor has other modulatory sites, in addition to its ion channel, that could potentially be used for safe but effective clinical intervention.[36]

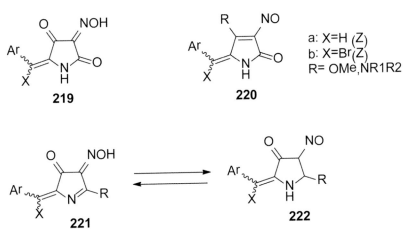

SCHEME 9.32 Synthesis of compound **222**.[36]

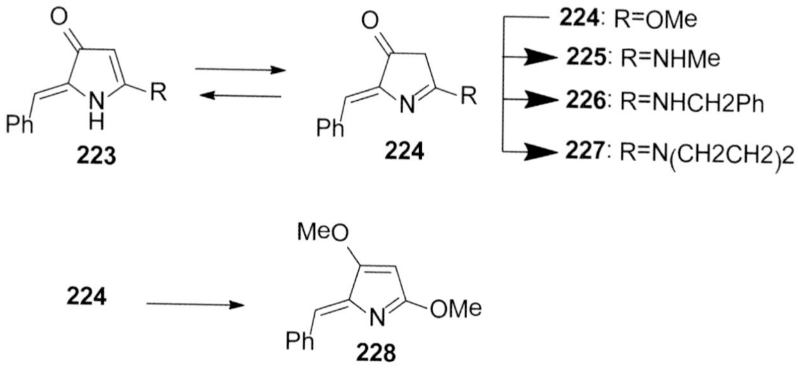

SCHEME 9.33   Synthesis of compound **228**.[36]

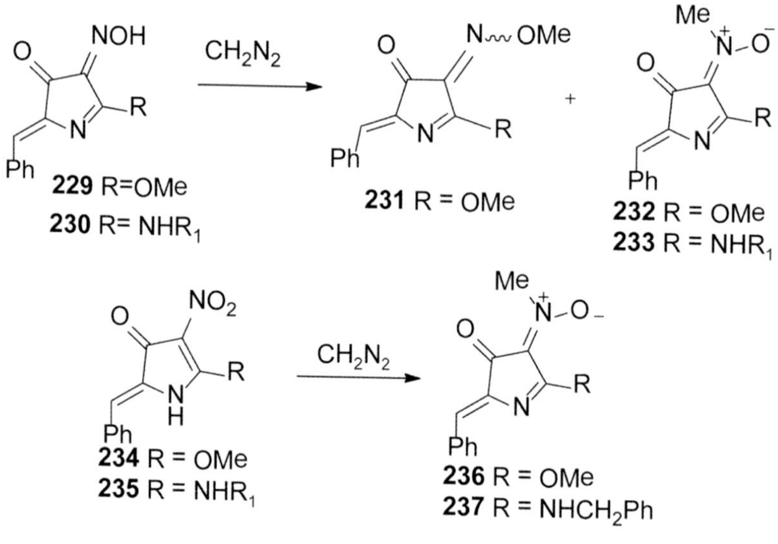

a: R₁=CH₂Ph; b: R₁=Ph; c: R₁=(4-Cl)Ph; d: R₁=(2-Cl)Ph

a: R_1=CH$_2$Ph; b: R_1=Ph; c: R_1=(4-Cl)Ph; d: R_1=(2-Cl)Ph

SCHEME 9.34   Synthesis of compounds **236** and **237**.[36]

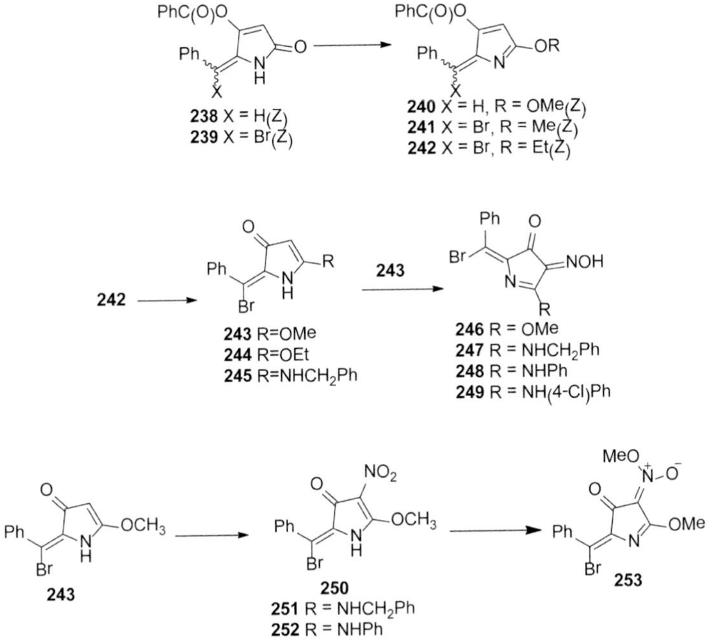

SCHEME 9.35 Synthesis of compound **253**.[36]

A large dosage of aspirin produces reversible hearing loss and tinnitus. These effects have been attributed to the salicylate ion, the active component of aspirin. Salicylate acts as a competitive antagonist at the anion-binding site of prestin, the motor protein of sensory outer hair cells. This provides an explanation for the hearing loss induced by aspirin. However, the molecular mechanism of salicylate-induced tinnitus remains obscure. One physiological basis of salicylate ototoxicity probably originates from altered arachidonic acid metabolism. Arachidonic acid potentiates NMDA receptor currents. The involvement of cochlear NMDA receptors in the occurrence of tinnitus have been noticed. Tinnitus was assessed with a behavioral test based on an active avoidance paradigm. Results showed that the occurrence of tinnitus Induced by salicylate can be suppressed by the application of NMDA antagonists into the cochlear fluids. The activation of NMDA receptors was linked to cyclooxygenase inhibition. Thus target cochlear NMDA receptors may present a therapeutic strategy for the treatment of tinnitus.[37]

NMDA receptor antagonists such as selfotel, aptiganel, eliprodil, licostinel, and gavestinel failed to show efficacy in clinical trials of stroke or traumatic brain injury. This failure has been attributed to the deficient properties of the molecules that entered human trials and to the inappropriate design of clinical studies. Glutamate may be involved in the acute neurodestructive phase that occurs immediately after traumatic or ischemic injury (excitotoxicity), but that, after this period, it assumes its normal physiological functions, which include promotion of neuronal survival. NMDA receptor antagonists failed stroke and traumatic brain injury trials in human beings because blockade of synaptic transmission mediated by NMDA receptors hinders neuronal survival. Recent clinical data suggest that chronic pain due to nerve or soft tissue injury may result in the sensitization of the CNS, mediated in part by the excitatory amino acids, glutamate, and aspartate.[38] In all examples presented here, NMDA-receptor antagonists with an affinity at the phencyclidine site have been shown to modulate pain and hyperalgesia but are limited by dose-limiting side effects. Thus, provided their therapeutic ratio is favorable, NMDA-receptor antagonists may be effective in the treatment of some types of chronic pain.[39]

A series of 1,3,5-alkyl-substituted cyclohexylamines were synthesized as ligands for the NMDA receptor PCP-binding site. Pure diastereomers with a defined configuration of the amino group were obtained. The optimal size of 1,3,5 substituents was determined for cyclohexylamines with an equatorial amino group in the lowest energy conformation using Hansch analysis. According to the data, the lipophilic part of cyclohexylamines does not discriminate between hydrophobic regions of the PCP-binding site but rather recognizes this site as a whole lipophilic pocket.[40]

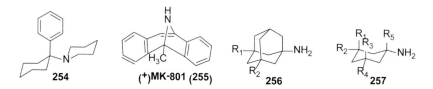

FIGURE 9.8   Chemical structure of PCP (**254**), MK-801 (**255**), 3,5-substituted amino adamantanes (**256**) and 1,3,5-substituted cyclohexylamines (**257**).[40]

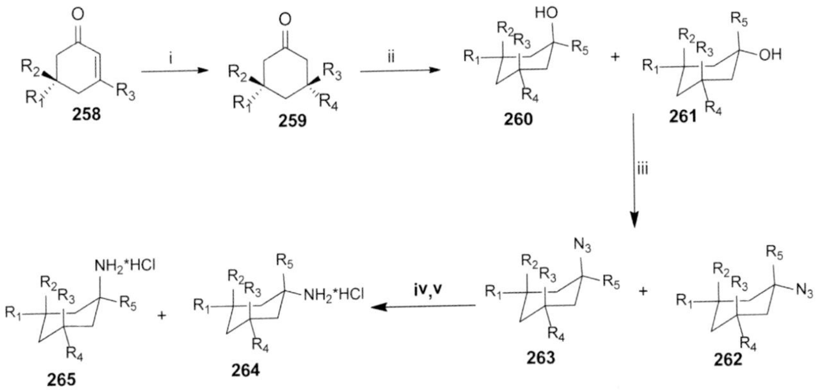

SCHEME 9.36 Synthesis of 1,3,5-substituted cyclohexylamines.
Reagents: (i) R_4–2CuMgX; (ii) R_5MgX; (iii) A: HN_3, $TiCl_4$; B: $TMSN_3$, BF_3·Et_2O; (iv) $LiAlH_4$; and (v) HCl.[40]

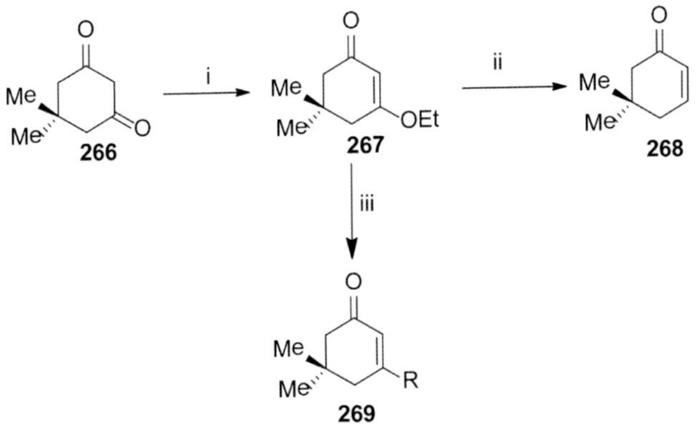

SCHEME 9.37 Synthesis of cyclohexen-2-ones.
Reagents and conditions: (i) EtOH, TsOH; (ii) $LiAlH_4$ then 10% H_2SO_4; (iii) RMgI then 5% H_2SO_4.[40]

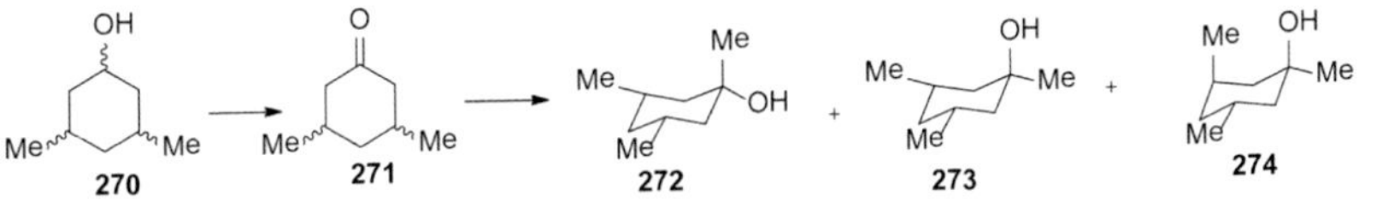

SCHEME 9.38 The synthesis of 1,3,5-trimethylcyclohexanols.
Reagents: (i) H_2SO_4, CrO_3 and (ii) Me–Mg–X.[40]

9.5   GLUTAMATE AND GLYCINE-BINDING LIGANDS

At CNS synapses, agonist binding to postsynaptic iGluRs results in signaling between neurons. NMDA receptors are a unique family of iGluRs that activate in response to the concurrent binding of glutamate and glycine.[41] Here, the process of agonist binding to the GluN2A (glutamate binding) and GluN1 (glycine binding) NMDA receptor subtypes using long-timescale unbiased molecular dynamics simulations. Positively charged residues on the surface of the GluN2A ligand-binding domain (LBD) assist glutamate binding via a "guided-diffusion" mechanism, similar in fashion to glutamate binding to the GluA2 LBD of AMPA receptors was investigated. Glutamate can also bind in an inverted orientation. Glycine, on the other hand, binds to the GluN1 LBD via an "unguided-diffusion" mechanism, whereby glycine finds its binding site primarily by random thermal fluctuations. Free energy calculations quantify the glutamate- and glycine-binding processes.[42]

Functional tetra-heteromeric NMDAR contains two obligatory GluN1 subunits and two identical or different non-GluN1 subunits that include six different gene products; four GluN2 (A–D) and two GluN3 (A–B) subunits. The heterogeneity of subunit combination facilities the distinct function of NMDARs. All GluN subunits contain an extracellular N-terminal domain and LBD, transmembrane domain, and an intracellular C-terminal domain. The interaction between the GluN1 and coassembling GluN2/3 subunits through the LBD has been proven crucial for defining receptor deactivation mechanisms that are unique for each combination of NMDAR. Modulating the LBD interactions has great therapeutic potential. In the present work, by amino acid point mutations and electrophysiology techniques, we have studied the role of LBD interactions in determining the effect of well-characterized pharmacological agents including agonists, competitive antagonists, and allosteric modulators. The results reveal that agonists (glycine and glutamate) potency was altered based on mutant amino acid side-chain chemistry and/or mutation site. Most antagonists inhibited mutant receptors with higher potency; interestingly, clinically used NMDAR channel blocker memantine was about three-fold more potent on mutated receptors than wild-type receptors. These results provide novel insights on the clinical pharmacology of memantine, which is used for the treatment of mild to moderate AD. In addition, these findings demonstrate the central role of LBD interactions that can be exploited to develop novel NMDAR based therapeutics.[43]

NMDAR exacerbated activation leads to neuron death through a phenomenon called excitotoxicity. These receptors are implicated in several neurological diseases and thus represent an important therapeutic target. We herein describe the study of enantiopure tryptophanol-derived oxazolopiperidone lactams as NMDA receptor antagonists. The most active hit exhibited an IC_{50} of 63.41 M in cultured rat cerebellar granule neurons thus being 1.5-fold more active than clinically approved NMDA antagonist amantadine.[44]

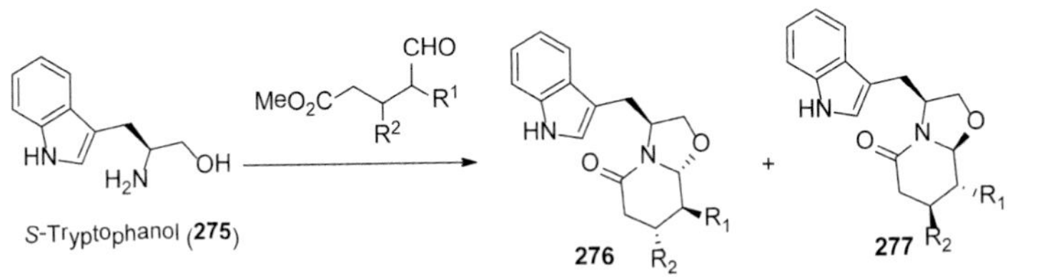

SCHEME 9.39(A) Synthesis of *S*-tryptophanol-oxazolopiperidones.
Reagents and conditions: 1.1 eq of oxo-esters, toluene, 16 h D, inert atmosphere, and Dean–Stark apparatus.[44]

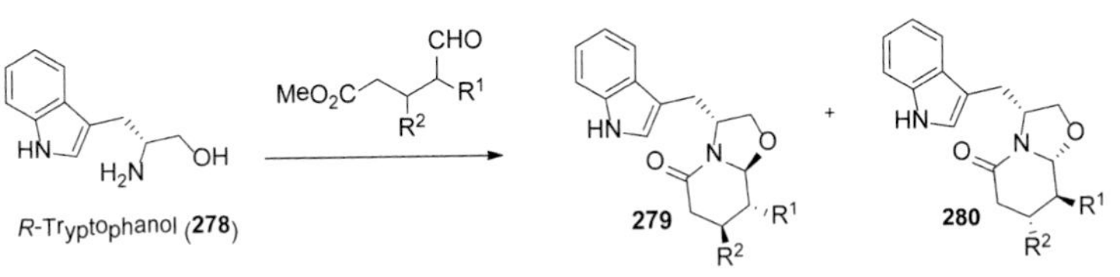

SCHEME 9.39(B) Synthesis of R-tryptophanol-derived oxazolopiperidones.
Reagents and conditions: 1.1 eq of oxo-esters, toluene, 16 h D, inert atmosphere, and Dean–Stark apparatus.[44]

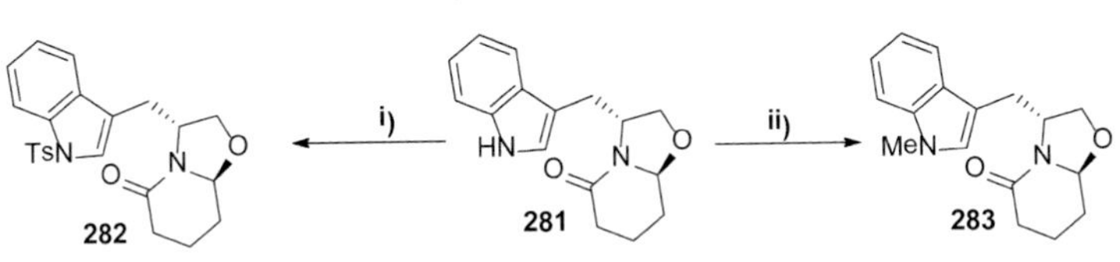

SCHEME 9.40 Synthesis of compounds **282** and **283**.
Reagents and conditions: (i) TsCl, CH_2Cl_2, NaOH (aq, 30% w/v), TBAI, 0°C, 16 h; (ii) NaH, MeI, DMF, 0°C.[44]

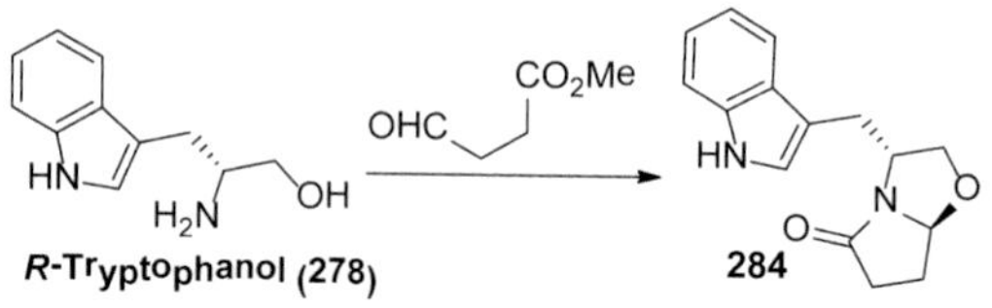

SCHEME 9.41   Synthesis of compound **284**.[44]

The identification of structurally novel analogs of ketamine and PCP, as NMDA receptor antagonists, with low-to-moderate potency at GluN2A and GluN2B receptors, is discussed. In particular, some examples, such as compounds 6 and 10, show decreased calculated lipophilicity, when compared to PCP, while retaining moderate activity. Moreover, the germinal aryl amino substituted lactam ring, as exemplified in compounds, constitutes a novel scaffold with potential application in the design of biologically active compounds.[45]

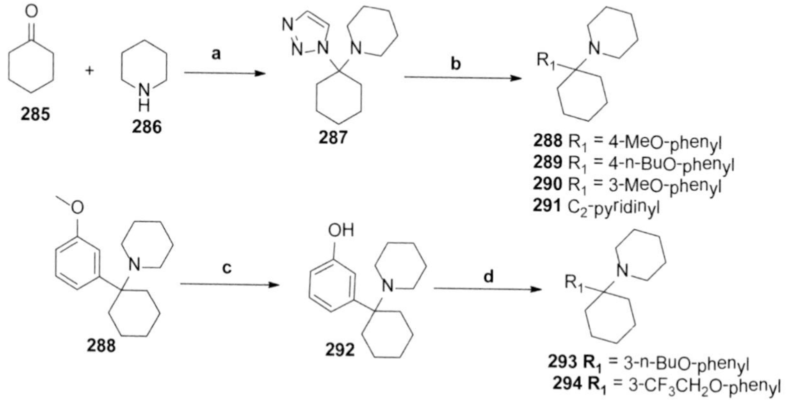

SCHEME 9.42   Synthesis of compound **318**.
Reagents and conditions: (a) 1,2,3-Triazole, toluene, 130°C, 12 h; (b) aryl magnesium bromide or aryl lithium, THF, −78°C, RT, 1–4 h; (c) −78°C, DCM, 3 h; (d) K_2CO_3, NaI, alkyl bromide or iodide, DMF, 80–120°C, 1–3 h.[45]

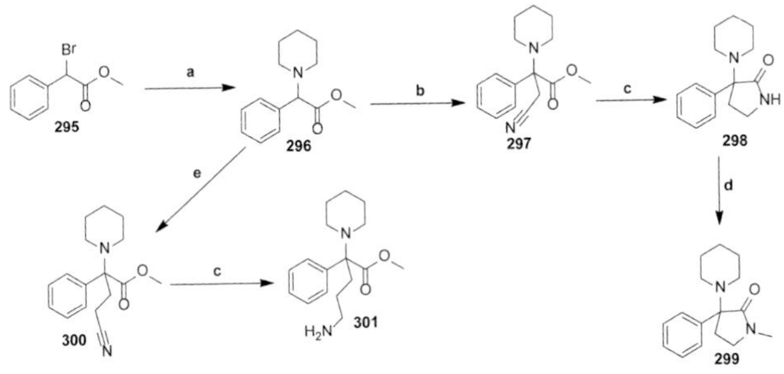

SCHEME 9.43   Synthesis of compound **299**.
Reagents and conditions: (a) Piperidine, RT, Et₂O, 20 h; (b) ICH₂CN, DIPA, *n*-BuLi in *n*-hexane 1.6 M, 78°C, THF, 2 h; (c) Raney Nickel, hydrogen, RT, 5 atm, MeOH, overnight; (d) MeI, KOH, TBAB, 0°C, RT, THF, 1 h; (e) Br(CH₂)₂CN, DIPA, *n*-BuLi in *n*-hexane 1.6 M, 30°C, THF, 3 h; (f) AcOH, 110°C, 7 h.[45]

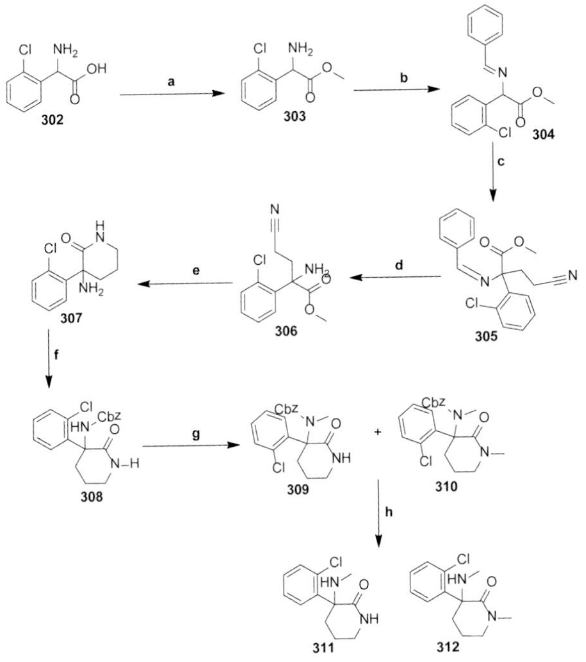

SCHEME 9.44   Synthesis of compound **311** and **312**.
Reagents and conditions: (a) SOCl₂, MeOH, RT, overnight; (b) NaOMe, PhCHO, MeOH, RT, overnight; (c) CH₂CHCN, KButO, ButOH, RT, overnight; (d) HCl 6 M, Et₂O, RT, 4 h; (e) COCl₂, NaBH₄, MeOH, 100°C, MW, 20 min for two cycles; (f) NaHCO₃, CbzCl, THF, RT, overnight; (g) MeI, NaH, DMF, 0°C, RT, overnight; and (h) TFA, 50°C, overnight, HPLC purification.[45]

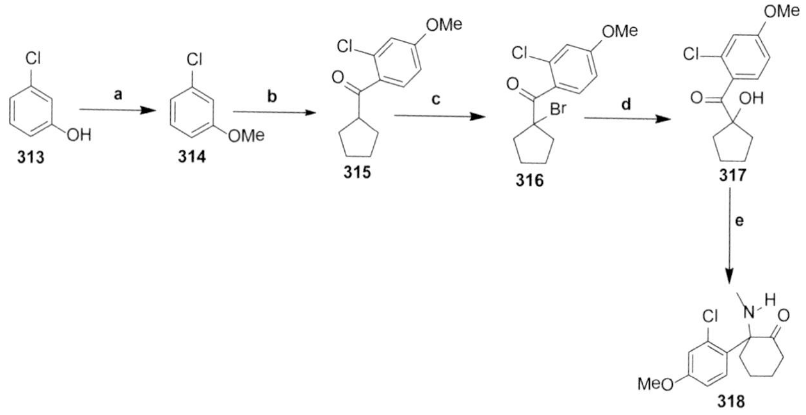

SCHEME 9.45   Synthesis of compound **318**.
Reagents and conditions: (a) K$_2$CO$_3$, MeI, DMF, RT, overnight; (b) cyclopentanecarbonyl chloride, AlCl$_3$, *n*-hexane, 40°C, 5 h; (c) Br$_2$, 1,4-dioxane, RT; (d) KOH, MeOH, RT, 2 h; (e) MeNH$_2$, MW, 165°C, 30 min.[45]

9.6   CONCLUSION

For all of the targets mentioned in this context, the selectivity of novel compounds remains a key feature that is just now under development. Additionally, it may be possible to modulate NMDA receptor function indirectly by altering signaling cascades that regulate NMDA receptors, such as those that induce phosphorylation of the channel; these types of strategies may have different outcomes versus direct and chronic inhibition of the channel. There has been much interest in targeting this glutamatergic system when developing new and promising drugs against neurodegenerative diseases.[46,47] The basis for this interest is the evidence supporting ketamine, an NMDA receptor agonist and antagonist's rapidly effective treatment of refractory epilepsy. Improvements to existing treatments for CNS diseases represent an unmet medical need, and NMDA receptors have become an important target for new therapeutic approaches. Progress in this area has been largely driven by the design and synthesis of subtype-selective NMDA antagonists which act at an allosteric site of the ATD without direct block of the ion channel pore. With the determination of the structure and molecular contacts of selective antagonists, a template is available for the design of molecules with improved potency and selectivity. Recent advances have not been limited to subtype-selective NMDA receptors. It is generally accepted that these ligands do not bind within the ATD, LBD, or ion channel pore, but instead at a novel site on the NMDA receptor complex. Though improvements in potency, selectivity, and drug-like properties are still needed, this class presents a new horizon for improvement of our understanding toward NMDA receptors and their pharmacology. This context provides detailed information related to design, synthesis, and pharmacophore available against NMDA receptor to treat neurodegenerative diseases.

ACKNOWLEDGMENTS

Authors are thankful to the Principal Dr. S. J. Surana, R. C. Patel Institute of Pharmaceutical Education and Research, Shirpur, Maharashtra (India) for providing necessary facilities.

KEYWORDS

- NMDA receptor
- neurodegenerative diseases
- synthesis
- glycine
- glutamate

REFERENCES

1. Wilkinson, J. L. Neurotransmitter Pathways of Central Nervous System. In *Neuroanatomy for Medical Students*, 2nd ed.; Butterworth Heinemann: Oxford, 1992; pp 265–270.
2. Rousseaux, C. G. A Review of Glutamate Receptors I: Current Understanding of Their Biology. *J. Toxicol. Pathol.* **2008**, *21*, 25–51.
3. Bowie, D. Ionotropic Glutamate Receptors and CNS Disorders. *CNS Neurol. Disord. Drug Targets* **2008**, *7* (2), 129–143.
4. Traynelis, S. F.; Wollmuth, L. P.; McBain, C. J.; Menniti, F. S.; Vance, K. M.; Ogden, K. K.; Hansen, K. B.; Yuan, H.; Myers, S. J.; Dingledine, R. Glutamate Receptor

Ion Channels: Structure, Regulation, and Function. *Pharmacol. Rev.* **2010**, *62* (3), 405–496.

5. Murata, S.; Kawasaki, K. Common and Uncommon Behavioural Effects of Antagonists for Different Modulatory Sites in the NMDA Receptor/Channel Complex. *Eur. J. Pharmacol.* **1993**, *239* (1–3), 9–15.

6. Obrenovitch, T. P.; Urenjak, J. Altered Glutamatergic Transmission in Neurological Disorders: From High Extracellular Glutamate to Excessive Synaptic Efficacy. *Progress Neurobiol.* **1997**, *51* (1), 39–87.

7. Parsons, C. G.; Danysz, W.; Quack, G. Glutamate in CNS Disorders as a Target for Drug Development: An Update. *Drug News Perspect.* **1998**, *11* (9), 523–569.

8. Danysz, W.; Parsons, C. G. Glycine and *N*-Methyl-*D*-Aspartate Receptors: Physiological Significance and Possible Therapeutic Applications. *Pharmacol. Rev.* **1998**, *50* (4), 597–664.

9. Paoletti, P.; Neyton, J. NMDA Receptor Subunits: Function and Pharmacology. *Curr. Opin. Pharmacol.* **2007**, *7*, 39–47.

10. Monaghan, D. T.; Irvine, M. W.; Costa, B. M.; Fang, G.; Jane, D. E. Pharmacological Modulation of NMDA Receptor Activity and the Advent of Negative and Positive Allosteric Modulators. *Neurochem. Int.* **2014**, *61*, 581–592.

11. Kalia, V.; Kalia, S. K.; Salter, M. W. NMDA Receptors in Clinical Neurology: Excitatory Times Ahead. *Lancet Neurol.* **2008**, *7*, 742–755.

12. Ruppa, K. B.; King, D.; Olson, R. E. NMDA Antagonists of GluN2B Subtype and Modulators of GluN2A, GluN2C, and GluN2D Subtypes: Recent Results and Developments. *Annu. Rep. Med. Chem.* **2009**, *47*, 89–102.

13. Ogden, K. K.; Traynelis, S. F. New Advances in NMDA Receptor Pharmacology. *Trends Pharmacol. Sci.* **2011**, *32* (12), 726–733.

14. Grazioso, G.; Moretti, L.; Scapozza, L.; De Amici, M.; De Micheli, C. Development of a Three-Dimensional Model for the *N*-Methyl-d-Aspartate NR2A Subunit. *J. Med. Chem.* **2005**, *48* (17), 5489–5494.

15. Agatonovic-Kustrin, S.; Kettle, C.; Morton, D. W. A Molecular Approach in Drug Development for Alzheimer's Disease. *Biomed. Pharmacother.* **2018**, *106*, 553–565.

16. Morelli, M. B.; Amantini, C.; Santoni, G.; Pellei, M.; Santini, C.; Cimarelli, C.; Marcantoni, E.; Petrini, M.; Del Bello, F.; Giorgioni, G.; Piergentili, A. Novel Antitumor Copper(II) Complexes Rationally Designed to Act Through Synergistic Mechanisms of Action, Due to the Presence of an NMDA Receptor Ligand and Copper in the Same Chemical Entity. *New J. Chem.* **2018**, *42*, 11878–11887.

17. Morris, P. J.; Moaddel, R.; Zanos, P.; Moore, C. E.; Gould, T.; Zarate C. A.; Thomas, C. J. Synthesis and *N*-Methyl-d-Aspartate (NMDA) Receptor Activity of Ketamine Metabolites. *Org. Lett.* **2017**, *19* (17), 4572–4575.

18. Alam, M. P.; Bilousova, T.; Spilman, P.; Vadivel, K.; Bai, D.; Elias, C. J.; Evseenko, D. John, V. A Small Molecule Mimetic of the Humanin Peptide as a Candidate for Modulating NMDA-Induced Neurotoxicity. *ACS Chem. Neuro.* **2017**, *9* (3), 462–468.

19. Rothan, H. A.; Amini, E.; Faraj, F. L.; Golpich, M.; Teoh, T. C.; Gholami, K.; Yusof, R. NMDA Receptor Antagonism with Novel Indolyl, 2-(1,1-Dimethyl-1,3 Dihydro-Benzo[*e*]Indol-2-Ylidene)-Malonaldehyde, Reduces Seizures Duration in a Rat Model of Epilepsy. *Sci. Rep.* **2017**, *7*, 45540.

20. Pereira, N. A.; Sureda, F. X.; Pérez, M.; Amat M.; Santos, M. M. Enantiopure Indolo [2,3-*a*] Quinolizidines: Synthesis and Evaluation as NMDA Receptor Antagonists. *Molecules* **2016**, *21* (8), 1027.

21. Kang, H.; Park, P.; Bortolotto, S. D. Brandt, T. Colestock, J. Wallach, G. L. Collingridge and D. Lodge, Ephenidine: A New Psychoactive Agent with Ketamine-Like NMDA Receptor Antagonist Properties. *Neuropharmacology* **2017**, *112*, 144–149.

22. Kaur, A.; Kaur, T.; Singh, B.; Pathak, D.; Buttar Singh, H.; Pal Singh, A. Curcumin Alleviates Ischemia Reperfusion-Induced Acute Kidney Injury Through NMDA Receptor Antagonism in Rats. *Renal Fail.* **2016**, *38* (9), 1462–1467.

23. Valverde, E.; Sureda, F. X. Vázquez, S. Novel Benzopolycyclic Amines with NMDA Receptor Antagonist Activity. *Bioorg. Med. Chem.* **2014**, *22* (9), 2678–2683.

24. Tamborini, L.; Pinto, A.; Mastronardi, F.; Iannuzzi, M. C.; Cullia, G.; Nielsen, B.; De Micheli, C. Conti, P. 3-Carboxy-Pyrazolinalanine as a New Scaffold for Developing Potent and Selective NMDA Receptor Antagonists. *Eur. J. Med. Chem.* **2013**, *68*, 33–37.

25. Li, N.; Liu, R. J.; Dwyer, J. M.; Banasr, M.; Lee, B.; Son, H.; Li, X. Y.; Aghajanian, G. Duman, R. S. Glutamate *N*-Methyl-d-Aspartate Receptor Antagonists Rapidly Reverse Behavioral and Synaptic Deficits Caused by Chronic Stress Exposure. *Biol. Psychiatry* **2011**, *69* (8), 754–761.

26. Hedegaard, M.; Hansen, K. B.; Andersen, K. T.; Bräuner-Osborne, H. Traynelis, S. F. Molecular Pharmacology of Human NMDA Receptors. *Neurochem. Int.* **2012**, *61* (4), 601–609.

27. Yoon, J. S.; Mughal, M. R.; Mattson, M. P. Energy Restriction Negates NMDA Receptor Antagonist Efficacy in Ischemic Stroke. *Neuromol. Med.* **2011**, *13* (3), 175.

28. Torres, E.; Duque, M. D.; López-Querol, M.; Taylor, M. C.; Naesens, L.; Ma, C.; Pinto, L. H.; Sureda, F. X.; Kelly, J. M. Vázquez, S. Synthesis of Benzopolycyclic Cage Amines: NMDA Receptor Antagonist, Trypanocidal and Antiviral Activities. *Bioorg. Med. Chem.* **2012**, *20* (2), 942–948.

29. Anver, H.; Ward, P. D.; Magony, A.; Vreugdenhil, M. NMDA Receptor Hypofunction Phase Couples Independent γ-Oscillations in the Rat Visual Cortex. *Neuropsychopharmacology* **2011**, *36* (2), 519.

30. Banerjee, A.; Schepmann, D.; Köhler, J.; Würthwein E. U.; Wünsch, B. Synthesis and SAR Studies of Chiral Non-Racemic Dexoxadrol Analogues as Uncompetitive NMDA Receptor Antagonists. Bioorg. Med. Chem. **2010**, *18* (22), 7855–7867.

31. Duque, M. D.; Camps, P.; Torres, E.; Valverde, E.; Sureda, F. X.; López-Querol, M.; Camins, A.; Prathalingam, S. R.; Kelly, J. M.; Vázquez, S. New Oxapolycyclic Cage Amines with NMDA Receptor Antagonist and Trypanocidal Activities. *Bioorg. Med. Chem.* **2010**, *18* (1), 46–57.

32. Childers, W. E.; Baudy, R. B. *N*-Methyl-d-Aspartate Antagonists and Neuropathic Pain: The Search for Relief. *J. Med. Chem.* **2007**, *50* (11), 2557–2562.

33. Large, C. H. Do NMDA Receptor Antagonist Models of Schizophrenia Predict the Clinical Efficacy of Antipsychotic Drugs? *J. Psychopharmacol.* **2007**, *21* (3), 283–301.

34. Zarrindast, M.; Jafari-sabet, M.; Rezayat, M.; Djahanguiri, B.; Rezayof, A. Involvement of NMDA Receptors in Morphine State-Dependent Learning in Mice. *Int. J. Neurosci.* **2006**, *116* (6), 731–743.

35. Poschenrieder, H.; Stachel, H. D.; Höfner, G.; Mayer, P. Novel Pyrrolinones as N-Methyl-d-Aspartate Receptor Antagonists. *Eur. J. Med. Chem.* **2005,** *40* (4), 391–400.

36. Lipton, S. A. Failures and Successes of NMDA Receptor Antagonists: Molecular Basis for the Use of Open-Channel Blockers like Memantine in the Treatment of Acute and Chronic Neurologic Insults. *NeuroRx* **2004,** *1* (1), 101–110.

37. Guitton, M.; Puel, J. L. Cochlear NMDA Receptors and Tinnitus. *Audiol. Med.* **2004,** *2* (1), 3–7.

38. Ikonomidou, C.; Turski, L. Why Did NMDA Receptor Antagonists Fail Clinical Trials for Stroke and Traumatic Brain Injury? *Lancet Neurol.* **2002,** *1* (6), 383–386.

39. Sang, C. N. NMDA-Receptor Antagonists in Neuropathic Pain: Experimental Methods to Clinical Trials. *J. Pain Symptom Manage.* **2000,** *19* (1), 21–25.

40. Jirgensons, A.; Kauss, V.; Kalvinsh, I.; Gold, M. R. W. Danysz, C. G. Parsons; Quack, G. Synthesis and Structure–Affinity Relationships of 1,3,5-Alkylsubstituted Cyclohexylamines Binding at NMDA Receptor PCP Site. *Eur. J. Med. Chem.* **1999,** *35* (6), 555–565.

41. Dickenson, A. H. A Cure for Wind Up: NMDA Receptor Antagonists as Potential Analgesics. *Trends Pharmacol. Sci.* **1990,** *11* (8), 307–309.

42. Yu, A.; Lau, A. Y. Glutamate and Glycine Binding to the NMDA Receptor. *Structure* **2018,** *26* (7), 1035–1043.e2.

43. Bledsoe, D.; Tamer, C.; Mesic, I.; Madry, C.; Klein, B. G.; Laube, B.; Costa, B. M. Positive Modulatory Interactions of NMDA Receptor GluN1/2B Ligand Binding Domains Attenuate Antagonists Activity. *Front Pharmacol.* **2017,** *8*, 229.

44. Pereira, N. A.; Sureda, F. X.; Esplugas, R.; Perez, M.; Santos, M. M. Tryptophanol-Derived Oxazolopiperidone Lactams: Identification of a Hit Compound as NMDA Receptor Antagonist. *Bioorg. Med. Chem.* **2014,** *24* (15), 3333–3336.

45. Zarantonello, P. Bettini, E.; Paio, A.; Simoncelli, C.; Terreni, S.; Cardullo, F. Novel Analogues of Ketamine and Phencyclidine as NMDA Receptor Antagonists. *Bioorg. Med. Chem.* **2011,** *21* (7), 2059–2063.

46. Kussius, C. L.; Popescu, A. M.; Popescu, G. K. Agonist-Specific Gating of NMDA Receptors. *Channels* **2009,** *4* (2), 78–82.

47. Ruppa, K. B.; King, D.; Olson, R. E. NMDA Antagonists of GluN2B Subtype and Modulators of GluN2A, GluN2C, and GluN2D Subtypes: Recent Results and Developments. *Annu. Rep. Med. Chem.* **2012,** *47*, 89–102.

CHAPTER 10

RECENT ADVANCES OF BENZIMIDAZOLE DERIVATIVES AS ANTI-HYPERTENSIVE AGENTS

KISHOR R. DANAO* and DEBARSHI KAR MAHAPATRA

Department of Pharmaceutical Chemistry, Dadasaheb Balpande College of Pharmacy, Nagpur 440037, Maharashtra, India

Corresponding author. E-mail: kishordanao1982@gmail.com

ABSTRACT

Benzimidazole (BZI) is an important pharmacophore privileged structure in medicinal chemistry. It is a heterocyclic aromatic organic compound which plays an important role in medical field owing to diverse pharmacological activities such as antimicrobial, antiviral, antidiabetic, antihypertensive, antiulcer, analgesic, antifungal, and anticancer activity. Hypertension is the chronic medical condition which is mainly responsible for cardiovascular diseases today. Targeting the AT1 receptors of Angiotensin-II with nonpeptide-based drugs which are otherwise called angiotensin receptor blockers (ARBs), led to the control of hypertension. The current chapter indicated the progress of BZI in exhibiting antihypertensive activity.

10.1 INTRODUCTION

The use of benzimidazole (BZI) dates many years back. It is a hetero-cyclic aromatic organic compound comprising of a bicycle with the fusion of benzene and imidazole.[1] It is an important pharmacophore and a privileged structure in medicinal chemistry which is known to play a very important role with plenty of useful therapeutic activities such as antiulcer, antihypertensive, analgesic, anti-inflammatory, antiviral, antifungals, anticancer, antibacterial, and anthelmintic.[2] Historically, the first BZI was prepared in 1872 by Hoebrecker, who obtained 2,5(or 2,6)-dimethyl BZI by the reduction of 2-nitro-4methylacetanilide.[3] BZI possesses numerous pharmacological activities out of many N-ribosyl-dimethyl BZI is a most prominent derivative which serve as an axial ligand for cobalt in vitamin B_{12}.[4] The heterocycle expresses a wide variety of pharmacological activities and is prominently seen in marketed drug formulations such as albendazole, omeprazole, astemizole, telmisartan, and so on[5] (Fig. 10.1).

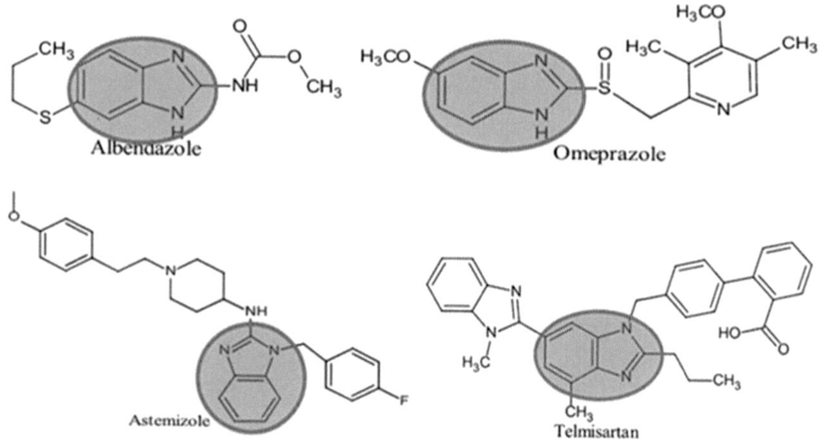

FIGURE 10.1 Benzimidazole scaffold in marketed products.

10.2 SYNTHESIS AND CHARACTERIZATION OF BENZIMIDAZOLES

The synthesis of BZI-based polyheterocycles draws the attention of pharmacists from last few decades as it functions as an important pharmacophore in medicinal chemistry and pharmacology.[6] It is produced traditionally by the condensation of ortho-phenylenediamine and formic acid or trimethyl orthoformate.[7] However, with the time-bound progress, several novel one-pot synthesis methods are reported. Some of the methods include heteroaromatic 2-nitroamines into bicyclic *2H*- BZIs by employing formic acid, iron powder, and NH_4Cl as additive; reaction of o-nitroanilines and alcohols in the presence of sodium sulfide and iron(III) chloride hexahydrate; NaH mediated reaction of carbonitriles and N-methyl-1,2-phenylenediamine; Ir-catalyzed annulation of imidamides with sulfonyl azides; copper-catalyzed multicomponent reaction of 2-haloanilines, aldehydes, and NaN_3; and so on.[8–10]

The molecule can be characterized predominantly by the spectroscopic techniques. The UV–Vis spectra of BZI present λ_{max} of 280 nm (ethanol), 274 nm (0.01 N HCl), and 277 nm (0.01 N NaOH). The marked shifts in the position and intensity of the absorption spectra are because of the difference in electron distribution between the charged and uncharged ions. The infrared spectra of BZI ring system have strong absorption band around 1400–1650 cm^{-1} for –C=N– stretching. It is very difficult to distinguish the C–H stretching vibrations occurring in the range of 3300–3100 cm^{-1} from the broad–NH stretching frequencies around 3300–2800 cm^{-1}. The molecule can be characterized by ^{1}H (proton) and ^{13}C (carbon) nuclear magnetic resonance (NMR). The chemical shifts of BZI have been manifested, at lower field δ 7.71 (C2-H), 7.67 (C4-H), 7.17 (C5-H), 7.24 (C6-H), and 7.32 ppm (C7-H) respectively. The overlapping signals ascribable to aromatic proton and –NH proton have been observed at δ 3.0–8.2 ppm, which are disappeared on D_2O addition. The chemical shift of C4-H and its deviation is because of various substituents to the magnetic anisotropy of the unsaturated nitrogen lone pair, which is removed when protonation occurs. The carbon-NMR presents BZI anion, BZI, and BZI cation in the range 116.41–143.88 ppm, 115.41–141.46 ppm, and 114.44–139.58 ppm, respectively, for the position 2, 4 to 9. The mass spectrum of BZIs exhibits molecular ion peak referred to as a base peak which corresponds with the molecular mass of the compound. It also shows an odd electron-ion m/z 91 (C_6H_5N) by the loss of hydrogen cyanide, which further loose acetylene to lead to another odd electron ion, m/z 65 (C_4H_3N) and not the second molecule of hydrogen cyanide.[11–12]

10.3 BENZIMIDAZOLES AS ANTIHYPERTENSIVES

Cardiovascular diseases are a cause of a significant number of mortalities among deaths reported due to various diseases. One of the most common ailments of the cardiovascular system is hypertension.[13] A patient as per guidelines is said to be hypertensive when blood pressure measures of 140/90 mm Hg (systolic/diastolic pressure). Enhanced blood pressure also involves slow degenerative changes of the vascular system of the body leading to hemorrhage of arteries of vital organs leading to serious fatal consequences.[14] Some of clinical strategies involved in the treatment of hypertension are diuretics, beta adrenergic blockers, aldosterone antagonist, and ACE inhibitors.[15] Imidazole is a planer five-member heterocyclic ring with 3C and 2N atoms in the ring where N is present in 1st and 3rd positions. Imidazole derivatives have occupied a unique place in the field of medicinal chemistry.[16] The incorporation of the imidazole nucleus is an important synthetic strategy in drug discovery. A large number of therapeutic agents have been synthesized from imidazole nucleus which has demonstrated considerable potency.[17] The development of BZI as an extension to imidazole has been found to profoundly enhance the pharmacological response.

Kumar et al. studied the antihypertensive potential of BZI derivative where compounds containing the ethyl group at position 2 gave a better result than the 2-phenyl. In the biphenyl ring, a carboxylic group at *ortho* position is necessary for pharmacological activity. The author concluded that substitution of tetrazolyl moiety at 2 position and amine group at the 5 position had the best pharmacological activity was found in the literature.[18]

Srinivasan et al. synthesized quinazoline containing BZI molecules with noteworthy blood pressure reducing potential. The electron-withdrawing and phenyl group at 2 and 7 positions have been found to be imperative for the activity.[19]

Sharma et al. developed a series of biphenyl linked tetrazole containing BZI compounds with active hypotensive perspective. The methoxylated derivative (substitution at 2 position) exhibited the highest activity with no prominent adverse effects.[20]

Datar et al. screened the antihypertensive prospects of amine-containing phenylated BZI compounds where ethyl containing derivative had the highest pressure reducing potential.[21]

Anisimova et al. studied the hypotensive characteristics of the N,N-dimethylethanamine containing BZI compounds. The 1,4-dihydroxymethylbenzene and 1,3-dihydroxymethylbenzene groups containing analogs demonstrated the highest activity.[22]

(1)

(2)

(3)

(4)

(5)

10.4 CONCLUSION

This chapter highlights that the BZI nucleus is a basic part of pharmaco-phore in modern drug discovery. The knowledge gained by various substi-tuted BZIs and heterocycles were found to be an effective antihypertensive agent. They are considered as the representative compound for the future discovery of rationally developed heteroatom containing antihypertensive agent owing to their simple synthetic procedure and easy analysis by UV, IR, NMR, and mass spectroscopy. Finally, it has been concluded that different substituted BZI derivatives have appreciable and selective action against angiotensin II-induced hypertension.

KEYWORDS

- benzimidazole
- scaffold
- heterocycle
- cardiovascular
- antihypertensive

REFERENCES

1. Maiti, B.; Chanda, K. Diversity Oriented Synthesis of Benzimidazole-Based Biheterocyclic Molecules by Combinatorial Approach: A Critical Review. *RSC Adv.* **2016**, *6* (56), 50384–50413.
2. Yadav, G.; Ganguly, S. Structure Activity Relationship (SAR) Study of Benzimidazole Scaffold for Different Biological Activities: A Mini-Review. *Eur. J. Med. Chem.* 2015, *97*, 419–443.
3. Keri, R. S.; Hiremathad, A.; Budagumpi, S.; Nagaraja, B. M. Comprehensive Review in Current Developments of Benzimidazole-Based Medicinal Chemistry. *Chem. Biol. Drug Des.* 2015, *86* (1), 19–65.
4. Rao, G. E.; Babu, P. S.; Koushik, O. S.; Sharmila, R.; Vijayabharathi, M.; Maruthikumar, S.; Prathyusha, R.; Pavankumar, P. A Review on Chemistry of Benzimidazole Nucleus and its Biological Significance. *Int. J. Pharm. Chem. Biol. Sci.* 2016, *6* (2).
5. Wang, M.; Han, X.; Zhou, Z.; New Substituted Benzimidazole Derivatives: A Patent Review (2013–2014). *Expert Opin. Ther. Pat.* 2015, *25* (5), 595–612.
6. Ingle, R. G.; Magar, D. D. Heterocyclic Chemistry of Benzimidazoles and Potential Activities of Derivatives. *Int. J. Drug Res. Technol.* 2017, *1* (1), 7.
7. P Barot, K.; Nikolova, S.; Ivanov, I.; D Ghate, M. Novel Research Strategies of Benzimidazole Derivatives: A Review. *Mini Rev. Med. Chem.* 2013, *13* (10), 1421–1447.
8. Li, J. J. Ed. *Name Reactions in Heterocyclic Chemistry*; John Wiley & Sons, 2004; Vol. 3.
9. Joule, J. A.; Mills, K. *Heterocyclic Chemistry*; John Wiley & Sons, 2008.
10. Katritzky, A. R.; Ramsden, C. A.; Joule, J. A.; Zhdankin, V. V. *Handbook of Heterocyclic Chemistry*; Elsevier, 2010.
11. Banwell, C. N.; McCash, E. M. *Fundamentals of Molecular Spectroscopy* (Vol. 851). McGraw-Hill: New York, 1994.
12. Pavia, D. L.; Lampman, G. M.; Kriz, G. S.; Vyvyan, J. A. *Introduction to Spectroscopy*; Cengage Learning, 2008.
13. Mahapatra, D. K.; Bharti, S. K. *Handbook of Research on Medicinal Chemistry: Innovations and Methodologies*; Apple Academic Press: New Jersey, 2017.

14. Mahapatra, D. K.; Bharti, S. K. Therapeutic Potential of Chalcones as Cardiovascular Agents. *Life Sci.* 2016, *148*, 154–172.
15. Mahapatra, D. K.; Bharti, S. K. *Medicinal Chemistry with Pharmaceutical Product Development*; Apple Academic Press: New Jersey, 2019.
16. Mahapatra, D. K.; Bharti, S. K. *Drug Design*; Tara Publications Private Limited: New Delhi, 2016.
17. Chhajed, S. S.; Upasani, C. D.; Wadher, S. J.; Mahapatra, D. K. *Medicinal Chemistry*; Career Publications Private Limited: Nashik, 2017.
18. Kumar, J. R.; Jawahar, L.; Pathak, D. P. Synthesis of Benzimidazole Derivatives: As Anti-Hypertensive Agents. *J. Chem.* 2006, *3* (4), 278–285.
19. Srinivasan, N.; Balaji, A.; Nagrajan, G.; Suthakaran, R.; Kumar, Y.; Jagdesh, D. *Asian J. Chem.* 2008, *20* (6), 4934–4936.
20. Sharma, M. C.; Kohli, D. V.; Sharma, S.; Sharma, A. D. Synthesis and Antihypertensive Activity of Some New Benzimidazole Derivatives of 4'-(6-Methoxy-2-Substituted-Benzimidazole-1-Ylmethyl)-Biphenyl-2-Carboxylic Acid in the Presences of BF3·OEt2. *Pelagia Res. Libr.* 2010, *1* (1), 104–115.
21. Datar, P. A.; Coutinho, E. C.; Srivastava, S. Comparative Study of 3D-QSAR Techniques on Angiotensin II Receptor (AT1) Antagonists. *Lett Drug Design Disc* 2004, *1*, 115–120.
22. Anisimova, V. A.; Kuz'menko, T. A.; Spasov, A. A.; Bocharova, I. A.; Orobinskaya, T. A. Synthesis and Study of the Hypotensive and Antiarrhythmic Activity of 2, 9-Disubstituted 3-Alkoxycarbonylmidazo [1, 2-a] Benzimidazoles. *Pharm. Chem. J.* 1999, *33* (7), 361–365.

CHAPTER 11

NATURAL AND SYNTHETIC PROP-2-ENE-1-ONE SCAFFOLD BEARING COMPOUNDS AS MOLECULAR ENZYMATIC TARGETS INHIBITORS AGAINST VARIOUS FILARIAL SPECIES

DEBARSHI KAR MAHAPATRA[1*], VIVEK ASATI[2], and SANJAY KUMAR BHARTI[3]

[1]Department of Pharmaceutical Chemistry, Dadasaheb Balpande College of Pharmacy, Nagpur 440037, Maharashtra, India

[2]Department of Pharmaceutical Chemistry, NRI Institute of Pharmacy, Bhopal 462021, Madhya Pradesh, India

[3]Institute of Pharmaceutical Sciences, Guru Ghasidas Vishwavidyalaya (A Central University), Bilaspur 495009, Chhattisgarh, India

*Corresponding author. E-mail: dkmbsp@gmail.com

ABSTRACT

Lymphatic filariasis, often termed as elephantiasis disease which has affected over 140 million people across the world. It spreads primarily through three pathogenic species *Wuchereria bancrofti*, *Brugia malayi*, and *Brugia timori* via vector species *Culex quinquefasciatus*, *Anopheles species*, *Aedes egyptii*, and *Mansonia annulifera/Mansonia uniformis*. The disease is quite common in the tropical regions with larger dominance in the continent of Asia, Africa, and South America. Pharmacotherapeutic through natural products may believe to offer better potency and reduced adverse effects. This chapter comprehensively highlighted vast chalcone (prop-2-ene-1-one) derivatives which modulated various antifilarial molecular targets such as *Setaria cervi* glutathione-S-transferase, *Brugia malayi* thymidylate kinase, and *Setaria cervi* ecto-protein tyrosine phosphatase. The simple C_6-C_3-C_6 system has been seen to significantly eradicate the based infections. The heterocycles (piperidine, pyrrolidine, benzotriazole, benzothiazole, furan, thiazole), electron donating groups, electron withdrawing groups, and sulfonamide moiety fused with the benzylideneacetophenone scaffold have been predominantly observed to inhibit the essential biological targets and thereby causing fatal paralysis to the virulent pathogens with no such adverse effects to the human body. At present, these molecules are at nascent stages and require further studies for the rational development into pharmaceutical products.

11.1 INTRODUCTION

Lymphatic filariasis, often termed as elephantiasis is a neglected tropical disease caused by round, coiled, and thread-like parasitic nematode worms belonging to the family Filariidae.[1] Out of the 100 reported species, only three species *Wuchereria bancrofti*, *Brugia malayi*, and *Brugia timori* have been found to be highly virulent. It is a painful and disfiguring disease which has a major social and economic impact.[2] It is majorly transmitted through mosquito species *Culex quinquefasciatus*, *Anopheles species*, *Aedes egyptii*, and *Mansonia annulifera/Mansonia uniformis*. These microscopic male worms are nearly 3–4 cm in length whereas the female worms are 8–10 cm in length nests in the human lymph, nodes, and vessels that are responsible for maintaining the blood and body fluid balance.[3]

The disease is quite common in the tropical regions with larger dominance in the continent of Asia, Africa, and South America. India, China, Southeast Asian nations are predominantly affected while North American nations are privileged.[4] Although the disease has affected over 140 million people across the world. Short-term to long-term travelers and immigration from endemic regions to several less severe regions have imposed a great threat.[5]. However, it is under continuous monitoring by the Centers for Disease Control and Prevention (CDC).

The lymphatic system is an essential component of the human body's immune system which helps in body fluid maintenance and fights infection.

When the infected mosquito bites a healthy individual, the microfilaria enters the lymphatics and nodes, where they develop into adult forms on the passage of time and in turn produce more microfilaria which worsens the condition.[6] When a new mosquito bites and sucks blood from the diseased state, the microfilaria present in the peripheral blood reaches the vector and on the further bite, it transmits the microfilaria in the next individual, there initiates the transmission cycle.[7] The active microfilaria circulates in the night and the blood samples through microscopic and serologic studies aids in the detection. It is a self-limiting disease until and unless reinfection occurs.[8]

Under asymptomatic conditions, subclinical manifestations such as proteinuria, haematuria, kidney damage, abnormally high levels of certain white blood cells (eosinophilia), lymphatic damage (lymphangitis), and so on are well known.[9] In early stages, it is usually characterized by high fever, headache, chills, skin lesions, extreme pain, and so on. With the progress in the disease, under lymphedema (swollen limbs), abnormally enlarged lymphatic vessels (varices), elephantiasis (swelling in legs), hydrocele (swelling in scrotum), swelling of the testes (orchitis), sperm ducts (epididymitis), sperm track (funiculitis), chronic lymph node swelling (lymphadenopathy), presence of lymphatic fluid in the urine (chyluria), lower extremities (legs below the knees), breast, vulva, abnormally thickening in skin, warty appearance, and so on are primarily affected.[10–11] It is chiefly a social stigma and the community often avoids and rejects the affected individuals, which distress their social life, workplace, and their family.

The nonpharmacological approach toward the management of this disease involves good hygiene along with physiotherapy to improve the flow of lymph. Pharmacological agents such as albendazole (400 mg), ivermectin (150–200 µg/kg), and diethylcarbamazine (6 mg/kg) finds application for the disease management.[12] These agents selectively work to kill the pathogen or inhibit their further reproductive process. Though, considerable side effects and adverse effects are seen in dominance on commencement of the therapy.[13] Accumulation of the dead worms in the bloodstream or lymph content drastically provokes abscesses and allergic reactions, therefore anti-inflammatory and antihistaminic classes of drugs are concurrently administered.[14] The treatment of lower extremities entails elevating and supporting through elastic stocking. Surgical approaches are employed in individuals to drain the fluid, adult worms, and developed calcifications when an excessive amount of fluid gets accumulated in the scrotum.[15]

11.2　DRUG DISCOVERY, DESIGN, AND DEVELOPMENT

The process of drug discovery and development is a long journey. It took several years to develop a fully functional product. The rational antifilarial drug design is a continuous process which has given this mankind several useful moieties such as diethylcarbamazine, ivermectin, albendazole, and so on along with their severe complications. Scientists have been working rigorously toward the enhancement of potency and a significant reduction in the adverse effects, though, nothing much has been achieved till date.[16]

Philosophers say Mother Nature has all the solution for every treacherous event which affects the mankind. About 75% of the drugs in market bear scaffold procured from nature or its analog is been utilized after suitable modifications. The acceptance of natural, herbal, nutraceutical, and plant-derived products among the masses over the centuries have made a subject of enormous concern. Likewise, through inspiration, numerous researchers are working on exploring the potential of unexplored classes of natural compounds with an immense pace. Natural products of flavonoid, flavonone, flavanol, isoflavone, chalcone, proanthocyanidin, anthocyanidin, and so on have been perceived to be emerging candidates for the future pharmacotherapeutics in the eradication of filariasis with less adverse effects.[17]

11.3　THERAPEUTIC TARGETS FOR ANTIFILARIAL ACTIVITY

For the development of any pharmacological product through the rigorous process of drug discovery, the knowledge of drug targets is very essential. The modern concept of structure-based drug design (SBDD) approach in the rational discovery of ligands bears complete information of the biological targets such as an enzyme, receptor, channel, and so on.[18] In a similar manner, the antifilarial drug development lies completely with the knowledge of the pathogens' biomolecular component(s). Basically, three molecular targets have been well known for the discovery of new therapeutically active molecules; glutathione-S-transferase, thymidylate kinase, and ecto-protein tyrosine phosphatase.

Glutathione-*S*-transferase (GST) is a ubiquitous enzyme that plays vital role in xenobiotic modification in the *Setaria cervi*, a zoonotic filarial species thereby offering resistance of high magnitude toward the incoming drug molecules. It catalyzes the nucleophilic conjugation of glutathione with electrophilic substrates to produce less reactive chemical species. The reduced form of the enzyme (GSH) interacts with the carboxylated drug to form active thiol esters and hydrolyzed further by GST to form inactive detoxified components. Inhibition of this target (GSH/GST system) will prevent detoxification of reactive intermediates produced from the active drug molecule, considerably decrease the cellular resistance, and will eventually lead to the death of pathogen.[19]

Brugia malayi thymidylate kinase (TK) is a ubiquitous enzyme located at the junction of *de novo* and salvage pathway of DNA synthesis in the pathogen. This enzyme play imperative role in the synthesis of pyrimidine that catalyzes thymidine-5′-monophosphate (dTMP) phosphorylation into thymidine-5′-diphosphate (dTDP) in the presence of adenosine triphosphate (ATP) and magnesium ion. This enzyme facilitates cellular proliferation and growth of the organism. Inhibition of this molecular target will hinder cellular growth and development and will ultimately lead to the death of the pathogen.[20]

The ecto-protein tyrosine phosphatase (PTP) of *Setaria cervi* is a crucial signal transduction enzyme located over the surface of several parasites which is responsible for the pathogenic nutritional uptake, signal transduction, disruption of the host actin filament, cellular differentiation, cellular adhesion, sensing of reacting oxygen species, cellular growth, and so on. Therefore, inhibition of this enzyme will lead to an acute reduction in the virulence.[21]

Therefore, inhibition of these molecular targets will produce complete reduction of pathogenic virulence, drastically reduces the drug resistance, prevent DNA formation, detoxify xenobiotics (drug), restricts cellular proliferation, and finally leads to death.

11.4 CHALCONE

Chalcone, also called benzylideneacetophenone having 1,3-diphenyl-2-propene-1-one scaffold (two aromatic nuclei are joined by a three-carbon α, β unsaturated carbonyl bridge) are the class of natural chromophoric compounds with multiple pharmacological activities such as antimicrobial, antifungal, antitubercular, antimalarial, antiretroviral, antileishmanial, antitrypanosomal, antiprotozal, anti-inflammatory, antinociceptive, antigout, anti-ulcer, antidiabetic, antihyperlipidemic, antihypertensive, antiplatelet, anti-obesity, antineoplastic, antimetastatic, anti-invasive, immunosuppressive, antioxidant, anti-fibrinogenic, anxiolytic, hypnotic, osteogenic, antihistaminic, and so on. It is known as an inhibitor of quinone reductase, xanthine oxidase, epoxide hydroxylase, tyrosine kinase, P-glycoprotein, p53 level, and produce antagonism of LTD_4. Nonpharmacological applications involve polymerization catalyst, scintillator, organic brightening agent, fluorescent whitening agent, artificial sweetener, insecticide, fluorescent polymers, and Fe(III) determination.[22–28]

They are the open chain intermediates in the aurones synthesis, precursors of flavonoids, and isoflavonoids. Chalcones and flavonoids are isomeric in nature and readily undergo interconversion in the presence of acids to form chalcone or bases to form flavonone formation.[29] The term "chalcone" was coined by Kostanecki and Tambor who first synthesized the product. Traditionally, the compounds are synthesized in the chemical laboratories by exploiting Claisen–Schmidt reaction where a condensation between benzaldehyde and acetophenone was performed by employing base (sodium/potassium hydroxide) as catalyst in 40% solution. Newer methods include irradiation with domestic microwave for the duration of 150–300 seconds employing the same chemicals.[30] They also act as Michael acceptors in Michael addition reactions. In the 21st century, chalcones have received adequate attention due to the simple structure, simple steps for the synthesis of diversely substituted analogs, a large number of hydrogen replacement domains, a vast opportunity for computational studies, and so on.[31] The benzylideneacetophenone scaffold serves as a template for the structural elucidation of flavonoid, coumarin, flavanone, and so on. Chalcones are also known to an ideal template for the synthesis of diverse heterocyclic compounds such as benzodiazepine, benzoxazepine, benzothiazepine, pyrazole, isoxazole, thiadiazole, pyrimidine, pyrazoline, and so on.[32]

11.5 CHALCONE (PROP-2-ENE-1-ONE) SCAFFOLD BEARING ANTIFILARIAL AGENTS

Awasthi et al. evaluated the filaricidal potential of chalcone-based molecules by their potential in inhibiting the *S. cervi* GST. Three analogs; 3-(4-chlorophenyl)-1-(4-piperidin-1-yl-phenyl)prop-2-en-1-one **(1)**, 1-(4-benzotriazol-1-yl-phenyl)-3-(4-methoxyphenyl)prop-2-en-1-one **(2)**, and 3-(4-methoxyphenyl)-1-(4-pyrrolidin-1-yl-phenyl)prop-2-en-1-one **(3)** were found to exhibit noteworthy *in vitro* inhibition of the detoxifying enzyme with IC_{50} values of 3 μM which lead to irreversible effect on viability and resulted in the death of adult parasite (Fig. 11.1).[33]

In a study, the compound **(3)** has been observed to produce a remarkable reduction of GSH, PTP, and PGHS levels along with a marked increase in the NO levels. A significant alteration in the proteomic expression and cytotoxic effect (irreversible inhibition in motility and viability) at 100 μM concentration has been detected. The inhibition of detoxification enzyme by the chalcone made the drug vulnerable to the parasite.[34]

In a similar screening, the PTP inhibitory perspective of compound **(3)** has been studied by Singh et al. where it was noticed that the molecule completely paralyzed the adult parasites by inhibiting the virulent enzyme with Km and Vmax of 2.574 μM and 206.3 μM Pi/h/two parasites, respectively. Against the microfilaria, the inhibition of the tyrosine phosphatase produced fatal death with Km and Vmax of 5.510 μM and 62.27 μM Pi/h/two parasites, respectively. Therefore, the biological target inhibition will produce an acute reduction of filarial infections.[35]

Sulfonamide chalcones have been recognized as potential antifilarial agents against *Brugia malayi*. The three derivatives **(4–6)** expressed IC_{50} values of < 5 μM by the inhibition of folate pathway which produced defects in the normal DNA formation in the pathogens. Authors concluded that lipophilic methyl moiety at the *para* position of terminal phenyl rings **(6)** presented the best filaricidal activity.[36] The compound **(6)** displayed anti-inflammatory activity along with antifilarial activity. The molecule increased the level of regulatory cytokines, IL-10 and TGF-β gene expression and also down regulated the TNF-α, IFN-γ, and iNOS in mice peritoneal exudate cells.[37]

Sashidhara et al. reported the *in vitro* antifilarial potential of novel chalcone-thiazole compounds against *B. malayi* microfilariae as well as adult worms, which provided a structural clue for the development of pharmacologically active heterocyclic hybrid. Two compounds (7–8) presented the highest promising activity. Compound (8) exhibited complete embryostatic effect and nearly half macrofilaricidal in B. malayi-jird (*Meriones unguiculatus*) and B. malayi- *Mastomys coucha* models.[38]

B. malayi TK inhibitors have been identified by Sashidhara and coworkers through *in vitro* validation and *in silico* docking techniques (MolDock docking model). The developed novel chalcone-benzothiazole hybrids (9–10) have been found to express notable antifilarial activities as distinguish from the IC_{50} values of 4.34 µM and 2.12 µM, respectively. The docking studies revealed that the most potent compound (10) radically bind with the pathogenic TK (−530 Kcal/mol) through His-70, Arg-77, Arg-98, Gly-103, and Thr-107, sparing the functional analog in human (−370 Kcal/mol) through Arg-76 and Gly-102.[39]

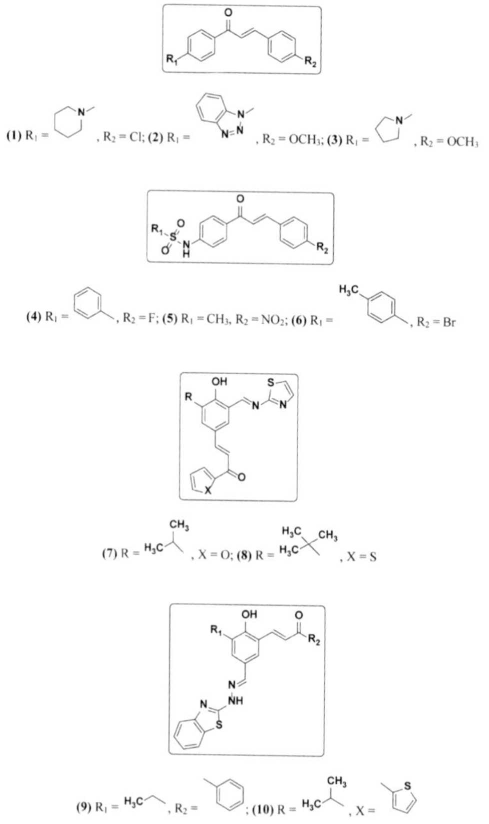

FIGURE 11.1   Chalcone-based antifilarial compounds.

11.6 CONCLUSION

The chapter highlighted vast chalcone (prop-2-ene-1-one) derivatives which modulated various antifilarial molecular targets such as *Setaria cervi* glutathione-S-transferase, *Brugia malayi* thymidylate kinase, and *Setaria cervi* ecto-protein tyrosine phosphatase. The simple C_6-C_3-C_6 system has been seen to significantly eradicate the based infections. The heterocycles (piperidine, pyrrolidine, benzotriazole, benzothiazole, furan, thiazole), electron donating groups, electron withdrawing groups, and sulfonamide moiety fused with the benzylideneacetophenone scaffold have been predominantly observed to inhibit the essential biological targets and thereby causing fatal paralysis to the virulent pathogens with no such adverse effects to the human body. At present, these molecules are at nascent stages and require further studies for the rational development into pharmaceutical products.

KEYWORDS

- chalcone
- anti-infective
- filariasis
- parasite
- inhibitor
- molecular targets

REFERENCES

1. Ramaiah, K. D.; Das, P. K.; Michael, E.; Guyatt, H. L. The economic burden of lymphatic filariasis in India. *Parasitol. Today* **2000,** *16* (6), 251–253.
2. Kumaraswami, V. The Clinical Manifestations of Lymphatic Filariasis. In *Lymphatic filariasis*; 2000, pp 103–125.
3. Ottesen, E. A. The Global Programme to Eliminate Lymphatic Filariasis. *Trop. Med. Int. Health* **2000,** *5* (9), 591–594.
4. Ottesen, E. A. The Welcome Trust Lecture: Infection and disease in Lymphatic Filariasis: An Immunological Perspective. *Parasitology* **1992,** *104* (S1), S71–S79.
5. Molyneux, D. H.; Zagaria, N. Lymphatic Filariasis Elimination: Progress in Global Programme Development. *Ann. Trop. Med. Parasitol.* **2002,** *96*, S15–S40.

6. Colledge, N. R.; Walker, B. R.; Ralston, S. H. *Davidson's Principles and Practice of Medicine*; Elsevier Ltd.: Amsterdam, 2010.

7. Lemke, T. L.; Williams, D. A. *Foye's Principles of Medicinal Chemistry*; Lippincott Williams & Wilkins: Philadelphia, 2012.

8. Beale, J. M.; Block, J. H. *Wilson and Gisvold's Textbook of Organic Medicinal and Pharmaceutical Chemistry*; Lippincott Williams & Wilkins: Philadelphia, 2011.

9. Craig, C. R.; Stitzel, R. E. *Modern Pharmacology with Clinical Applications*; Lippincott Williams & Wilkins: Philadelphia, 2004.

10. Taylor, M. J.; Hoerauf, A.; Bockarie, M. Lymphatic Filariasis and Onchocerciasis. *Lancet* **2010,** *376* (9747), 1175–1185.

11. Ottesen, E. A. Immunopathology of Lymphatic Filariasis in Man. *Springer Sem. Immunopathol.* **1980,** *2* (4), 373–385.

12. Brunton, L.; Parker, K.; Blumenthal, D.; Buxton, I. *Goodman & Gilman's Manual of Pharmacology and Therapeutics*; The McGraw-Hill: New York, 2008.

13. Katzung, B. G.; Masters, S. B.; Trevor, A. J. *Katzung's Basic and Clinical Pharmacology*; McGraw-Hill Education: New York, 2012.

14. Golan, D. E. *Principles of Pharmacology: The Pathophysiologic Basis of Drug Therapy*. Lippincott Williams & Wilkins: Philadelphia, 2008.

15. Ottesen, E. A.; Duke, B. O.; Karam, M.; Behbehani, K. Strategies and Tools for the Control/Elimination of Lymphatic Filariasis. *Bulletin World Health Organ.* **1997,** *75* (6), 491.

16. Mahapatra, D. K.; Bharti, S. K. *Drug Design*; Tara Publications Private Limited: New Delhi, 2016.

17. Mahapatra, D. K.; Bharti, S. K. Eds. *Handbook of Research on Medicinal Chemistry: Innovations and Methodologies*. Apple Academic Press: New Jersey, 2017.

18. Chhajed, S. S; Upasani, C. D; Wadher, S. J; Mahapatra, D. K. *Medicinal Chemistry*. Career Publications Private Limited: Nashik, 2017.

19. Strange, R. C.; Spiteri, M. A.; Ramachandran, S.; Fryer, A. A. Glutathione-S-Transferase Family of Enzymes. *Mutat. Res./Fundam. Mol. Mech. Mutagen.* **2001,** *482* (1), 21–26.

20. Doharey, P. K.; Suthar, M. K.; Verma, A.; Kumar, V.; Yadav, S.; Balaramnavar, V. M.; Rathaur, S.; Saxena, A. K.; Siddiqi, M. I.; Saxena, J. K. Molecular Cloning and Characterization of Brugia Malayi Thymidylate Kinase. *Acta Tropica* **2014,** *133*, 83–92.

21. Andreeva, A. V.; Kutuzov, M. A. Protozoan Protein Tyrosine Phosphatases. *Int. J. Parasitol.* **2008,** *38* (11), 1279–1295.

22. Mahapatra, D. K.; Bharti, S. K.; Asati, V. Anti-Cancer Chalcones: Structural and Molecular Target Perspectives. *Eur. J. Med. Chem.* **2015,** *98*, 69–114.

23. Mahapatra, D. K.; Bharti, S. K.; Asati, V.. Chalcne Scaffolds as Anti-Infective Agents: Structural and Molecular Target Perspectives. *Eur. J. Med. Chem.* **2015,** *101*, 496–524.

24. Mahapatra, D. K.; Asati, V.; Bharti, S. K. Chalcones and their Therapeutic Targets for the Management of Diabetes: Structural and Pharmacological Perspectives. *Eur. J. Med. Chem.* **2015,** *92*, 839–865.

25. Mahapatra, D. K.; Bharti, S. K.; Asati, V. Chalcone Derivatives: Anti-Inflammatory Potential and Molecular Targets Perspectives. *Curr. Top. Med. Chem.* **2017**, *17* (28), 3146–3169.

26. Mahapatra, D. K.; Bharti, S. K. Therapeutic Potential of Chalcones as Cardiovascular Agents. *Life Sci.* **2016**, *148*, 154–172.

27. Mahapatra, D. K.; Bharti, S. K.; Asati V. Recent Perspectives of Chalcone Based Molecules as Protein Tyrosine Phosphatase 1B (PTP-1B) Inhibitors. In *Medicinal Chemistry with Pharmaceutical Product Development*; Mahapatra, D. K., Bharti, S. K., Eds.; Apple Academic Press: New Jersey, 2019.

28. Mahapatra, D. K.; Bharti, S. K.; Asati V. Perspectives of Chalcone Based NFκβ Inhibitors as Anti-Inflammatory Agents. In *Pharmacological Perspectives of Low Molecular Weight Ligands*; Mahapatra, D. K., Bharti, S. K., Eds.; Apple Academic Press: New Jersey, 2019.

29. Sahu, N. K.; S. Balbhadra, S.; Choudhary, J.; V. Kohli, D. Exploring Pharmacological Significance of Chalcone Scaffold: A Review. *Curr. Med. Chem.* **2012**, *19* (2), 209–225.

30. Singh, P.; Anand, A.; Kumar, V. Recent Developments in Biological Activities of Chalcones: A Mini Review. *Eur. J. Med. Chem.* **2014**, *85*, 758–777.

31. Zhuang, C.; Zhang, W.; Sheng, C.; Zhang, W.; Xing, C.; Miao, Z. Chalcone: A Privileged Structure in Medicinal Chemistry. *Chem. Rev.* **2017**, *117* (12), 7762–7810.

32. Matos, M. J.; Vazquez-Rodriguez, S.; Uriarte, E.; Santana, L. Potential Pharmacological uses of Chalcones: A Patent Review (from June 2011–2014). *Expert Opin. Ther. Pat.* **2015**, *25* (3), 351–366.

33. Awasthi, S. K.; Mishra, N.; Dixit, S. K.; Singh, A.; Yadav, M.; Yadav, S. S.; Rathaur, S. Antifilarial Activity of 1, 3-Diarylpropen-1-One: Effect on Glutathione-S-Transferase, a Phase II Detoxification Enzyme. *Am. J. Trop. Med. Hyg.* **2009**, *80* (5), 764–768.

34. Rathaur, S.; Yadav, M.; Singh, N.; Singh, A. Effect of Diethylcarbamazine, Butylated Hydroxy Anisole and Methyl Substituted Chalcone on Filarial Parasite Setaria cervi: Proteomic and Biochemical Approaches. *J. Proteom.* **2011**, *74* (9), 1595–1606.

35. Singh, N.; Heneberg, P.; Rathaur, S. Presence of Ecto-Protein Tyrosine Phosphatase Activity is Vital for Survival of Setaria Cervi, a Bovine Filarial Parasite. *Parasitol. Res* **2014**, *113* (10), 3581–3589.

36. Bahekar, S. P.; Hande, S. V.; Agrawal, N. R.; Chandak, H. S.; Bhoj, P. S.; Goswami, K.; Reddy, M. V. R. Sulfonamide Chalcones: Synthesis and In Vitro Exploration for Therapeutic Potential against Brugia malayi. *Eur. J. Med. Chem.* **2016**, *124*, 262–269.

37. Bhoj, P.; Togre, N.; Bahekar, S.; Goswami, K.; Chandak, H.; Patil, M. Immunomodulatory Activity of Sulfonamide Chalcone Compounds in Mice Infected with Filarial Parasite, Brugia malayi. *Indian J. Clin. Biochem.* **2018**, 1–5.

38. Sashidhara, K. V.; Rao, K. B.; Kushwaha, V.; Modukuri, R. K.; Verma, R.; Murthy, P. K. Synthesis and Antifilarial Activity of Chalcone–Thiazole Derivatives against a Human Lymphatic Filarial Parasite, Brugia malayi. *Eur. J. Med. Chem.* **2014**, *81*, 473–480.

39. Sashidhara, K. V.; Avula, S. R.; Doharey, P. K.; Singh, L. R.; Balaramnavar, V. M.; Gupta, J.; Misra-Bhattacharya, S.; Rathaur, S.; Saxena, A. K.; Saxena, J. K. Designing, Synthesis of Selective and High-Affinity Chalcone-Benzothiazole Hybrids as Brugia Malayi Thymidylate Kinase Inhibitors: In vitro Validation and Docking Studies. *Eur. J. Med. Chem.* **2015**, *103*, 418–428.

CHAPTER 12

DNA: AN IMPORTANT COMPONENT OF LIFE

ANAMIKA SINGH[1] and RAJEEV SINGH[2*]

[1]Department of Botany, Maitreyi College, University of Delhi, New Delhi

[2]Department of Environmental studies, Satyawati College, University of Delhi, New Delhi

[*]Corresponding author. E-mail: 10rsingh@gmail.com

ABSTRACT

Nucleic acids are the basic molecules of life and it is an important mark of a living cells. It can produce exact replicas of them and that's why they maintain continuity of life. Small gene is present on chromosomes and these genes are made up of nucleic acids. These nucleic acids are found to be major components and are present on chromosomes. Nucleic acids have coded information and instructions which is used for making a complete organism. Elemental analysis of nucleic acids showed the presence of phosphorus, along with C, H, N, and O. Nucleic acid is actually a polymer made up of monomer units are nucleotides. Living cells have two types of nucleic acids: deoxyribonucleic acid (DNA) and ribonucleic acid (RNA). DNA helps in transfer of genetic characteristics from parent to child and it is found in nucleus of the cell. RNA is present in all part of the cell and it's mainly functions in cellular protein synthesis. The nucleic acids (DNA and RNA) are considered as the "molecules of heredity."

12.1   INTRODUCTION

Friedrich Miescher (1844–1895) was a student of eminent German chemist, Felix Hoppe-Seyler. He purified nuclein and all proteins were completely removed; later it was clear that the genetic material was an acid and referred to as nucleic acid. Deoxyribonucleic acid (DNA) and ribonucleic acid (RNA) are mainly composed of nucleic acid and it has components like nitrogenous bases, sugar moiety, and phosphorus acid.

1. **Nitrogenous Bases:** They are organic compounds (carbon based) having nitrogen containing ring structure. Nitrogenous bases are derived from purine and pyrimidines.

    a. **Purines:** They are heterocyclic compounds that contain pyrimidines ring and an imidazole ring fused together. The two purine bases are adenine and guanine and both are found in DNA (Table 12.1). Guanine was first isolated from guano bird that is why it is named guanine.

    b. **Pyrimidines:** Pyrimidine bases consist of six membered rings with two nitrogen atoms. The pyrimidine bases are cytosine, thymine, and uracil. Thymine is found in DNA while cytosine is found in both RNA and DNA. Uracil is found in only RNA. Sometimes tRNA will contain some thymine as well as uracil (Table 12.2).

Conformation of pyrimidine is planar while purine is puckered. Cytosine, thymine, uracil, guanine, and adenine are more soluble because they have many polar groups that are available for hydrogen bonding. Due to the presence of aroma, ring pyrimidines and purines can all absorb UV light and that is the reason we can easily measure DNA and RNA concentration in a sample.

2. **Sugar Moiety:** In nucleic acid two tyes of sugars are found and both are pentose sugar found in DNA and RNA. It is present in their close five number ring "β-furanose" from and of β-configuration. These two sugars are **deoxyribose** and ribose. Five-carbon pentose sugar in DNA is called **deoxyribose**, while in RNA, the sugar is **ribose**. These two are very similar in structure with only one difference the second carbon of deoxyribose has hydrogen

TABLE 12.1 Chemical Structure and Details of Purines.

Name	Formula	Chemical name	Nature	Molecular weight	Melting point	Structure
Adenine (A)	C5H5N5	6-Amino Purine	White crystalline purine base	135.13 g/mol	360–365°C	
Guanine (G)	C5H5ON5	2-Amino-6-oxyPurine	Colorless, insoluble crystalline substance	151.129 g/mol	360°C	

TABLE 12.2   Chemical Structure and Details of Pyrimidines.

Name	Formula	Chemical name	Nature	Molecular weight	Melting point	Structure
Cytosine (C)	C5H6O2N5	2-Oxy-4-amino pyrimidine	White crystalline	111.1 g/mol	320–325°C	
Thymine (T)	C5H6O2N2	2,4-dioxy-5-methyl pyrimidine	White crystalline	126.13 g/mol	316–317°C	
Uracil (U)	C4H4O2N2	2,4-dioxy pyrimidine	White crystalline	112.10 g/mol	338°C	

while in ribose hydroxyl group is present. The carbon atoms of a nucleotide's sugar molecule are numbered as 1′, 2′, 3′, 4′, and 5′ (1′ is read as "one prime") shown in the figure. In a nucleotide, the sugar occupies a central position, with the base attached to its 1′ carbon and the phosphate group (or groups) attached to its 5′ carbon (Fig. 12.1).

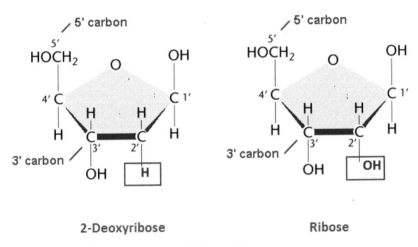

2-Deoxyribose   Ribose

FIGURE 12.1   Showing structure of DNA and RNA sugar.

3. **Phosphate:** Next important component is phosphate (Fig. 12.2). In a nucleotide, single or upto chain of three phosphate groups are attached to the 5′ carbon of the sugar. This complete structure is now called as nucleotide. When the nucleotide joins the growing DNA or RNA chain, it loses two phosphate groups.

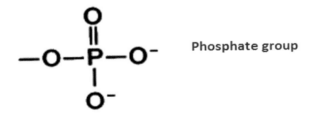

Phosphate group

FIGURE 12.2   Showing phosphate structure.

So, in a chain of DNA or RNA, each nucleotide has just one phosphate group. Monovalent hydroxyl groups and one divalent oxygen atom all are linked to pentavalent phosphorous atom. The base is joined covalently (at N1 of pyrimidines and N9 of purines) and the phosphate is esterified to the 5′-carbon. The N-glycosyl bond is formed by removal of the elements of water (a hydroxyl group from pentose and hydrogen atom from the base).

Nucleosides: These are the structures formed by covalent addition of ribose or 2-deoxyribose sugar to a nitrogenous base (A, T, G, C) is called as nucleoside. Carbon number 1 of the sugar is attached to nitrogen 9 of a purine base or to nitrogen 1 of a pyrimidine base forming beta-N glycosydic bond. The names of purine nucleosides end in -osine and the names of pyrimidine nucleosides end in -idine. For example, adenosine, guanosine, thymidine, and cytidine (Fig. 12.3).

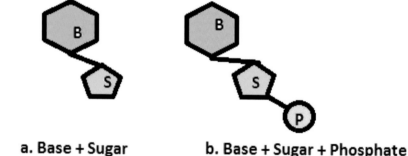

a. Base + Sugar   **b. Base + Sugar + Phosphate**

FIGURE 12.3   Showing (a) nucleosides and (b) nucleiotides structure.

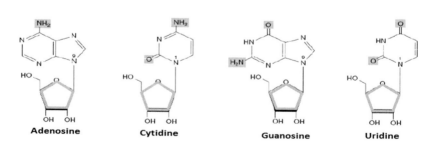

FIGURE 12.4   Showing different nucleosides.

Nucleotides: It is formed by joining phosphoric acid to a nucleoside at the C5′ or the C3′. The phosphate bonds with ester linkage to carbon 5′ of the sugar. If more than one phosphate is present, then they form acid anhydride linkages to each other. For example 3′–5′ cAMP indicates that a phosphate is in ester linkage to both the 3′ and 5′ hydroxyl groups of an adenosine molecule and forms a cyclic structure (Fig. 12.5). Adenosine monophosphate (AMP), cytidine diphosphate (CDP), deoxy guanosine triphosphate (dGTP), cyclic adenosine monophosphate (3′–5′ cAMP), and deoxy thymidine triphosphate (dTTP) are few nucleotides.

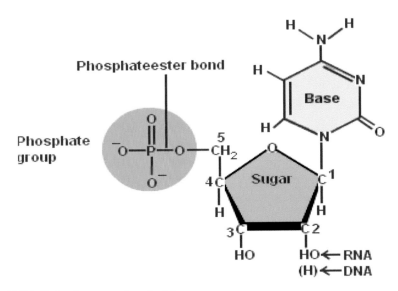

FIGURE 12.5   Structure of nucleotide.

Few nucleotides join together and form a chain of nucleotides called as polynucleotide chain. This structure is directional and having two ends and both the ends are different to each other. Starting point is 5′ end and the 5′ phosphate group of the first nucleotide in point lies sticks out. At the other end, called the 3′ end, the 3′ hydroxyl of the last nucleotide is exposed at the end. DNA sequences are usually written in the 5′ to 3′ direction; it shows that nucleotide at the 5′ end comes first and the nucleotide at the 3′ end comes last. As new nucleotides are added to a preexisted strand of DNA or RNA and the strand grow at its 3′ end, with the 5′ phosphate of an incoming nucleotide attaching to the hydroxyl group at the 3′ end of the chain. This makes a chain with each sugar joined to its neighbors by a set of bonds called a phosphodiester linkage (Fig. 12.5). Phosphodiester linkages 3' OH of the (deoxy) ribose of one nucleotide is linked to the 5' OH of the (deoxy) ribose of the next nucleotide via a phosphate. The phosphate is in an ester linkage to each hydroxyl, that is, a phosphodiester group links two nucleotides.

Nucleic Acid Types:
Nucleic acids are macromolecules formed by smaller units known as nucleotides. In nature two types of nucleiotides are present **DNA** and **RNA**. DNA is the most common genetic material found in living organisms from single-celled organism to multicellular mammals. RNA is genetic material of some viruses but never DNA and RNA both. DNA is found mainly in the chromatin of the cell nucleus while RNtoplasm (90%) and very small in nucleous (10%). In the below section we will study DNA and RNA in detail.

DNA: Nucleus is the place where DNA is found both in plants and animals (eukaryotes). In case of bacteria cell like prokaryotes DNA is found in the form of nucleoid. In eukaryotes, DNA is long, linear pieces called chromosomes while in prokaryotes it is circular (ring shaped) in nature. A chromosome may contain tens of thousands of genes, each providing instructions on how to make a particular product needed by the cell.

DNA is found in every living cell in an organism and it can form exact copies (except for the gametes). Two helically intertwined backbones made up of alternating phosphate and deoxyribose (sugar) molecules supporting internal base pairs adenine (A) paired with thymine (T) cytosine (C) paired with guanine (G) (Fig. 12.6). DNA is found in two different helix form right handed and left handed. On the basis of this DNA are of three forms: A, B, and Z form. Right handed helix and most common form found in all living cells is known as B form DNA.

Watson and Crick Model: Watson and Crick proposed a model of DNA structure. It provides a support and explanation for the Chargaff's base composition data. In the Watson and Crick model two right-handed helical polynucleotide chains forms a double helix around a central axis. The two strands are antiparallel, means their 3'–5' phosphodiester links are in opposite directions. The bases are stacked inside the helix in a plane perpendicular to the helical axis. These two strands are held together by hydrogen bonds formed between the pairs of bases. Adenine (A) and

Thymine (T) are connected together by two hydrogen bonds while Cytosine (C) and Guanine (G) by three hydrogen bonds.

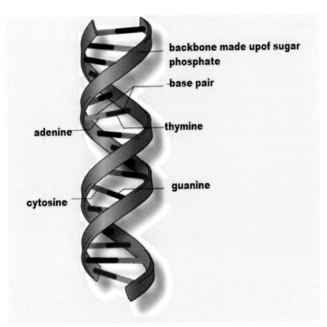

FIGURE 12.6   Structure of double helical DNA.

Hydrophobic interactions are the second bond type formed between the stacked bases and help to maintain the double helical structure of DNA. As per this model, the distance between the stacked bases is 3.4 Å (0.34 nm), a turn of the double helix is completed in 34 Å (3.4 nm), a length that corresponds to 10 nucleotide residues. The double helix has a mean diameter of ~20 Å (2.0 nm), and two grooves are formed; a deep or major and a shallow or minor groove.

B-DNA: It represents an average conformation of DNA, based on fiber diffraction studies. Dimensions of B-form (the most common) of DNA is 0.34 nm between bp, 3.4 nm per turn, about 10 bp per turn 1.9 nm (about 2.0 nm or 20 Å) in diameter (Table 12.3).

As per Watson–Crick B-DNA structure specific structure of B-DNA, major and minor grooves are formed. The major groove is wider as compared to the minor groove in DNA Figure 12.5. Major groove is the site where specific amino acid (proteins) interacts. Purine N7 and C6 groups while pyrimidine C4 and C5 groups are facing into the major groove. It provides specific contacts with amino acids in DNA-binding proteins. Some amino acids bind to the minor groove also. Amino acids act as source of H donors and acceptors to form hydrogen bond with nucleotide.

A-DNA: It was first discovered by fiber-diffraction studies of DNA at "low" (75%) relative humidity. It is also a right-handed Helices DNA. Under dehydrating conditions, and certain purine stretches will favor an A-conformation. A stretch of four purinies or pyrimidines in a row are able to form a local A-DNA helix. So it might be possible that certain stretch is having A form while others is having B form. The main difference is A form of DNA is wider as compared to B and Z form because the size of minor groove and major groove is almost of same size. In A-DNA is less stable as compared to B, it shows more rigidity due to presence of off-center base B-form. Base pair tilting in A-DNA is higher as compared to B-DNA (Table 12.3) stacking. There are about 11 bp per turn for A-DNA, compared with about 10 bp per turn for the B-DNA.

TABLE 12.3   Comparative Analysis of A, B, and Z DNA.

	B form	A form	Z form
Helix sense	Right handed	Right handed	Left handed
Base pairs per turn	10	11	12
Vertical rise per bp	3.4 Å	2.56 Å	19 Å
Rotation per bp	+36°	+33°	−30°
Helical diameter	19 Å	19 Å	19 Å

Z-DNA: It is left-handed helix and it was the first DNA to be crystallized as an oligomer d(GCGCGC). Its structure is not a smooth helical, but zig zag like. That is why its name is Z-DNA. The Z-helix is narrower than the A-and B conformations, and it has 12 bp per turn (Table 12.3). The nucleotide bases are flipped upside down, relative to the phosphate backbone, in Z-DNA when compared with A-DNA and B-DNA. Biology of A, B, and Z-DNA.

A-form helices are common for DNA–RNA hybrids, as well as for double-stranded RNA; in addition, the A-conformation is favored in triplex DNA. A transition from B-DNA to A-DNA has been postulated to occur during transcription, where the RNA–DNA hybrid would be more stable in the A-conformation. A-DNA also plays a role in some processes that do not involve RNA. For example, in sporulating bacteria, there is a protein which can bind to DNA in the B-conformation and induce a change to the A-DNA helix. Z-DNA, the minor groove is deep and narrow, and the major groove is almost nonexistent (Fig. 12.7).

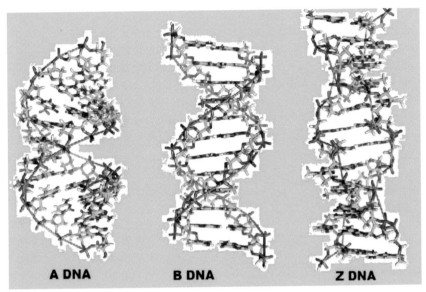

A DNA   **B DNA**   **Z DNA**

FIGURE 12.7   Showing structure of three DNA forms.

Chargaff's Rules:
Chargaff (1950) made some rules on the basis of his observations on the bases and components of DNA. These observations are called Chargaff's base equivalence rule.

(i) The amount of purine and pyrimidine base pairs are in equal amount, like adenine + guanine = thymine + cytosine. [A + G] = [T + C], that is, [A+G]/[T+C] = 1

(ii) Molar amount of adenine is always equal to the molar amount of thymine. Similarly, molar concentration of guanine is equaled by molar concentration of cytosine.
[A] = [T], that is, [A]/[T] = 1; [G] = [C], that is, [G]/[C] = 1

(iii) Phosphate and sugar deoxyribose occur in equimolar proportions.

(iv) A–T and C–G base pairs are rarely equal to each other.
(v) The ratio of [A + T]/[G + C] is variable but constant for a specific species, this ratio is used to identify the source of DNA. It is low in primitive organisms and higher in advanced ones.

DNA is a major source of genetic information and it transfers from one generation to another so it must be highly stable. Aromatic stacking and hydrogen bonding are mainly responsible for the stability of DNA. Aromatic stacking is actually a weak noncovalent force caused by overlapping of p-orbitals also known as pi stacking. The pyrimidine and purine bases, which bond parallel to each other in DNA, participate in aromatic stacking this is due to the overlap of their p-orbitals. Hydrogen bonding is the main structural feature and millions of hydrogen bonds are formed in DNA. These hydrogen bonds can be easily broken during replication.

12.2   CONCLUSION

DNA is a polynucleotide. DNA functions as storage for genetic information. Enzymes DNA polymerase is used to catalyze the synthesis of DNA in the 5′ to 3′ direction. DNA double helix strand orientated in the opposite direction. Nature of DNA is acidic due to the phosphate groups between each 2′ deoxyribose. Primary structure of DNA contains sequences of adenine, guanine, cytosine, and thymine. Secondary structure is a double helical structure stabilized by hydrogen bonding between base pairs. Tertiary structure is nucleic acids super coil and wrap around histones (proteins). Eukaryotic cell's DNA is found in nucleus of cell while in prokaryotes it is found in the form of nucleoid.

KEYWORDS

- deoxyribose nucleic acid
- nitrogenous bases
- phosphate
- disulphate bond
- phosphodiester bond

REFERENCES

Calladine, C. R.; Drew, H. R. *Understanding DNA, The Molecule & How it Work*; Academic Press, 1992, ISBN 0-12-155086-9.

Frank-Kamenetskii, M. D. *Unravelling DNA*; VCH Publishers, 1993, ISBN 1-56-081617.

Bates, A. D.; Maxwell, A. *DNA Topology;* Oxford University Press, IRL Press, In Focus Series, 1993, ISBN 0-19-963349-5.

Sinden, R. R. *DNA Structure and Function;* Academic Press, 1994, ISBN 0-12-645750-6.

CHAPTER 13

BIOINFORMATIC INSIGHTS ON MOLECULAR CHEMISTRY

CHIN KANG CHEN[1], HERU SUSANTO[2*], and LEU FANG-YIE[3]

[1]*The Indonesian Institute of Sciences, Indonesia*

[2]*Tunghai University, Taichung, Taiwan*

[3]*University of Brunei, Bandar Seri Begawan, Brunei*

Corresponding author. E-mail: heru.susanto@lipi.go.id

ABSTRACT

This report is exclusively concentrating on how information system, technology, and science, such as bioinformatics, can be related to one another. This will also present an in-depth understanding on how information system, technology can be used in conducting any scientific research with examples, to be shown in the content section, on the importance of studying bioinformatics, how data will be analyzed, and recent projects that are related to this topic.

13.1 INTRODUCTION AND BACKGROUND

13.1.1 INFORMATION SYSTEM

In an organization, they usually deal with large amount of data. In order for the organization to organize and analyze the enormous data in a convenient and fastest way is by using information system (IS). Many big companies, such as eBay, Amazon, and Alibaba also use information system. Information is widely used in any organization nowadays. IS is a software that is used to collect, store, and process data. It is also used to spread information and feedback will be provided for it to meet an objective. People often mistake data with information. Data are raw facts that are used for reference. Information, however, is a collection of data that can be used to answer question as well as problem-solving (Paul Zanderbergen). IS's primary purpose is to collect raw data and transform it into information that will be beneficial for decision making.

The three main roles of an IS are: It supports competitive advantage and decision making, supports business decision making, and supports business processes and operations. For each role, it has its own level where it operates. For support competitive advantage and decision making, it works on a strategic level, whereas support business decision making works on tactical level and support business process and operations works on operational level. With regard to the type of IS, there is not only one type of IS. In fact, it varies depending on the usage of the information in an organization. Decision support system is one type of IS. Often, it is used for decision making where the system will analyze and works on existing data that will project statistical prediction and data model. Transaction process systems allowed multiple transactions, such as collecting, processing, storing, displaying, modify or canceling transaction, at one time. Management ISs mainly focus on processing the data from transaction process in order to make it useful for business decisions according to specific problems. Office automation systems concerned on office tasks as it will control the organization's flow of information. Executive ISs create conceptual information, such as strategic and tactical decisions, to satisfy the senior management. Expert system is said to be a set of computer programs that can imitate human expert.

In science, it is difficult to find the results of relationships between genetic variability, diseases, and treatment responses where it usually come out as uncertain and inconsistent. However, there are systems, such as Fuzzy Arden Syntax or the probabilistic OWL reasoner Pronto, which can be used to increase the size of the classical rule engines. Such systems are examples of decision support systems. It must be associated with specialists and international bodies so it would affect the clinical practices efficiently. The system must be directly interconnected with the IS of the hospital, so there are existing workflows when handling information gathered from electronic patient records and clinical laboratories.

13.1.2   *INFORMATION TECHNOLOGY*

Information Technology (IT) is a computer technology that consists of hardware, software, computer network, users and the internet. IT enables organization to collect, make their work organize, and analyze data that helps them achieve their objectives. IT personnel main focuses on certain area there are business computer network, database management, information security, software development, and also sciences field. In bioscience, IT is generally used for automated data collection, statistical study of data, internet-accessible shared databases, modeling and simulation, imaging and visualization of data and investigation, internet-based communication among researchers, and electronic dissemination of research results. For instance, IT is used for automated gene sequencers, which use robotics to process models and computers to manage, store, and retrieve data, have made potential the rapid sequencing of the human genome, which, in turn, has resulted in first time expansion of genomic databases. Shared internet-accessible databases are important in paleontology, and models, as well as databases, are of significant use in population biology and ecology, and genomics are influencing many fields in biology. Furthermore, IT can be unique tools from the scientific tools, for instance, microscopes or physics accelerators, which are commonly used in the scientific process, such as data gathering. In addition, IT supports in hypothesis formation that is the first stage to gather observations about the problem examined in biological study, research design, collection of data, data analysis, and communication of scientific result.

In other science fields, IT also helps in analyzing subsurface creations, mapping, and modeling complex systems. For example, seismic data, used to measure earthquakes, were traditionally recorded on paper or film but today they are recorded digitally, making it possible for the researches to analyze the data swiftly. Furthermore, internet connection allows many researchers to obtain and contribute data for large problem. In several area of sciences, imaging and visualization become important because it can give clear modeling that helps the researchers understand biological systems such as tissues, organisms, and cells.

The role of IT toward software is that it helps the software to communicate with the hardware to input data, process data, and give the output. The communication between software and hardware can be defined when collecting and processing signal detected by laboratory equipment, example charged-couple devices, spectrophotometers that is used to measure the amount of light reflected or absorbed from a sample object and other devices that can be connected to a computer via an analog to digital. Computer-aided algorithms are being used to examine the behavior of thousands of genes at a time and are creating a foundation of data for building integrated models of cellular processes. Molecular biologists and computer scientists have experimented with various computational methods established in intellect artificial, including knowledge-based and expert systems, qualitative simulation, and artificial neural networks and other mechanical learning techniques. These methods have been applied to problems in data analysis, creation of databases with advanced retrieval capabilities, and modeling of biological systems. Practical outcomes have been obtained in finding active genes in genomic sequences, assembling physical and genetic maps, and predicting protein structure. IT has proved to be of conspicuously great importance on different areas of bioscience.

13.1.3 BIOINFORMATICS

Bioinformatics is the application of computer technology in managing any biological information and their management. This application is extensively being used to analyze specifically on biological and genetic information based on living things, both in plants and animals. Essentially, it has been used in many applications, such as studying human disease, managing biological information, managing ISs for molecular biology management, and other related fields. In other terms, such as biologically, it is conceptualizing the study of molecules, composed with informatics techniques, combination of computer science, applied math, and statistics in the sense of physical chemistry that are worked together.

Previously, the use of traditional methods for studying diseases mostly observed at single factors but present technologies help in studying multiple factors at the same time, together with each and every possible variables. The application of bioinformatics methods also being used to undo the fundamental molecular biology of the disease and move toward personalized medicine which involves understanding these diseases and transfer to new and more fitting treatment regimes.

The purpose of studying bioinformatics is any biological data will be organized in a specified database and this will help researchers to access or even enter any new related entries accordingly. Another, it is a useful tool in developing the resources with the aid of data analysis, and lastly, this tool is able to develop, implement computational algorithms and other software tools that help in understanding, interpreting, and analyzing any biological data that serve the humankind in a meaningful manner. Moreover, the computational tools are efficient for interpreting the results for biological research or can be applied on protein, cell, and gene research, on discovering any new drugs development or even herbicide-resistant crop combination.

The importance of bioinformatics application simply involves melding biology with computer science, the use of genomics information in understanding human disease and the identification of new molecular targets for drug discovery on a large scale. The use of bioinformatics is mostly in analyzing biological and genetic information which is associated with biomolecules on a large-scale, discipline in molecular biology areas from structural biology, genomics to gene expression studies applied to gene-based drug discovery, and development genomic information resulting from the Human Genome Project. Experts and researchers furthermore practice bioinformatics application in studying the sequences of genomes that appeared both in plants and animals in the field of agricultural studies, advancement in genomics technologies throughout the years from the 1950s until now, genome sequencing apparently involves in genetic databases for patients, next-generation sequencing technology that allows researchers to study complex genomics research, analyze genome-wide methylation or DNA-protein interactions, the study of microbial diversity in the environments and in human.

Toward the end of this report, it will show on how biological databases of commercialization on bioinformatics, biotechnology, and bioterrorism give an impact to this new field of research and development for business purposes and current issues assist to this.

13.2   APPLICATIONS OF BIOINFORMATICS

13.2.1   GENOMICS, BIOMEDICINE, AND MICROBIOLOGY

According to Ma and Liu (2015), genomics is a large-scale data acquisition, technological advancements that involve genome structures, evolution, and variations. Genomics origin can be traced as far back to the 19th century from the work of Gregor Mendel. However, in the middle of the 19th century, the progress of IS and IT was not as advanced as it is today. It is important to remember that genomics is an essential area of bioinformatics, as well as understanding its roles in the milestones of biological and molecular discovery. For instance, in Human Genome Project, an international scientific research project with goals to determine what makes up human DNA and its physical and functional characteristics, understanding heredity, understanding diseases, its role in pushing the innovation in genomic technologies, and many more. Another view on genomics is that the main concept of genome informatics was to analyze, process, and interpret all aspects of DNA in order to come up with a more defined and accurate information on biological structure and components of DNA (Chen, 2015). All things considered, genomics is evolving duly because IT and IS keep on improving throughout the years. Owing to this, the world is progressing at a much faster pace, namely in biomedicine and microbiology, and the knowledge that it brought had or are still being used to broaden our views on molecular mechanisms in the spreading, treating, curing, and preventing the development of diseases.

Almost every year, new drugs are being discovered or improved to better serve their purpose in curing, treating, and preventing health issues all around the world. Bioinformatics acts as the main agent for its progression due to its vast collection of advanced tools for managing a large volume of data, as well as to help interpret, predict, and analyze clinical and preclinical data. As biological technologies progress, so does the data it produces and this often leads to a massive boom in database collection. Useful data could be proven to be useless without a proper system or tools to access it accurately and thus it is imperative to have computational tools that can search and integrate significant information. Development of bioinformatics resources has shown that it is essential in screening valuable data for effective drug solution in a profitable and timely manner. As an example, Array Comparative Genomic Hybridization method has been used globally for DNA analysis on normal and pathological clinical samples to check for the DNA copy number gain and loss across the chromosomes (Leung et al., 2012). In addition, the current proteomic analysis that uses MS-based technology is progressively used for identifying molecular network targets and is responsible for many discoveries in profiling correlations in the pathogenesis of certain human illnesses. Through this analysis and method, integration of the connections between proteomics and metabolomics platforms can increase the dynamic and potency of the drug treatment solution.

Adverse drug reactions (ADRs) are often caused by all-purpose drugs that exist in today's market. Most people would prefer these types of drugs due to their economic status and often due to their state of living. Personalized medicine could provide the needed solution to these circumstances. Yan (2013) argued that through the development of pharmacogenomics and systems biology, personalized medicine could aid in the advancement of reductionism-based and disease-centered curative methods to systems-based, correlative and human-centered care. Developing further understanding between genotypes and phenotypes from analyzed data of genomic analysis through data integration methods help connect an efficient clinical and laboratory data flow. By implementing a translational informatics support into data mining techniques, knowledge discovery, and electronic health records, better diagnostic and treatment selection can bring a more suitable medication for the right people. A good translational bioinformatics will aid in establishing a powerful platform to connect various knowledge scopes for translating numerous biomedical data into predictive and preventive medicine (Yan, 2013). Altogether, this will bring about an ideal personalized medicine that is less costly, reduce errors and risks, diminish ADRs, and overcome the therapeutic obstruction.

According to Wu et al. (2012) Cancer is one of the most prevalent and profound diseases that could occur at anytime and anywhere in the body. Its development is explained as an uncontrollable genetic mutation of cells in the body of organisms whereby it drastically affected the metabolism, loss in genes, and promotion of invasive tumor growth, metastases, and angiogenesis (Mount, 2005). Multiple factors, such as the period, severities, drug resistance, cell origins, locations, and affectability, can be the causes for poor diagnoses and therapies result for the cancer patient. However, over the years, the results from advanced and accurate clinical bioinformatics and uses of new systems clinical medicine have helped improve the results of cancer treatment and diagnosis all around the world. Adoptive immunotherapy (gene therapy) commonly used for cancer treatment, uses the technology of genetic modification whereby T cells with antitumor antigen receptors or chimeric antigen receptor are used, duly because they can target antigens expressed on tumor cells (Morgan et al., 2013). In recent times, the use of Semantic Web technology enables better understanding of high throughput clinical data and establish quantitative semantic models gathered from Corvus (data warehouse providing systematic interface to numerous forms of Omics data) rooted from systematic biological knowledge and by application of SPARQL endpoint (Holford et al., 2011). In addition, application of new biomarkers strategies in cancer bioinformatics has become more popular in monitoring progress of the disease and its response to therapy. It is expected to coordinate with clinical informatics that includes patient inputs such as complaints, history, therapies, symptoms and signs, medical examinations, biochemical analysis, imaging profiles, and other valid inputs. All in all, the expected result would provide more accurate interpretable signatures and, therefore helps, in better diagnosis and cancer solutions for specific patients.

The world's population is continuously booming and is expected to reach 11 billion by the year 2100 and this brings about new challenges in managing disease outbreaks. A rise of infectious diseases by new viruses and drug-resistant bacteria are the tendencies of disease outbreaks. Over the last 2 decades alone, new virus strains have kept the world in constant fear of deadly outbreaks threats: Swine flu pandemic, SARS (severe acute respiratory syndrome), HIV (human immunodeficiency virus), and AIDS (acquired immune deficiency syndrome), malaria, tuberculosis and, more recently, Zika Virus. Steps in bottling more outbreaks have been initiated throughout the globe but, more importantly, the sharing of knowledge on how it came to be and the proper exploitation methods to discover the viruses' weaknesses has proven to be a better front in battling outbreaks. Next-generation genome sequencing has aided the advancement of biotechnologies and tools by providing new insight into viral distinctiveness, allows in-depth sampling and provides bigger capacity for automation and thus providing new data interpretation on what could be done or changed to the characterization of viral quasi-species (Kijak et al., 2013). Bioinformatics package named Nautilus, by Kijak et al. (2013), which runs on several operating systems, represents new sets of tools to support better data analysis to facilitate the application of next-generation sequencing and allowing better insight on HIV genome characterizations throughout the population and its evolution. Nevertheless, the rapid occurrences of antimicrobial resistance in micro-organisms cannot be diminished simply by continuous biological studies but also through a global understanding in public members to always keep a hygienic environment and in practices, as well as awareness, wherever and whenever they are. This method is the main preventative method for generally, all kinds of microbial infections, duly because producing a constantly evolving medicine and treatment to fight against a rapidly- evolving antimicrobial resistance illnesses will take higher health care expenditures and is time-consuming for all sides. The risk of death from resistant micro-organisms is much higher than that of the same nonresistant micro-organisms.

13.2.2 BIOLOGICAL DATABASE

Database is seen as a major tool for storing biological data for public use. Relational database concept of computer science and information retrieval concept of digital libraries is implemented to fully interpreted biological database. Gene sequence, attributes, textual descriptions, and ontology classification are stored in biological database. The data mentions are categorized as semistructured data that later can be displayed in tables form, key delimited record, and XML structure. The common method of cross-referencing is often used by database accession number.

A biological database can be defined as the collection of biological data collected during live-experiment and computation operation and analysis. Biological data should be organized properly to enable easy data operations such as manipulation, deletion, and calculation. The aim of the database must follow two principles that are accessible and can be used in both single and multiuser system environment.

Databases commonly can be grouped into primary, secondary, and composite databases. Primary databases include data that is gathered during experiment, such as nucleotide sequences and three-dimensional structure. It is often called as archival databases. The data gathered resulted from experiment of researchers all around the world, GenBank, DNA database of Japan (DDBJ), SWISS-PROT (Fig. 13.1). Secondary databases are derived from analysis of the first hand (primary) data such as sequences and secondary structure. The result of secondary databases is usually in the form of conserved sequences, signature sequences, and active site residues of protein. Curated database is another term for secondary databases. Some of the database was created and hosted by the researchers themselves at their own laboratories, such as SCOP, CATH, and PROSITE that was developed in Cambridge University, University College of London, and Stanford University accordingly.

The first databases were created in 1956, which was after the insulin protein sequence available, which was the first protein to be sequenced. The content of the insulin sequence includes just 51 residues that characterized the sequence. After Insulin protein, the first nucleic acid sequence of Yeast tRNA with 77 bases was discovered 4 years after, which was in 1960. Three-dimensional structure was also studied as well as the creation of the first protein structure database with only 10 entries in 1972. Currently, the Protein Data bank has grown to store more than 10,000 entries.

Since protein sequence databases were maintained on individual laboratories, SWISS-PROT protein sequence started to exist, which was categorized as consolidated format database, which began in 1986. Database functionality was also expanded not only with the capabilities of handling data, sophisticated queries facilities, and bioinformatics analysis function were also implemented in modern databases.

Similar to general databases, biological database can also be categorized into two groups: Sequence structure databases and pathway databases. Sequence structure databases mainly focus on nucleic acid sequence and protein sequence whereas pathway databases will only focus on protein.

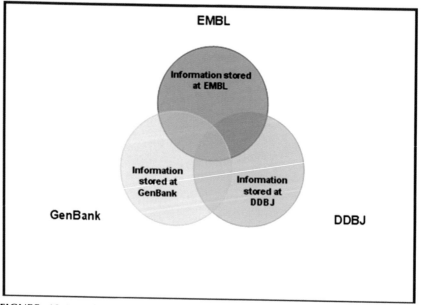

FIGURE 13.1 Information stored at GenBank, EMBL, and DDBJ is shared with each database daily.

13.2.2.1 SEQUENCE DATABASES

Sequence databases categorized as the most frequently used databases and some of the databases in sequence databases are marked as the best biological databases. GenBank is one of the examples of widely used sequence databases. GenBank focuses on DNA and Protein Sequence.

GenBank is classified as one of the most widely used sequence biological databases. The name refers to the DNA sequence databases of the National Center for Biotechnology Information (NCBI). GenBank's data are mainly made up of sequences submitted by individual laboratories and data interchange from international nucleotide sequence databases, European Molecular Biology laboratory (EMBL) and DDBJ (Priyadarshi, 2014).

13.2.2.2 STRUCTURE DATABASES

To fully be able to understand the protein function, knowledge of protein structure, molecular interaction and mechanism must be understood completely. The Protein Data Bank (PDB) is the worldwide repository of experimentally which classified the protein structure, nucleic acids, and complex assemblies, including drug-target complexed (Chun-Nan Hsu, 2015). The PDB was created in Brookhaven National Laboratories during 1971. It mainly contained information on molecular structure of macromolecules from X-Ray crystallography, NMR method. Currently, Research Collaboratory for Structural Bioinformatics plays huge role of maintaining PDB. One of the features of PDB mainly is it allows user to display and present data either in plain text or through a molecular viewer using JMOL.

13.2.2.3 PATHWAY DATABASES

The growth of metabolic databases through metabolic study pathway will fulfill the need and enhance the development of system biology. One of the popular pathway databases is KEGG. KEGG refers to The Kyoto Encyclopedia of Genes and Genomes. KEGG databases is the center of information toward system analysis of gene function and connecting genomic information with higher-order functional information. KEGG consists of three

databases namely PATHWAY, GENES, and LIGAND. PATHWAY databases are responsible for storing the higher-order functional information.
These informations include the computerized knowledge on molecular
interaction networks. These data are often encoded by coupled genes on
the chromosome that is crucial for predicting gene functions. The GENES
databases consist of the collection of genes catalog and sequence of genes
and protein produced by the Genome Project. The third database LIGAND
kept information regarding the chemical compound and chemical reaction,
which is important to cellular processes.

13.2.2.4   THE COMMERCIALIZATION OF BIOINFORMATICS

The success of development in combining both computer technology
and biomedicine has helped scientists to become more efficient and
productive with the ability to predict the upcoming trend of bio solution
with the help of bioinformatics. With the advancement of bioinformatic
technology widely being exploited, the opportunity of commercialization
in unquestionable. However, many investors were reluctant to invest on
bioinformatics sector due to its history of invest during the late 1990s,
which resulted in high loss. Despite the loss being made, in 2002, Philip
Green, a biologist in University of Washington, wanted to decipher human
genome with more accurate reading of DNA letter. Celera-made machine
was the only tool he used that was supplied by Applied Biosystems. Due
to the lack of functionality of this software, he then designed his own
software to cater the needs of his project. As a result, Green's innovation
is categorized as industry standard and its source code is available without
the need of paying.

13.2.2.5   ISSUES OF COMMERCIALIZATION

The advancement of technology made a huge role in the success of bioinformatics where computer tools are being used for managing biological
information and computational biology that is used to identify the molecular component of living things. The involvement of computer technology
in biological area also introduces the studies of principle and operation of
data manipulation and data analysis of biomolecules, structure or composition or various materials, such as nucleic acids and product genes, such

as protein. Research and data gathering on biological field involving lab experimental where Mathematical operations and computation are used to obtain meaningful information from meaningless data especially in genomics. Computers have been used as the backbone in bioinformatics and eventually became one of the major tools in storing biological data and compare with the existing data set that provide important useful input for computer-user researcher that biologist usually gathers during their hands-on laboratory experiment saves a lot of time and resources. Cost of laboratory has been cut-down since the use of computer and software where most of the operation and experiments are done via computer with the help of special-purpose software.

The popularity of using open-source software has increased over the year, which has affected bioinformatics companies. Open-source software can be defined as a computer software freely available to the public. In general, it is a free software that can be freely copied, distributed, modified and manufactured. Characteristics of open source are there should be no discrimination to people, groups, or endeavor, the license distribution should be costless and general to every product and the license must be restriction-free of other software and technology-neutral. The Linux system is one of the great examples of open-source software with a major success. Bioinformatics firm finds it hard to gain profit due to this open-source software movement.

13.2.3 GENOMICS SEQUENCING IN AGRICULTURAL STUDIES

Another application of bioinformatics, scientist has taken advantage of, is in agriculture field in which the sequences of the plants and animals genomes offer great advantages for the agricultural. Moreover, this can be utilized for the genes within these genomes and their purpose, producing healthier plants. Tools of bioinformatics play a significant role in providing information about the genes that occurred in the genome of these species. These appliances have also made it possible to predict the purpose of various genes and factors affecting these genes. The information offered about the genes by the tools makes the scientists produce enhanced species of plants that have drought, herbicide, and pesticide resistance in them. In other words, bioinformatics plays a significant role that allows agriculture to enhance the food (plant) nutrient and improve crops that are capable to manage poor soil growing conditions and poor weather.

The relative genetics of the plant genomes has proved that the structure of their genes has continued more well-preserved in excess of evolutionary time than was previously thought. These results propose that evidence achieved from the prototypical crop schemes can be recycled to recommend progres to other food crops. *Arabidopsis thaliana* and *Oryza sativa* (rice) are samples of comprehensive vegetation genomes.

"*Bacillus thuringiensis*" genes that can manage a few important nuisances have been effectively relocated to maize, potatoes, and cotton. This innovative facility of the vegetation to battle insect attack defines that the total of insecticides being utilized can be lessened and, therefore, the nutritional quality of the crops is greater than before.

Similarly, scientists have just flourished in transmitting protein sequence into rice with bioinformatics to upsurge levels of iron, Vitamin A, and other micronutrients. Scientists have injected a gene from yeast into the tomato and the outcome is a plant whose fruit go extended on the vine and has a lengthier lifespan.

Moreover, with technology, it supports to cultivate in subordinate soils and sturdy drought. The advancement has been completed in agricultural cereal diversities that have greater leniency for soil alkalinity, iron toxicities, and free aluminum. These diversities will let food production to be resilient in poorer soil parts, consequently adding new land to the global production base. Furthermore, research is in improvement to harvest crop diversities adept of enduring concentrated water conditions.

13.3 EVALUATION/OPINION

13.3.1 BIOTERRORISM

One type of threat that is possible due to the invention of bioinformatics is bioterrorism. Bioterrorism refers to terrorism involving the intentional release or dissemination of biological agents. These agents are bacteria, viruses, or toxins, and maybe naturally occurring or human-modified (Wikipedia, 2016). These activities may result in illness and even death toward people, animals, and plants. These substances and agents are common in our natural environment; however, the properties of these agents can be altered to allow it to be more resistant to medicines and antibodies.

The main source of bioterrorism agents and substances disperse through air, water supply, and food supply. Terrorists may use these biological substances due to its detection difficulties which the symptoms can only appear after several days or hours. Bioinformatics is covering to open-access that can be easily accessed by anyone. These enable people with bad intention to access biological data structure and analysis can be easily learned and altered to create a new virus. Due to this issue, there will be a contradicting view on making bioinformatic freely available and strictly to only specific intention for it not to fall to the wrong hand. Bioterrorism agent falls into three categories: Category A, Category B, and Category C. Category A includes high-priority agents, such as organisms or toxins, which can cause harm because it can easily spread from person to person. It also may cause death, panic, and social destruction that requires special action for public health. Category B is the second-highest priority because it is fairly easy to disperse with minimal cause of death. Category C is the highest priority agent and it can be used to engineer for mass spreading. These types of agents can be easily available, constructive, and disperse without any restriction.

The effect of this category can result in major impact of morbidity, mortality, and health. The use of bioterrorism and biological warfare long existed during 600 BC where the spread of diseases from animal and contaminating enemies' water supplies became one of their enemy's strategies. These strategies have continued and also being practiced during European wars, American Civil wars, and even now. During middle age, infectious patients became very valuable which is perceived as a weapon. Siege of Caffa is one of the examples where the Tartar force was infected with an epidemic of plague which then spread to the city. This resulted in a plague outbreak that caused The Genoese forces to retreat. Epidemic plague continued to spread all over Europe, the near East, and North Africa in the 14th century. This event is considered as one of the worst cases involving public health.

Another example on the use of biological weapons was during March 1995 where Sarin gas was used to attack the Tokyo Subway system by the Aum Shinrikyo. Before this event, the group had attempted three attacks, which was unsuccessfully executed with the use of anthrax and botulinum toxin. The members also tried to gain Ebola viruses in Zaire in the year 1992. However, the project had been uncovered by the Japanese forces; unfortunately, the only evidence caught was insufficient to be made public. Until now, the biological weapon project created by Aun Shinrikyo remained a mystery.

With the advancement of technology and biological breakthrough, it is quite hard to detect any bioterrorism activities. The creation of new virus and diseases has increased over a decade with the return of viruses that were long gone coming back to life. The cause and source of this virus remained uncertain, whether from natural sources or from bioterrorists. To be classified between those two are low in possibilities with the need of deep examination, analysis, and taking into account multiple perspectives such as current environment, original and current structure of molecules.

13.4   ADVANTAGES AND DISADVANTAGES

Bioinformatics makes the information accessible and shared in comparison with traditional biological records where the developing tools make it easy to send, receive, and share information. For example, electronic medical records (EMR) reduce the opportunities of error that are caused by obstruction and other researcher's conflicts during the manual data entry process after data collection on paper-based. Besides that, it also supports to eliminate the manual task of extracting data from charts or filling out specified datasheets. The data stored can be obtained directly from the EMR. By referring to EMR, the researchers did not need to examine or observe the task again Bioinformatics has grown rapidly, it produced into subdisciplines, such as in chemistry, named as cheminformatics also neuroinformatic, which is related to gathering data across all scales, and neuroscience level to understand the complex function of brain and work toward treatments for brain-related illness and immunoinformatic, it uses informatics techniques to study about molecules of the immune system.

Usually, the organizations, such as Antigen Discovery, Rasa Life Science Informatics, and LabCentrix, that use bioinformatics is storing large amount of data or, in other words, big data which means it contains both structured and unstructured data that is hard to process if the organization uses traditional database and software techniques, as the data are large. Examples of big data are patient's information, types of disease, and DNA. Hence, by applying bioinformatics, this can be done easily as it can store a huge amount of data.

From the definition of bioinformatics, it is said that bioinformatics uses computer technology. Since bioinformatics involved technology, thus, it can be a threat to the organization using it as people nowadays know how to create computer threats and use for crime. Hence, bioinformatics can simply be hacked by computer hackers. Hackers are usually people who know programing really well and use the capability to break into someone's computer. There are different types of hackers such as white hat, black hat, gray hat, script kiddie, hacktivist, and phreaker. For bioinformatics, the organization has to be cautious about black hat hacker, that is, identity theft. Identity theft is when a person steals someone's information (such as name or date of birth) without their consent and take advantage of it in order to get goods or services. Since bioinformatics contains a lot of confidential information, it is important for the organization to secure that information cautiously. One way to overcome this problem would be to encrypt all sensitive files, where each file will be secured with a password or key and only people who know it can decrypt and get access to the file.

Bioinformatics interface seems to be unattractive, the designing of the tools has to be user-friendly, where people can easily understand it and cope with it. To have a user-friendly interface, it can make the researchers analyze the information more efficiently and effectively to convert the information into knowledge. Other than that, users must be properly trained to use bioinformatics tools to prevent difficulties. This would be a tough situation for developing regions as training and knowledge is required, which may also require time and financial support. For example, in Ghana, they suffer months, and sometimes, years of drought, resulting agriculture is almost impossible to succeed. Although, bioinformatics might help them to grow plants, they may not be familiar with the system, hence, know any single thing about the technology.

All and all, bioinformatics is important yet the biggest challenge to look out the molecular biology society nowadays is to make sense of the wealth of data that has been produced by the genome sequencing projects. With the advent of new tools and databases in molecular biology, researchers are now enabled to carry out research not only at genome level but at proteome, transcriptome, and metabolome levels. Therefore, incisive computer tools must be improved to accept the extraction of meaningful biological information.

13.5 CONCLUSIONS

In conclusion, the applications of bioinformatics are widely being used, from single traditional methods in handling genomic studies to more advanced methodologies toward the improvements in biological studies. Understanding that the vast collection of bioinformatics tools and technologies that exist to serve different purposes is also vital to the advancement in IT and IS and vice versa. Bioinformatics help in improving the ways of biological research and provide innovative ways, for instance, the use of databases to store any biological information together with more advanced software tools and computational algorithms. these databases are mostly related to micro-organisms that are being stored in the computer memory. In business studies, the research on scientific fields gives opportunities for businesses to broaden their opportunities in making profits, for instance, the invention of new medicines, drug developments, and so forth.

In the world of biomedicine and microbiology, IT and IS of bioinformatics have provided numerous resources and tools into new drug discovery, personalized and preventive medicine. Moreover, the successes in cancer treatment via gene therapy are also gradually increasing, owing to the next-generation sequencing techniques and technologies. Not only for cancer but also for other known diseases, such as HIV and AIDS.

On the other hand, databases are also being widely used in bioinformatics applications. The relational database concept of computer science and information retrieval concept is implemented to fully interpret biological database. The aims of the database are basically can be accessible and can be used in both single and multiuser system environment. Several types of databases are provided for each and different purposes such as for protein development, human brain studies, diseases, drug discoveries and development, and also in agricultural studies in both plants and animals. These data can be seen as highly accessible and reliable for other researchers and scientists, not only that, it has data integration and even they can add new findings or even update as it is easy to use. Scientists and researchers are also being trained in handling databases.

Meanwhile, with bioinformatics, vegetations can successfully grow for agricultural community. The tools used can help the plants to withstand drought season or poor weather conditions, enhance the nutrition quality, resilient to pest and poor soil environment.

Finally, even though the bioinformatics applications are widely being used for more advanced technological developments, there are pros and cons not only in biological manner but also in business manner. As stated, these are being handled properly and their usage is being improved throughout the years.

KEYWORDS

- molecular chemistry
- biomolecular chemistry
- bioinformatics
- information systems
- biomedicine
- biological database

REFERENCES

Almunawar, M. N.; Anshari, M.; Susanto, H.; Chen, C. K. How People Choose and Use Their Smartphones. In *Management Strategies and Technology Fluidity in the Asian Business Sector*; IGI Global, 2018, pp 235–252.

Almunawar, M. N.; Anshari, M.; Susanto, H. Adopting Open Source Software in Smartphone Manufacturers' Open Innovation Strategy. In *Encyclopedia of Information Science and Technology*; 4th ed; IGI Global: Hershey, Pennsylvania, USA, 2018; pp 7369–7381.

Almunawar, M. N.; Susanto, H.; Anshari, M. The Impact of Open Source Software on Smartphones Industry. In *Encyclopedia of Information Science and Technology*; 3rd ed; IGI Global: Hershey, Pennsylvania, USA, 2015; pp. 5767–5776.

Almunawar, M. N.; Anshari, M.; Susanto, H. Crafting Strategies for Sustainability: How Travel Agents Should React in Facing a Disintermediation. *Oper. Res.* **2013**, *13* (3), 317–342.

Almunawar, M. N.; Susanto, H.; Anshari, M. A Cultural Transferability on IT Business Application: iReservation System. *J. Hosp. Tour. Technol.* **2013**, *4* (2), 155–176.

Benson, D. A.; Karsch-Mizrachi, I.; Lipman, D. J.; Ostell, J.; Sayers, E. W. GenBank. *Nucleic Acids Res.* **2009**, 38(suppl_1), D46-D51

Biological Database. Retrieved from Wikipidea: https://en.wikipedia.org/wiki/Biological_database (accessed May 8, 2015).

Castro, D. The Role of Information Technology in Medical Research. *Inform. Technol. Inn. Foundation* **2009**.

Chen, R. On Bioinformatic Resources. *Genom. Proteom. Bioinf.* **2015**, *13* (1), 1–3. http://dx.doi.org/10.1016/j.gpb.2015.02.002.

Holford, M.; McCusker, J.; Cheung, K.; Krauthammer, M. A Semantic Web Framework to Integrate Cancer Omics Data with Biological Knowledge. *BMC Bioinf.* **2011**, *13* (Suppl 1), S10. http://dx.doi.org/10.1186/1471-2105-13-s1-s10.

Huang, Y.-H. A Case Study of the Protein Data Bank. *Citing a Data Repository,* 2015

Iranbaksh, A.; Seyyedrezaei, S. H. The Impact of Information Technology in Biological Sciences. *Procedia Comput. Sci.* **2011**, *3,* 913–916.

Kumar, D. Information Technology: Roles, Advantages and Disadvantages. *Int. J. Adv. Res. Comput. Sci. Software Eng.* **2014**, *4* (6) 1020–1024.

Kanehisa, M. KEGG: Kyoto Encyclopedia of Genes and Genomes. *Nucleic Acid Res.* **2000**, *28* (1), 27–30.

Kijak, G.; Pham, P.; Sanders-Buell, E.; Harbolick, E.; Eller, L.; Robb, M. et al. Nautilus: A Bioinformatics Package for the Analysis of HIV Type 1 Targeted Deep Sequencing Data. *AIDS Res. Hum. Retrovir.* **2013**, *29* (10), 1361–1364. http://dx.doi.org/10.1089/aid.2013.0175.

Leu, F. Y.; Ko, C. Y.; Lin, Y. C.; Susanto, H.; Yu, H. C. Fall Detection and Motion Classification by Using Decision Tree on Mobile Phone. In *Smart Sensors Networks*; Academic Press, Elsevier: 2017; pp 205–237.

Leu, F. Y.; Liu, C. Y.; Liu, J. C.; Jiang, F. C.; Susanto, H. S-PMIPv6: An Intra-LMA Model for IPv6 Mobility. *J. Netw. Comput. Appl.* **2015**, *58*, 180–191.

Leung, E.; Cao, Z.; Jiang, Z.; Zhou, H.; Liu, L.; Network-based Drug Discovery by Integrating Systems Biology and Computational Technologies. *Brief. Bioinform.* **2012**, *14* (4), 491–505. http://dx.doi.org/10.1093/bib/bbs043.

Luscombe, N.; Greenbaum, D.; Gerstein, M. *What is Bioinformatics? An Introduction and Overview*; Department of Biophysics and Biochemestry, Yale University: New Haven, USA, 2011.

Luscomber, N. M.; Greenbaum, D.; Gerstein, M. Yearbook of Medical Bioinformatics. *Bioinf. Intr. Overv.* **2001**, 87–88.

Liu, J. C.; Leu, F. Y.; Lin, G. L.; Susanto, H. An MFCC-based Text-independent Speaker Identification System for Access Control. *Concurr. Comp. Pract. E.* **2018**, *30* (2), e4255.

Ma, D.; Liu, F. Genome Editing and Its Applications in Model Organisms. *Genom., Proteom. Bioinf.* **2015**, *13* (6), 336–344. http://dx.doi.org/10.1016/j.gpb.2015.12.001.

Morgan, R.; Chinnasamy, N.; Abate-Daga, D.; Gros, A.; Robbins, P.; Zheng, Z. et al. Cancer Regression and Neurological Toxicity Following Anti-MAGE-A3 TCR Gene Therapy. *J. Immunother.* **2013**, *36* (2), 133–151. http://dx.doi.org/10.1097/cji.0b013e3182829903.

Mount, D. Using Bioinformatics and Genome Analysis for New Therapeutic Interventions. *Mol. Cancer Ther.* **2005**, *4* (10), 1636–1643. http://dx.doi.org/10.1158/1535-7163.mct-05-0150.

Oliva, A.; Rendy, L.; Racheal, B.; Janet, W. Bioinformatics Modernization and the Critical. *Drug Inform.* **2008**, 273–279.

Priyadarshi, M. B. Sequence Databases. Retrieved from Biotech Articles: http://www.biotecharticles.com/Bioinformatics-Article/Bioinformatics-Sequence-Databases-3278.html (accessed Nov 10, 2014).

Raunakms. What is Bioinformatics? - A General Perspective, 2010. Retrieved from https://raunakms.wordpress.com/2010/06/05/what-is-bioinformatics-%E2%80%93-a-general-perspective/ (Feb 22, 2016).

Susanto, H.; Chen, C. K.; Almunawar, M. N. Revealing Big Data Emerging Technology as Enabler of LMS Technologies Transferability. In *Internet of Things and Big Data Analytics Toward Next-Generation Intelligence*; Springer: Cham, 2018; pp 123–145.

Susanto, H. Cheminformatics—The Promising Future: Managing Change of Approach Through ICT Emerging Technology. *Applied Chemistry and Chemical Engineering: Principles, Methodology, and Evaluation Methods*; 2017, Vol. 2, p 313.

Susanto, H. Biochemistry Apps as Enabler of Compound and DNA Computational: Next-Generation Computing Technology. *Applied Chemistry and Chemical Engineering: Experimental Techniques and Methodical Developments*; 2017; Vol. 4, p 181.

Susanto, H. Electronic Health System: Sensors Emerging and Intelligent Technology Approach. In *Smart Sensors Networks*; 2017; pp 189–203.

Susanto, H.; Chen, C. K. Information and Communication Emerging Technology: Making Sense of Healthcare Innovation. In *Internet of Things and Big Data Technologies for Next Generation Healthcare*; Springer, Cham, 2017; pp 229–250.

Susanto, H.; Almunawar, M. N.; Leu, F. Y.; Chen, C. K. Android vs iOS or Others? SMD-OS Security Issues: Generation Y Perception. *Int. J. Technol. Diffus.* **2016,** *7* (2), 1–18.

Susanto, H. Managing the Role of IT and IS for Supporting Business Process Reengineering. *J. Systems Information Technol.* **2016.**

Susanto, H.; Kang, C.; Leu, F. Revealing the Role of ICT for Business Core Redesign, *Information System & Economics eJournal* **2016.**

Susanto, H.; Almunawar, M. N. Security and Privacy Issues in Cloud-Based E-Government. In *Cloud Computing Technologies for Connected Government*; IGI Global, 2016, pp 292–321.

Susanto, H.; Almunawar, M. N. Managing Compliance with an Information Security Management Standard. In *Encyclopedia of Information Science and Technology*; 3rd ed; IGI Global: Hershey, Pennsylvania, USA, 2015; pp 1452–1463.

Susanto, H.; Almunawar, M. N. *Information Security Management Systems: A Novel Framework and Software as a Tool for Compliance with Information Security Standard*; CRC Press: Canada, 2018.

Susanto, H.; Chen, C. K. Macromolecules Visualization Through Bioinformatics: An Emerging Tool of Informatics. *Appl. Phys. Chem. Multidisc. Approaches*; 2018; p 383.

Susanto, H.; Chen, C. K. Informatics Approach and its Impact for Bioscience: Making Sense of Innovation. *Applied Physical Chemistry with Multidisciplinary Approaches*; 2018; p 407.

Susanto, H. Smart Mobile Device Emerging Technologies: An Enabler to Health Monitoring System. *Kalman Filtering Techniques for Radar Tracking*; 2000, 241.

Toomula, N.; Kumar, A.; Kumar, D. S.; Bheemidi, V. S. Biological databases-integration of life science data. *J. Comput. Sci. Syst. Biol.* **2012,** *4,* 87–92.

Wu, D.; Rice, C.; Wang, X. Cancer Bioinformatics: A New Approach to Systems Clinical Medicine. *BMC Bioinform.* **2012,** *13* (1), 71. http://dx.doi.org/10.1186/1471-2105-13-71.

Yan, Q. Translational Bioinformatics Support for Personalized and Systems Medicine: Tasks and Challenges. *Transl. Med.* **2013,** *03* (02). http://dx.doi.org/10.4172/2161-1025.1000e120.

CHAPTER 14

BIOINFORMATICS: PROGRESS, TRENDS, AND CHALLENGES

HERU SUSANTO[1,2,3*], CHIN KANG CHEN[4], and LEU FANG-YIE[2]

[1]The Indonesian Institute of Sciences, Indonesia

[2]Tunghai University, Taichung, Taiwan

[3]University Technology of Brunei, Bandar Seri Begawan, Brunei

[4]University of Brunei, Bandar Seri Begawan, Brunei

*Corresponding author. E-mail: heru.susanto@lipi.go.id

ABSTRACT

In today's society, bioinformatics research puts a great emphasis on answering "when," "what if," and "why" questions with the help of information system and technology, and some researchers had argued that it could be the key factor in facilitating and attaining an efficient decision-making in medical research. Hence, the main purpose of this chapter is to explore the application of information system in biological world and to study the extent to which technology could bring opportunities as well as challenges in science. Also, this chapter will examine the importance and evolution of bioinformatics over the past decades.

14.1 INTRODUCTION

With the current deluge of data, computational methods have become indispensable to biological investigations. Originally developed for the analysis of biological sequences, bioinformatics now encompasses a wide range of subject areas including structural biology, genomics, and gene expression studies. Additionally, nowadays biological data is proliferating rapidly. With the advent of the World Wide Web and fast Internet connections, the data contained in these databases and a considerable amount of special purpose programs can be accessed quickly and efficiently from any location in the world. As a consequence, computer-based tools now play an increasingly significant role in the advancement and development of biological research. Hence, this chapter will investigate the relationship between information system and science as well as the consequences and implication of technology in supporting medical research.

14.1.1 INTRODUCTION TO INFORMATION SYSTEM AND TECHNOLOGY

Information systems is a part of information technology. It has been well defined in terms of two perspectives: one relating to its purpose, the other relating to its structure. From a functional perspective, an information system is a technologically implemented medium for the purpose of recording, storing, and disseminating linguistic expressions as well as for the supporting of inference making. While from a structural perspective, an information system consists of a collection of people, processes, data, models, technology, and partly formalized language, forming a cohesive structure which serves some organizational purpose or function.

However, they also can be defined as a set of interconnected components that assemble (or retrieve), process, store, and allocate information in order to support decision-making and control in an organization. In addition to this, information systems may also aid in helping workers in analyzing problems, visualize complex subjects, and create new products.

14.1.1.1 THE GENERAL IMPORTANCE OF INFORMATION SYSTEM IN SCIENCE

Due to the availability of large data sets of digital medical information, the use of informatics to improve healthcare and medical research has made possible where they provide a new trail for investigation and medical discovery. This is because informatics focuses on developing new and effective methods of using technology to process information.

In today's society, informatics is being applied at every stage of health-care from basic research to care delivery and includes many special-izations such as bioinformatics, medical informatics, and biomedical informatics.

The field of bioinformatics has exploded within the past decade to keep pace with advancements and development in molecular biology and genomics research where researchers could use bioinformatics to obtain an effective understanding of complex biological processes which includes examining DNA sequences or restructuring protein structures.

Furthermore, informatics has also had huge impact on the field of systems biology as systems biology could uses computer modeling and mathematical simulations to predict how complex biological systems will behave. National Institute of Health has claimed that researchers have created models to simulate tumor growths. By applying the computer models in the study, researchers can obtain a better and more comprehen-sive understanding of how diseases affect an entire biological system in addition to the effects on individual component.

The use of informatics to improve healthcare and medical research has been made possible due to the availability of large datasets of digital medical information. This is due to the development a new trail for investigation and medical research. Informatics highlights on improving a new and effective method of using technology to process information. In today's society, informatics is being applied at all healthcare phases from elementary study to care delivery, including a considerable amount of specializations such as bioinformatics, medical informatics, and biomedical informatics.

Within this past decade, the study of bioinformatics has exploded. This is to keep pace with progression and development in molecular biology and genomics research. Thus, researchers could use bioinformatics to obtain an effective understanding and knowledge of complex biological processes which includes examining DNA sequences or modifying the protein structures.

Furthermore, the prediction of how complex biological systems will behave also influenced the development of informatics as it had a huge impact on the field of systems biology and systems biology could uses computer modeling and mathematical simulation. National Institute of Health has claimed that researchers have created models to simulate tumor growths. Therefore, researchers can obtain a better and more comprehensive understanding on how diseases may affect an entire biological system in addition to the effects on individual components by applying the computer models in the study.

14.1.2 THE RELATIONSHIP BETWEEN INFORMATION SYSTEM AND BIOINFORMATICS

According to Cannataro, et al. (2009), bioinformatics is the application of computational tools and techniques to the management and analysis of biological data. Over the past few decades, rapid developments in genomic and other molecular research technologies and developments in information technologies have combined to produce a tremendous amount of information related to molecular biology. The primary goal of bioinformatics is to increase the understanding of biological processes.

Bioinformatics develops algorithms and biological software of computer to analyze and record the data related to biology including the data of genes, proteins, drug ingredients, and metabolic pathways. A study has concluded that the creation and analysis of group of sequences, large data sequences, and adding new modules for visual representation of input data and output results on the Microsoft windows platform is the field of science in which biology, computer science, and information technology merge to form a single discipline (Santhaiah, 2014). Biological data is in need of certain storage house in which the data can be stored, organized, and manipulated. Thus, biological software and databases provide the scientists and researchers this opportunity, enabling them to extract data from these database efficiently and effectively.

Bioinformatics can be considered to be the combination of several scientific disciplines that include biology, biochemistry, mathematics, and computer science. This is due to the availability of enormous amounts of public and private biological data and compelling need to transform biological data into useful information and knowledge. Additionally, understanding the correlations, structures, and patterns in biological data are the most important task in bioinformatics. Thus, the knowledge and understanding obtained from these disciplines could be sensibly used for applications that cover drug discovery, genome analysis, and biological control. Furthermore, it involves the use of computer technology and statistical methods to manage and analyze a huge volume of biological data regarding DNA, RNA and protein sequences, protein structure, gene expression profiles, and protein interactions.

14.1.2.1   AIMS FOR BIOINFORMATICS

There are three aims in using bioinformatics. Firstly, bioinformatics is used as a data organizer in a way that it allows researchers to access existing information as well as making new entries of fresh data. However, information stored in bioinformatics databases will not be useful unless they are analyzed, which extend the purpose of bioinformatics. Secondly, bioinformatics is also used as developing tools and resources to analyze the information. For example, sequence of a particular protein needs more than a simple text-based search and program which needed to be supported by biologically significant match. Additionally, this development process needs an expertise which not only is required in computational expert, but also needed in understanding of a medical research. The third aim of bioinformatics is to use the developing tools in analyzing the data and interpreting the result in a biologically meaningful manner. Traditionally, biological studies are conducted on individual system and comparison process. With the help of bioinformatics system, the analysis process can be conducted globally with large range data available and aim of open common principle across many systems.

14.1.2.2   THE PROGRESS OF BIOINFORMATICS

Grid infrastructures played an important role in the recent decade as supporting scientific computer-based analysis. However, the increasing complexity of bioinformatics resulted in finding new solutions to speed up computational time. Grid infrastructure is not completely satisfactory in terms of providing services and managing data that are reliable for presenting bioinformatics.

Another key issue is represented by the fact that the grid is offering poor chances to customize the computational environment. In fact, it is quite common in computational biology to make use of relational data-bases and/or web-oriented tools to perform analyses, store output files, and visualize results, which are difficult to exploit without having administration rights on the used resources. Another related problem derives from the huge amount of bioinformatics packages available in different programing environment (such as R, Perl, Python, and Ruby) that typically require many dependencies and fine-tuned customizations for the various users.

These are the reasons why cloud computing is the best solution. Computation is moving from in-house computing infrastructure to cloud computing delivered over the internet. Cloud computing provides cheap, reliable large scale of data where small size organization can get the same information as well-funded organization. Bioinformatics grew as the rising of the use of the internet which allowed creation and shared large biological data and offered rapid publication of research results. The internet also provides the researchers to supercomputing system that are complex such as grid infrastructure.

14.2   THE APPLICATION OF BIOINFORMATICS

Some of the grand area of research in bioinformatics includes:

14.2.1   SEQUENCE ANALYSIS

It is the most primitive operation in computational biology where the operation includes finding which part of the biological sequences are alike and which part differs during medical analysis and genome mapping processes. Hence, the sequence analysis implies subjecting a DNA or peptide sequence to sequence alignment, sequence databases, repeated sequence searches, or other bioinformatics methods on a computer.

14.2.2   ANALYSIS OF MUTATIONS IN CANCER

The arrangement of the genomes of affected cells is complex where a huge sequencing strength is needed to identify previously unknown point mutations in a variety of genes in cancer. By producing specialized automated systems, a management sheer volume of sequence data could be produced and managed, and they create new algorithms and software in order to compare the sequencing results to the growing collection of human genome sequences and germline polymorphisms. Another type of data that requires novel informatics development is the analysis of lesions found to be recurrent among many tumors.

14.2.3 MODELING BIOLOGICAL SYSTEMS

Modeling biological systems is significant in biology system and mathematical biology, where computational systems biology aims to develop and use efficient algorithms, data structures, visualization, and communication tools for the integration of large quantities of biological data with the goal of computer modeling. It involves the use of computer simulations of biological systems, including cellular subsystems such as the networks of metabolites and enzymes, signal transduction pathways, and gene regulatory networks to both analyze and visualize the complex connections of these cellular processes.

14.2.4 HIGH-THROUGHPUT IMAGE ANALYSIS

Computational technologies are used to accelerate and facilitate the processing, quantification, and analysis of a considerable amount of high-information content biomedical images. Additionally, modern image analysis systems enhance an observer's ability to make measurements from a large or complex set of images. A fully developed analysis system may completely replace the observer. Biomedical imaging is becoming more important for both diagnostics and research. Some of the examples of research in this area are clinical image analysis and visualization, inferring clone overlaps in DNA mapping, and bioimage informatics.

14.2.5 DRUGS DISCOVERY

Traditionally, pharmaceutical companies may only be attracted in introducing new drugs when any well-known pharmaceutical company had successfully developed them. However, in today's society, company has invested heavily on approaches that can speed up the development process. The pressure of producing drugs in short period of time with a high standard of safety concern has resulted in extremely enhancing interest of the researchers in bioinformatics. Bioinformatics acts as an identification of biological candidate and could be the storage of information. Drugs only can be produced if the drug target is studied and identified. For example, human genome sequence information can be found in the system that can help in drug making process.

14.2.6 PREVENTION AND TREATMENT OF DISEASES

Bioinformatics is a scientific discipline that deals with earning, analyzing, distributing, processing, and storing of biological information. It uses scientific knowledge such as algorithm, computer science in order to understand the biological significance of a wide variety of data. With this, it enables researchers to find new strategies to look for clues in the prevention and treatment of diseases. Bioinformatics has turned into a key ingredient with the alliance of genomics, proteomics, and drugs in today's world.

In fact, bioinformatics owes its creation to the need to handle large amounts of data produced by these "-omic" technologies (genomics, proteomics, and more recently metabolomics). This method of information is generated by high-performance methods such as gene sequencing, DNA microarrays, and mass spectroscopy. For this reason, bioinformatics can be called a transverse activity because it is applicable to all the subsectors of biotechnology and life sciences. However, its main application is biomedicine. Bioinformatics manages and decodes "-omic" data and it facilitates the translational medicine concept by helping to distribute information throughout the entire healthcare value chain. This covers the discovery and analyzing of genes, the protein structures coded by these genes, and the design of molecules and drugs to counter these proteins, up to their clinical application, which is where bioinformatics is leading a role in the development of specific medicine.

14.2.7 STUDYING GENETIC DISEASE

There is a growing market in the use of microarrays for studying diseases associated with genetic characteristics. The widespread acceptance of this technique is driving demand for a more user-friendly version of the software and bioinformatics companies are supporting this idea in their latest product developments. The big pharma companies are using systems biology in their drug discovery processes. For example, Novartis has created Novartis Biologics: a new division that incorporates bioinformatics at all levels of the drug-creation value chain. Programers have recently developed an extended markup language exclusively for systems biology, called Systems Biology Markup Language (SBML).

This language makes it possible to integrate the software applications of different providers. As a result, bioinformatics is also moving toward standardization of the language used for developing software. This will accelerate the production of new applications and utilities by small (non-industrial) developers, using an open-source environment. In fact experts expect that within a few years all legacy applications in bioinformatics will be available via the internet and will run in ordinary browsers. Consequently, it will be important for bioinformatics companies to adapt their existing products for online use or to develop new applications that are suitable for this purpose.

14.3   THE BENEFITS OF USING INFORMATION SYSTEM IN BIOINFORMATICS

Bringing together large data sets of medical data and tools to analyze the data offers the potential to enlarge the research capabilities of researchers where they could use this vast source of biological and clinical data to discover and develop new treatments and better understand illnesses. Pharmaceutical companies could use the biomedical data to create drugs targeted at specific populations. Furthermore, healthcare providers can use the data to better inform their treatments and diagnoses (Castro, 2009).

Etheredge as cited in Castro (2009) claimed that applying informatics to healthcare creates the possibility of enabling "rapid learning" health applications to aid in biomedical research, effectiveness research, and drug safety studies. For example, using this technology, the side-effects from drugs newly introduced to the market can be monitored in real time, and problems, such as those found with the recently withdrawn prescription drug Vioxx, can be identified more quickly. Moreover, the risks and benefits of drugs can be studied for specific populations yielding more effective and safer treatment regimens for patients.

Etheredge had concluded that using rapid learning techniques can not only improve patient safety, but also can lead to substantial improvements in the quality and cost of care by turning all of the raw digital data into knowledge where these rapid learning health networks can enable doctors and researchers to better practice evidence-based medicine. Evidence-based medicine is the use of treatments judged to be the best practice for a certain population on the basis of scientific evidence of expected benefits and risks.

14.4 THE LIMITATIONS OF INFORMATION SYSTEM IN BIOINFORMATICS

However, achieving the vision of an intelligent and fully connected health research infrastructure has not yet been realized. While various pilot projects have shown success and have demonstrated the potential benefits that can emerge from a ubiquitous deployment of informatics in health research, many technical obstacles still need to be overcome. Doolan as cited in Castro (2009) believes that these obstacles include making data accessible, connecting existing data sources, and building better tools to analyze medical data and draw meaningful conclusions. Much medical research data is not accessible electronically.

Achieving the widespread use of electronic health records is a necessary requirement for creating the underlying data sets needed for bioinformatics research. Access to the electronic health records of large populations will help researchers apply informatics to various problems including clinical trial research, comparative effectiveness studies, and drug safety monitoring. However, collecting medical data in electronic format is only the first step. Interoperability poses a substantial challenge for biomedical research. This is because the vast amount of electronic medical data cannot fully be utilized by researchers because the data resides in different databases. Even when the organizations that collect and distribute biomedical data are willing to share data, incompatible data formats or data interfaces can create challenges for analyzing data across multiple data sets.

Thus, Stein as cited in Castro (2009) claims that researchers wishing to use multiple data sets must devote significant resources simply to manage the differences between the data and, as a result, have fewer resources available for working with the data.

Highly trained workers that are familiar with life sciences are needed to be able to maintain the system in bioinformatics. In addition, researchers will also need to be trained that may cost the organization.

14.5   THE EVOLUTION OF BIOINFORMATICS

Bioinformatics deals with computer management and analysis of biological information: genes, genomes, proteins, cells, ecological systems, medical information, robots, and artificial intelligence as there are many applications of bioinformatics from the combination of computer and biology. The evolution of technology helps in supporting bioinformatics in discovering diseases and application in forensics using software packages and bioinformatics tools. For example, the evolution of technology by bioinformatics such as IIlumina next-generation sequencing (NGS) to provide accurate sequencing. NGS technology can provide valuable and useful information for a better understanding in health and diseases.

The use of bioinformatics can also be useful in determining the order of the four chemical building blocks called bases that make up the DNA molecule. This is because the sequence provides scientists regarding what kind of genetic information is carried in a particular DNA segment. Moreover, the sequence data can highlight the changes in a gene that may cause disease.

14.5.1   FORENSIC DNA AND BIOINFORMATICS

Bioinformatics and forensic DNA are fundamentally characterized by both study and draw their techniques from statistics and computer science which facilitate in solving the problems in law and biology. It could be useful to identify victim or suspect with personal relatedness to other individuals are the two major focus of forensic DNA analysis. It is a common event in forensic analysis especially by crime and investigation unit or CSI by looking at close connections, for example, paternity disputes, suspected incest case, corpse identification, alimentary frauds (e.g., OGM, poisonous food, etc.), semen detection on underwear for suspected infidelity, insurance company fraud investigations when the actual driver in a vehicle accident is in question, criminal matters, and autopsies for human identification following accident investigations. All of these problems may be solved by using bioinformatics methods (Lucia and Pietro, 2007).

Also, genetic tests have been widely used for major catastrophic events such as terrorist attacks, airplane crash, and tsunami disaster. It can be used for mass-fatality identification and forensics evidences. Personal identification relies on identifiable characteristics as the human body has a personal identity that is unique biologically (such as blood, saliva, DNA) and physiological difference (such as fingerprints, eye irises and retinas, hand, palms, and facial geometry), and also behaviorally different (such as body posture, habits, signature, keystroke dynamics, and lip motion and combination of physiological and dynamical characteristics such as the voice).

Hence, genetic testing results are integrated with the information collected by multidisciplinary teams composed of medical examiners, forensic pathologists, anthropologists, forensic dentists, fingerprint specialists, radiologists, and experts in search and recovery of physical evidence. Officers could have access to the personal information where biological data can be obtained from hospital records and behavioral data may be collected from banks or office document such as fingerprint or signature just by looking at the database.

Therefore, the application of genetic testing in large scale tissue sampling and long-term DNA preservation plays an important role in mass fatalities which have been recently labelled (Lucia and Pietro, 2007). Thus, DNA has become the most important personal identification characteristic because all genetic differences whether being expressed regions of DNA (genes) or some segments of DNA have characteristic of a person, DNA poses coding pattern of inheritance which can be monitored and can be used as markers.

14.5.2 BIOINFORMATICS AND CANCER

According to the Cancer Research UK (2012), cancer is one of the leading cause of death worldwide where 14.1 million cases of cancer were recorded and about 8.2 million death of worldwide cancer was estimated in 2012. A leading cause of cancer is when any malignant growth or tumor is caused by abnormal and uncontrolled division due to the changes of DNA in cell by mutation. Also, errors in the genes may cause this abnormal behavior to be cancerous. These changes develop when exposed to a certain type of cancer-causing substances.

In the era of post-genome, age holds phenomenal promise for identifying the mechanistic bases of organismal development, metabolic processes, and diseases. Bioinformatics research will lead to a wide understanding at the regulation of gene expression, protein structure determination, comparative evolution, and drug discovery. Presently, 2D gel protein pattern can be easily analyzed using bioinformatics technology where these software applications possess user-friendly interfaces that are incorporated with tools for linearization and merging of scanned images.

New techniques and new collaborations between computer scientists, biostatisticians, and biologists are required in today's research. There is a need to develop and integrate database repositories for the various sources of data being collected, to develop tools for transforming raw primary data into forms suitable for public dissemination or formal data analysis, to obtain and develop user interfaces to store, retrieve, and visualize data from databases and to develop efficient and valid methods of data analysis (Bensmail and Haoudi, 2003).

Cancer DNA sequencing using NGS provides a better information and offered less time consuming compared to NGS using gel structure. With NGS, researchers can perform whole-genome studies, targeted gene profiling, tumor normal comparisons. Therefore, it is easy to detect tumor and DNA fragments with detailed quantitative measurements from the database.

Furthermore, the prediction of genes is likely to be linked to a new developed disease or a modified version of old disease that evolves or mutates. The use of bioinformatics can be easily recognized and related genes that are similar to any function or characteristic from an original gene such as the similarity in percentage of DNA sequence. The highest challenge is to identify enormous markers of DNA as the application of molecular links to diseases will continue to face technological as well as biological and algorithm challenges. The human body consists of very complicated and diverse features because it is continually evolving and responding to changes.

As for using bioinformatics to replicate, the structure of new DNA structure provides a challenge in technology. This is because other interrelationship such as cells that may not be visible through the microscopic view. Thus, the already designed computer frameworks or databases may not cope with the expanding in network-level measurements and information.

14.5.3 ETHICAL ISSUE

According to Johnson (1999), "computer ethics has followed computer technology in its evolution, and for the same reason computer ethics as a separate discipline will disappear in the near future. In fact, when computing becomes a mature technology, the problem of its (urgent) ethical and social impacts due to policy vacuums (according to Moor, 1985) will diminish, and using computers as a means of achieving some goals will become part of ordinary human action."

What he said was, as time changes from period to period, technology changed. He believes that when the technology changes, the ethics of computer also changes when there is an adaptation of easily accessible technology.

Another citation from Johnson "Once the new instrumentation is incorporated into ethical thinking, it becomes the presumed background condition ... What was for a time an issue of computer ethics becomes simply an ethical issue. Copying software becomes simply an issue of intellectual property. Selling software involves certain legal and moral liabilities. Computer professionals understand they have responsibilities. Online privacy violations are simply privacy violations. So, as we come to presume computer technology as part of the world we live in, computer ethics as such is likely to disappear."

14.5.4 INFECTIOUS DISEASES ETHICS

The emphasis of human bioethics in the 1950s and 1960s coincided with a widespread in particular area and time (but, with hindsight, unwarranted and dangerous) belief that the problems of infectious diseases had been solved by sanitation, immunization, and antibiotic therapy. The much-quoted pronouncement that "it is time to close the book on infectious disease" is usually attributed to former US Surgeon General William Stewart. Although there appears to be no evidence that he ever actually said this, "the sentiment was certainly widely shared" at the time (Sassetti and Rubin, 2007). This widespread complacency remained largely unchallenged throughout most of the 20th century. It was dispelled by the unfolding of HIV pandemic and the plethora of other emerging and re-emerging infectious diseases that followed (or in some cases preceded) it, but it had already contributed to the gross neglect of infectious diseases by bioethicists (Smith et al., 2004; Francis et al., 2005; Selgelid and Selgelid, 2005).

AIDS was a rare exception, but many of the ethical issues is raised—confidentiality, discrimination, patient's' rights, and sexual freedom—and were not specifically related to its status as an infectious disease. Belatedly, this neglect is now being addressed; infectious diseases have at last come to the attention of bioethicists. During the 21st century, public health ethics has become a rapidly growing subdiscipline of bioethics, and much of the public health ethics literature has focused on infectious disease in particular. In addition to AIDS, attention has especially focused on severe acquired respiratory syndrome (SARS), pandemic influenza planning, and issues related to bioterrorism (Reid, 2005; Thompson et al., 2006; Miller et al., 2007).

There has also been a debate about the ethics of issues such as intellectual property rights, relating to antimicrobial agents and their implications for the access to essential treatment of infectious diseases (Gupta et al., 2005) and the relationship between marketing of antimicrobials and the emergence of antibiotic resistance (Selgelid, 2007).

By the citation of the researchers, it can be argued that using bioinformatics technology can make it more efficient and much more reliable. But it might as well give the people a negative impact such as the confidentiality as well as the consent of the participants.

14.6 EXAMPLES OF BIOINFORMATICS IN INFORMATION CONCEPT SYSTEM

Generally, information system concept in bioinformatics has the same aim, and hence has similar flow of procedure. It organizes data which all users had input and access existing data, analyze each input, and interpret the results in a biological manner.

14.6.1   EBI

The European Bioinformatics Institute (EBI), is a research and services center in bioinformatics. This database provides researchers with molecular biology, genetics, medicine, biotechnology, and industries related to pharmaceutical and chemicals.

There are various ways for data entry. Data input can be done via web, accessing their website or via Sequin, a developed tool accessed via an FTP server; or via e-mail to users whose internet access is through e-mailing services.

Data inputted by users are then analyzed whether there are new data or existing data. For instance, a sample of an unknown virus shows similar signs and symptoms as an existing virus. This data is then compared to each other and produces a result to which it is further elaborated and understood to be interpreted by the user.

14.6.2   PANCANRISK

PanCanRisk is a European project which aims to identify cancer vulnerability and clinical management via bioinformatics. With this, they are able to predict the treatments to cancer as the cancer genome sequencing is very challenging to be understood.

The company intend to give a deliberate, cross-disciplinary structure for a superior comprehension, joining and utilization of tumor clinical information in the assessment of the large number of hereditary variations, and changes included in growth vulnerability for the immediate advantage of disease patients.

Similar to that of EBI, PanCanRisk uses existing data to compare newly provided sample and look for varieties of genotypes vulnerable of getting cancer.

14.6.3   GENOGRAPHIC

It is an anonymous, non-medical, non-profitable project, sponsored by National Graphic Society and Waitt Family foundation which helps with migratory history of the human species, and all results will be placed in the public domain following scientific peer publication.. The project will be able to compile the data in collaboration with the indigenous and traditional people globally. This will study historical DNA patterns from contributors worldly to better recognize our anthropological genetic heritages. All results are published and accessible to the public.

14.6.4 GEMINI

It is a flexible software for exploring all forms of human genetic variation. It is designed for reproducibility and flexibility for biologists and researchers with a standard framework for medical genomics. Gemini incorporates genetic variation with a various and adjustable set of genome annotations into a unified database to enable interpretation and data exploration.

Among many bioinformatics service providers and softwares, these are the four which stands out and yet still have improvement that can be done. The development not only will take time but also it will be very costly as well. Most of the concerns raised along with the advancement of the system is the purchase of the machines required to run such experiments for researchers and students majoring in bioinformatics.

14.7 OPINION

We believe that bioinformatics deals with computer management and analysis of biological information: genes, genomes, proteins, cells, ecological systems, medical information, robots, and artificial intelligence as there are many applications of bioinformatics from the combination of computer and biology. The evolution of technology helps in supporting bioinformatics in discovering diseases and application in forensics using software packages and bioinformatics tools. Also, we believe that information system could be the key factor in facilitating and attaining an efficient decision-making in medical research as the knowledge and understanding obtained from bioinformatics could be sensibly used for applications that cover drug discovery, genome analysis, and biological control.

14.8 CONCLUSION

In conclusion, with the current deluge of data, computational methods have become indispensable to biological investigations. Thus, bioinformatics tools hold a huge potential for use in medical research and clinical practice as the analysis of genetic information offered by bioinformatics and the study of systems behavior with detailed mathematical models may lead to huge benefits for drug development and personalized healthcare. Also, the research and education in life sciences are increasingly dependent on bioinformatics and advanced information system to support the evidence using large set of data.

KEYWORDS

- molecular chemistry
- bioinformatics
- information systems
- correlation
- models

REFERENCES

Almunawar, M. N.; Anshari, M.; Susanto, H.; Chen, C. K. How People Choose and Use Their Smartphones. In *Management Strategies and Technology Fluidity in the Asian Business Sector*; IGI Global, 2018, pp 235–252.

Almunawar, M. N.; Anshari, M.; Susanto, H. Adopting Open Source Software in Smartphone Manufacturers' Open Innovation Strategy. In *Encyclopedia of Information Science and Technology, Fourth Edition*; IGI Global, 2018, pp 7369–7381.

Almunawar, M. N.; Susanto, H.; Anshari, M. The Impact of Open Source Software on Smartphones Industry. In *Encyclopedia of Information Science and Technology, Third Edition*; IGI Global, 2015, pp 5767–5776.

Almunawar, M. N.; Anshari, M.; Susanto, H. Crafting Strategies for Sustainability: How Travel Agents Should React in Facing a Disintermediation. *Operational Res.* **2013**, *13*(3), 317–342.

Almunawar, M. N.; Susanto, H.; Anshari, M. A Cultural Transferability on IT Business Application: iReservation System. *J. Hospitality Tourism Technol.* **2013**, *4*(2), 155–176.

Bensmail, H.; Haoudi, A. Postgenomics: Proteomics and Bioinformatics in Cancer Research. *BioMed Res. Int.* **2003**, *4*, 217–230.

Cancer Research UK. Worldwide cancer statistics, 2014. Retrieved from http://www. cancerresearchuk.org/health-professional/worldwide-cancer-statistics

Cannataro, M.; Santos, R. W.; Sundnes, J. Bioinformatics' Challenges to Computer Science: Bioinformatics Tools and Biomedical Modeling, Part I, LNCS, 2009, pp. 807–809.

Ibmcom. *Ibmcom*, 2016 Retrieved on 20 February, 2016, from http://researcher.watson. ibm.com/

Katara, P. Role of Bioinformatics and Pharmacogenomics in Drug Discovery and Development Process, Center for Bioinformatics, IIDS, University of Allahabad, 2013.

Lucia, B.; Pietro, L. Forensic DNA and Bioinformatics. *Brief in Bioinform.* **2007**, *8*(2), 117–128.

Luscombe, N. M.; Greenbaum D.; Gerstein M. *Ebiacuk*, 2001. Retrieved 20 February, 2016, from https://www.ebi.ac.uk/luscom be/docs/imia_review.pdf

Luscombe, N. M.; Greenbaum, D.; Gerstein, M. What is Bioinformatics? An Introduction and Overview, Department of Molecular Biophysics and Biochemistry Yale University New Haven, USA, 2001.

Paila, U.; Chapman, B. A.; Kirchner R.; Quinlan A. R. GEMINI: *Integrative* Raza K / *Indian J. Comput. Sci. Eng.* **2013**, *1* (2), 114–118.

Reid, L. Diminishing Returns? Risk and the Duty to Care in the SARS Epidemic. *Bioethics* **2005**, *19*(4), 348–361.

Rodriguez-tomé, P. EBI Databases and Services. *Mol. Biotechnol.* **2001**, *18* (3), Retrieved 20 February, 2016, from http://link.springer.com/article/10.1385%2FMB%3A18%3A3 %3A199.

Santhaiah, C.; Reddy, R. M. Role of Computers in Bioinformatics by Using Different Biological Datasets. *J. Comput. Eng. (IOSR-JCE)* **2014**, *16* (2), 2278–8727.

Leu, F. Y.; Liu, C. Y.; Liu, J. C.; Jiang, F. C.; Susanto, H. S-PMIPv6: An Intra-LMA Model for IPv6 mobility. *J. Network Comput. Appl.* **2015**, *58*, 180–191.

Leu, F. Y.; Ko, C. Y.; Lin, Y. C.; Susanto, H.; Yu, H. C. Fall Detection and Motion Classification by Using Decision Tree on Mobile Phone. *Smart Sensors Networks* **2017**, 205–237.

Liu, J. C.; Leu, F. Y.; Lin, G. L.; Susanto, H. An MFCC-Based Text-Independent Speaker Identification System for Access Control. *Concurr Comp. Pract and E.* **2018**, *30*(2), e4255.

Susanto, H. Cheminformatics—The Promising Future: Managing Change of Approach Through ICT Emerging Technology. *Applied Chemistry and Chemical Engineering, Volume 2: Principles, Methodology, and Evaluation Methods.* 2017, 313.

Susanto, H. Biochemistry Apps as Enabler of Compound and DNA Computational: Next-Generation Computing Technology. *Applied Chemistry and Chemical Engineering, Volume 4: Experimental Techniques and Methodical Developments.* 2017, 181.

Susanto, H. (2017). Electronic Health System: Sensors Emerging and Intelligent Technology Approach. *Smart Sensors Networks.* 2017, 189–203.

Susanto, H.; Chen, C. K.; Almunawar, M. N. Revealing Big Data Emerging Technology as Enabler of LMS Technologies Transferability. In *Internet of Things and Big Data Analytics Toward Next-Generation Intelligence*; Springer, Cham, 2018, pp 123–145.

Susanto, H.; Almunawar, M. N. *Information Security Management Systems: A Novel Framework and Software as a Tool for Compliance with Information Security Standard.* CRC Press, 2018.

Susanto, H.; CHEN, C. K. Macromolecules Visualization through Bioinformatics: An Emerging Tool of Informatics. *Appl. Phys. Chem. Multidisciplinary Approaches.* **2018,** 383.

Susanto, H.; Chen, C. K. Informatics Approach and Its Impact for Bioscience: Making Sense of Innovation. *Appl. Phys. Chem. Multidisciplinary Approaches.* **2018,** 407.

Susanto, H. Smart Mobile Device Emerging Technologies: An Enabler to Health Monitoring System. *Kalman Filtering Techniques for Radar Tracking.* **2000,** 241.

Susanto, H.; Chen, C. K. Information and Communication Emerging Technology: Making Sense of Healthcare Innovation. In *Internet of Things and Big Data Technologies for Next Generation Healthcare*; Springer: Cham, 2017.

Susanto, H.; Almunawar, M. N.; Leu, F. Y.; Chen, C. K. Android vs iOS or Others? SMD-OS Security Issues: Generation Y Perception. *Int. J. Technology Diffusion (IJTD).* **2016,** *7*(2), 1–18.

Susanto, H. Managing the Role of IT and IS for Supporting Business Process Reengineering, 2016.

Susanto, H.; Kang, C.; Leu, F. Revealing the Role of ICT for Business Core Redesign, 2016.

Susanto, H.; Almunawar, M. N. Security and Privacy Issues in Cloud-Based E-Government. In *Cloud Computing Technologies for Connected Government*; IGI Global, 2016, pp 292–321.

Susanto, H.; Almunawar, M. N. Managing Compliance with an Information Security Management Standard. In *Encyclopedia of Information Science and Technology, Third Edition*; IGI Global, 2015, pp 1452–1463.

Valencia, A. Bioinformatics: Biology by Other Means. **2002,** *18* (12), 1551–1552.

Yao, J.; Zhang, J.; Chen, S.; Wang, C.; Levy, D.; Liu, C. A Mobile Cloud with Trusted Data Provenance Services for Bioinformatics Research, Information Engineering Laboratory, CSIRO ICT Centre, Australia, 2013.

CHAPTER 15

INSIGHTS INTO THE NATURAL HYPOGLYCEMIC PRINCIPLES: TRANSLATING TRADITIONAL MOLECULAR TARGET KNOWLEDGE INTO MODERN THERAPY

SATYAENDRA K. SHRIVASTAVA* and SUMEET DWIVEDI

Department of Pharmacognosy and Biotechnology, Swami Vivekanand College of Pharmacy, Indore 452020, Madhya Pradesh, India

Corresponding author. E-mail: skshrivastava@svcp.ac.in

ABSTRACT

The chapter highlights the principles, fundamentals, applications, merits, demerits, formulae, and procedures of Ayurveda and traditional knowledge. The content exclusively focuses on modern pharmacognostic approaches and linking with the traditional knowledge. The chapter signifies the current status, prevalence, general aspects, understanding the concept from Ayurvedic point of view, and demography of diabetes mellitus (DM). In addition to it, the role of modern herbal therapy, Ayurvedic crude drugs, Indian medicinal plant with antihyperglycemic attributes, marketed antidiabetic formulations, etc. are comprehensively emphasized. The chapter will provide information of the antidiabetic plant extracts and products utilizing both modern approach and inspiration from the traditional Ayurvedic principles.

15.1 INTRODUCTION

Ayurveda, "the science of life" is a very comprehensive system of healing which is the most ancient system of medicine with a history of over 3000 years old. The word Ayurveda is composed of two Sanskrit terms, viz, "ayus" meaning life and "veda" meaning knowledge. Ayurveda is an eternal science of holistic healing and healthy living. It defines life as the intelligent coordination of body, senses, mind, and soul, with the totality of life and the concept of health/illness is recognized as the state of harmony/disharmony between them. Caraka has defined Ayurveda as the "science through the help of which one can obtain knowledge about the useful and harmful types of life (*hita* and *ahita ayus*), happy and miserable types of life, things which are useful and harmful for such types of life, the span of life as well as the very nature of life." From this definition, Ayurveda emphasizes not only leading a life which is full of happiness and which implies a personal attitude but also leading a life which will be useful to society as a whole. Ayurveda forms an important component of health care in India which is based upon century's old observation, rich in traditional wisdom and with its own strong basic principles and philosophy as its skeleton and body. As per concepts of Ayurveda, every material of Earth is made up of five basic elements, which are *prithvi* (Earth), *jal* (water), *tej* (fire), *vayu* (air), *aakash* (space) which is true for both plants as well as human beings providing their interface (Lad, 2002; Ayurvedic Pharmacopoeia of India, 2001, 2001a; Dev, 1999).

15.2 CONCEPT OF AYURVEDA

According to Ayurveda, the human body is composed of three fundamental elements called dosas, dhatus, and malas. The dosas govern the physiochemical and physiological activities of the body, while dhatus enter into the formation of the basic structure of a body cell and perform some specific actions. Malas are substances partly utilized in the body and partly excreted in a modified form after performing their physiological functions. These three elements are said to be in a dynamic equilibrium with each other for the maintenance of health and any imbalance of their relative preponderance in the body results in disease and decay. "Dosas" are mainly three known as *vata* (air), *pitta* (fire), and *kapha* (water). When these three are in a state of equilibrium along with properly functioning dhatus, malas, sense organs with a pleasant state of mind and spirit is considered as positive health and imbalance in the above factors results in disease (Mukherjee, 2001, 2006).

Ayurvedic formulations are those which are prepared in accordance with the formulae and procedures described in above authoritative texts such as *Arogya Kalpadruma, Arka Prakasha Ayurveda Samgrahka, Bhaisajya Ratnavali, Bharati Bhaisjya Ratnavali, Bava Prakasha, Brihat Nighantu Ratnakara, Rasa Chandanshu, Rasa Yoga Samgraha, Rasendra Sar Samgraha, Rasa Pradipka, Sahasrayoga, Sarvayoga Chikitsa Ratnam, Sharangadhra Samnita Siddna Bhaishajya, Manimala, Siddha Yoga Samgarha, Sushruta Samnita, Vaidhya Chintamani, Vaidyaka Shabda Sindhu, Vaidyaka Chikitsa Sar, Vasaya jiwash, Vasayka Rajeeyam, Yoga Patnakara, Yoga Tarangni, Yoga Chintamani, Kashyapa Samhita, Bhela Samhita, Vishwantha Chikitsa, Virada Chikitsa, Ayurveda Chintamani, Abhinava Chintamani, Ayurveda Ratnakar, Yoga Ratna Samgraha, Ramamrsita, Dravyaguna nighantu, Rasamanjari,* and *Bangasena*. Different solvents (menstrum) used in preparations of Ayurvedic formulations are water, oils, milk, ghee, cows urine, and so on. The use of sweetening agents, binding agents, colorants, flavoring principles, and other adjuvants are also very common in Ayurvedic preparations. With an objective of obtaining maximum therapeutic benefit and making the formulation palatable, different pharmaceutical process is prescribed in Ayurveda.

15.3 AYURVEDIC HERBAL MEDICINES

Ayurveda, the traditional Indian medicine remains the most ancient yet living traditions. It is a great tradition with sound philosophical, experiential, and experimental basis. Increased side effects of chemical drugs, failure of the allopathic system of medicine in various chronic ailments, a high cost of new drugs, microbial resistance and emerging diseases are some reasons for public interest in complementary and alternative medicines. The global acceptance of Ayurveda is gearing up and there has been a steep rise in the demand for medicinal plants from India. The western population is looking for natural remedies which are safe and effective. It is documented that 80% of the world's population has faith in traditional medicine, particularly herbal drugs for their primary health care (Humber,

2002; Dubey, 2004). The focus on the plant-based research has been in existence for many years in India and rest of the world. Large numbers of plants have been tested for pharmacological effect (Vaidya, 1994, 1997; Bhatt, 1996; Aswal, 1996; Gupta, 1994; Dhanukar, 2000). Herbal preparations which have drawn widespread acceptability as therapeutic agents include analgesics, anti-inflammatory, antidiabetic, lipid-lowering agent, hepatoprotective, antihypertensive, and antimicrobial agents. Some of the herbal drugs which have received pharmacological and clinical support for their therapeutic claims are listed in Table 15.1.

TABLE 15.1 Ayurvedic Crude Drugs with Proven Therapeutic Claims.

S. no.	Plants	Part	Effective components	Therapeutic claims
	Adhatoda vasica	Root, leaf	Vasicine	Bronchodilator
	Phyllanthus amarus	Whole plant	Phyllanthin	Antidiabetic
	Andrographis paniculata	Root, leaf	Andrographolide	Hepatoprotective
	Asparagus racemosus	Root	Shatavarin-1	Anti-abortifacient
	Azadirachta indica	Bark	Gedunin	Antimalarial
	Ocimum sanctum	Whole plant	Ocimin	Anti-inflammatory
	Bacopa monnieri	Aerial	Baccosides	Memory enhancer
	Butea frondosa	Seed, leaf, bark	Palasonin	Anti-helmintic
	Hibiscus vitifolius	Whole plant	Eugenol, carvacol	Analgesics
	Centella asiatica	Aerial	Asiaticosides	Psychotropic, skin diseases
	Curcuma longa	Rhizome	Curcumin	Anti-inflammatory, antibacterial
	Eugenia jambolana	Seed, fruit pulp	Antimellin,	Antidiabetic
	Gymnema sylvestre	Root, leaf	Gymnemic acid	Antidiabetic
	Holarrhena antidysenterica	Bark, seed	Conessine steroidal alkaloids	Anti-dysenteric
	Momordica charantia	Fruit, leaf	Steroidal glycosides	Anti-diabetic
	Picrorhiza kurroa	Root	Picroside, kutcoside	Hepatoprotective
	Psoralea corylifolia	Seed	Psoralen, bakuchiol	Anti-leucoderma

TABLE 15.1   *(Continued)*

S. no.	Plants	Part	Effective components	Therapeutic claims
	Pterocarpus marsupium	Stem, bark	(-)- Epicatechin	Anti-diabetic
	Trigonella foenum-graecum	Seed	Trigonelline, fenugreekine	Anti-diabetic
	Digitalis purpurea	Leaves	Digitoxin, digoxin	Cardiotonic
	Strychnos nuxvomica	Seed	Strychnine loganin	CNS stimulant
	Salix alba	Bark	Salicin	Antipyretic
	Gautheria procumbens	Leaves	Gautherin	Anti-inflammatory
	Rauwolfia serpentina	Root	Reserpine	Antihypertensive
	Vinca rosea	Whole plant	Vincristine, Vinblastine	Anticancer
	Taxus baccata	Leaves	Taxol, taxine	Anticancer
	Tribulus terrestris	Fruits	Tribuloside	Diuretic
	Commiphora wightti	Whole plant	Guggulsterones	Hypolipidemic

15.4   DEMERITS OF AYURVEDA IN MODERN APPROACH

Standardization of Ayurvedic/herbal drugs involves many obstacles because synthetic drugs have well-defined structure, established assays, standard analytical parameters, and reference standard for comparison. Therefore, quality control is not a problem for the synthetic drug. There are several obstacles in the standardization of Ayurvedic/herbal product. The obstacles like the identity of various plants, deliberate adulteration of plant material, problems in storage and transport. There are many problems in developing quality control methods as mentioned below:

- Herbal drugs are usually mixtures of many constituents.
- Selective analytical methods or compounds are not available commercially.
- Plant materials are chemically and naturally variable.
- The sources and quality of raw materials are variable.
- The methods of harvesting, drying, storage, transportation.

- The methods of processing (mode of extraction and polarity of extracting solvent, instability of constituents, etc.)

15.5 DIABETES MELLITUS (DM)

Ayurveda (In Sanskrit "knowledge of life" or "knowledge of longevity") is one of the most ancient traditions of India and it has now spread beyond India to other countries like, Sri Lanka, Malaysia, Mauritius, South Africa, Japan, Russia, Europe, and North America (Elder, 2004; Hankey, 2005; Patwardhan, 2010; Vaidya, 2001). Herbs are commonly used for treatment in Ayurveda. Indian health care consists of various systems of medicines and Ayurveda still remains dominant compared to modern medicine, particularly for treatment of a variety of chronic disease conditions. Considerable research on pharmacognosy, chemistry, pharmacology, and clinical therapeutics has been carried out on Ayurvedic medicinal plants (Patwardhan, 2004). The Ayurvedic Pharmacopoeia of India is especially rich in herbal treatments for diabetes (Ayurvedic Pharmacopoeia of India, 2008). Ethnobotanical studies of traditional herbal remedies used for diabetes around the world have identified more than 1200 species of plants with hypoglycemic activity although only a few of them have been scientifically studied (Ajgaonkar, 1979; Yoshiharu, 1994; Alarcon, 2000; WHO, 2005; Vaidya, 1979). Medicinal plants used to treat hypoglycemic or hyperglycemic conditions are of considerable interest for ethnobotanical community as they are recognized to contain valuable medicinal properties in different parts of the plant and a number of plants have shown a varying degree of hypoglycemic and antihyperglycemic activity.

India is endowed with the traditional wealth of medicines as is evident from the fact that the "Shushruta-Samhita," the ancient repository, differentiated between genetically and the acquired forms of diabetes and recommended different treatments for the two types of diabetes (Grover, 2002). In India, plants have long been used for the empirical treatment of diabetes (Pulok, 2006; Vaidya, 2008). The hypoglycemic activity of a large number of these plants have been evaluated and confirmed in different animal models (Preston, 1985; Portha, 2007; Frode, 2008). DM was well known to the ancient founders of Ayurveda, as judged from the detailed descriptions of the disease in the classic texts like Charaka-Samhita, Sushruta-Samhita, and Bhrigu-Samhita, and so on. (Satyavati,

1989; Dhanukar, 2000). It means, "Madhumeha" is a disease in which a patient passes sweet urine and exhibits sweetness all over the body, that is, in sweat, mucus, breath, blood, and so on (Ashtang Hridayam, 2000; Subbalakshmi, 2001). DM is described in Ayurveda as madhumeha kshaudrameha which literally means "excessive urine with a sweet taste like honey," or dhatupak janya vikriti which means a disease caused by a defective metabolism leading to derangement in body tissue (seven dhatus) transformation process (Subbalakshmi, 2001; Dwivedi, 2007).

Historically, Ayurvedic texts have described 20 types of urinary disorders (pramehas) based on the predominant doshas (10 kaphaja, 6 pittaja, and 4 vataja urinary disorders) and physical characteristics of the urine (e.g., volume, color, odor, taste, sediments, solid particles, presence of seminal fluid, and mucus). The urine is discharged in excessive quantities and is generally turbid. DM is one of these pramehas that may occur in any of the three (vata, kapha, or pitta) body constitutions. The Ayurvedic approach to DM management includes lifestyle dietary interventions, exercise, and a variety of hypoglycemic herbs and herbal formulas depending upon the predominant dosha. Cleansing procedures are unique to the Ayurvedic approach to DM. However, the Ayurvedic clinical description of DM, etiology, diagnosis, prognosis, and recommended lifestyle changes are basically similar to those described in Western medicine (Vaidya, 1971).

15.6   PREVALENCE OF DIABETES MELLITUS

Diabetes is an iceberg disease, which is rapidly increasing and the prevalence is a significant cause of concern (Frank et al., 2003). DM is one of the main threats to human health in the 21st century (Pradeepa and Mohan, 2002). According to WHO (1997), the global prevalence of type 2 diabetes, will more than double from 135 million in 1995 to 200 million by 2025. It has been projected that the global prevalence of T2DM is on the increase, the degree of which differ between countries and ethnic groups within the country. According to Sridhar et al. (2005), the total number of people worldwide with type 2 diabetes in 2000 was more than 176 million. By the year 2030, the number is estimated to rise to 370 million. In 2025, the worldwide prevalence of diabetes among adults is expected to increase by 35% and total diabetics by 122%. It is also estimated that the countries with the largest number of diabetics in 2030 will be India

(80.9 million), followed by China (42 million), and the United States (30 million). Type 2 diabetes affects 15 million people in the United States and approximately 150 million diabetics around the world. Diabetes is said to be the seventh leading cause of death in the United States (Ornish, 2004). DM is a growing epidemic in both developed and developing countries. The spectacular increase in the incidence and prevalence of this chronic disease is destined to have an enormous impact on mortality, morbidity, and health care resources. The global number of people with DM is expected to be at least 220 million in 2010 reaching 324 million by 2025 (Jayakumar and Nisha, 2005).

The world prevalence of diabetes among adults (aged 20–79 years) was estimated to be 6.4%, affecting 285 million adults, in 2010, and will increase to 7.7% and 439 million adults by 2030 (Shaw et al., 2010). Globally, diabetes prevalence is similar in men and women but it is slightly higher in men <60 years of age and in women at older ages (International Diabetes Federation, 2006). According to Shaw et al. (2010), India had 50.8 million diabetic subjects in the year 2010 and this number would increase to 87 million by the year 2030 (Table 15.2). The top 10 countries based on the number of sufferers are India, China, the United States, Indonesia, Japan, Pakistan, Russia, Brazil, Italy, and Bangladesh. Demographic and epidemiological evidence suggest that in the absence of effective intervention of diabetes will continue to increase its frequency worldwide. Thus, prevention of diabetes and its consequences is not only a major challenge for future but essential, if health for all is to be an attainable target.

TABLE 15.2 Top 10 Countries with Diabetic Population Aged Between 20–79 Years in the Year 2010 and Predicted Values for the Year 2030.

Ranking	2010		2030	
	Country	No. of adults with diabetes (millions)	Country	No. of adults with diabetes (millions)
	India	50.8	India	87.0
	China	43.2	China	62.6
	the United States	26.8	the United States	36.0
	Russian Federation	9.6	Pakistan	13.8
	Brazil	7.6	Brazil	12.7

TABLE 15.2   *(Continued)*

Ranking	2010		2030	
	Country	No. of adults with diabetes (millions)	Country	No. of adults with diabetes (millions)
	Germany	7.5	Indonesia	12.0
	Pakistan	7.1	Mexico	11.9
	Japan	7.1	Bangladesh	10.4
	Indonesia	7.0	Russian Federation	10.3
	Mexico	6.8	Egypt	8.6

Nearly 25% of Indian city dwellers (the subpopulation most at risk) have not even heard of diabetes (Mohan et al., 2007). According to the Diabetes Atlas of International Diabetes Federation (IDF, 2009) India has 40.9 million people with diabetes followed by China with 39.8 million diabetics. As for the projections, in 2035 India will top the list with 69.9 million diabetics (The Hindu, 2006). India had the largest number of persons with diabetes with 23 million cases in 2000, rising to 57 million by the year 2025 (Hilarg, 2003). One out of the four individuals will be an Indian diabetic in the world while three out of four will be from the developing countries (RSSDI, 2007; Chandaraju, 2005). Recent studies show that up to 10% of India's urban population and 2% of the rural population above the age of 15 years has diabetes (Elizabeth and Makol, 2005). Alberti (2001) points out that T2DM in urban Indian adults had increased from less than 3% in the 1970s to greater than 12% by 2000 while in rural population it has increased to 7%. Indians are more susceptible to diabetes, particularly when they are exposed to affluent lifestyles. It is postulated that intake of high calorie and highly milled refined foods in association with sedentary life may be responsible for the higher prevalence of diabetes in urban Indians and migrant Indians.

World Health Organization estimates that diabetes in India would increase to 57.2 million in 2025, from 30 million in 2002 and India will become the diabetic capital of the world (Alberti, 2001). Prasad (2002) cautions that 21 million Indians are presently suffering from diabetes; India's contribution to the diabetic global population would be a whopping 60 million by 2010. The epidemiological survey has revealed the prevalence of T2DM in semi-urban areas to be almost the same as urban areas, but only 2.9% in tribal (Podsedek, 2007). India is considered as the diabetic paradise of the world, in view of the high prevalence of DM in the country. The approximate prevalence in an urban area is around 13.5% and in rural, it is around 3% (Paulose, 2005). Bhattacharjee (2004) reports that India has the largest number of diabetic patients in the world. Diabetes prevalence in urban India range from 16 to 20% and in rural, it is about 4%. As high as 63% of diabetics in India are not aware of the fact of disease and hence exposed to diabetes-related complications. The prevalence of DM is showing a rising trend in Kashmir valley, lifestyle changes, and aggressive control of the risk factors is urgently needed to tame this trend. The prevalence of DM was 6.05%, with known DM being 4.03% of the study population and undiagnosed DM being 2.02% subjects (Ahmad et al., 2011).

15.7 UNDERSTANDING DIABETES FROM AYURVEDIC PRINCIPLES

The major signs and symptoms of DM described in classic Ayurvedic texts consist of honey-like sweetness of urine, thirst, polyphagia, tiredness, obesity, constipation, burning sensation in the skin, seizures, insomnia, and numbness of the body. Boils, wounds, and abscesses are often difficult to heal in a diabetic patient and are recognized in Ayurveda. All these symptoms are very similar to those currently described in Western medicine. Ayurvedic physicians also use modern diagnostic chemical analysis of urine and blood for confirmation. The etiology of DM in Ayurveda is multifactorial. DM may be a familial trait, and overweight (fat-meda) patients with this diagnosis may be engaged in a lethargic lifestyle and unhealthy diet (e.g., idle sitting, excessive sleep, overeating sweet and fatty food items, and lack of physical exercise) (Crawford, 1999; Vaidya, 1989, 2004; Mishra, 2004).

Ayurveda divides DM into two categories:

- Genetic (sahaja), occurring in young age from the very beginning of life that has some similarities with juvenile diabetes or insulin-dependent diabetes; and
- Acquired (apathyaja) due to an unhealthy lifestyle that occurs in old age and obese people and has similarities with type 2 DM.

In addition, Charak Samhita (100–400 A.D.) describes two types of DM: one that occurs in very underweight people (krsa prameha) and one that occurs in obese people (sthula). The former DM requires restorative (santarpan) treatment along the line of insulin treatment and the later requires fat-reducing (apatarparna) treatment (Sharma, 1998; Bhaishajya Ratnawali, 1985). Type 2 DM has even greater involvement of genetic factors than type 1 DM, but no specific gene has been linked to DM to account for the role. There is no evidence available to show the role of autoimmunity in type 2 DM. The two major problems in type 2 DM are the reduced secretion of insulin from beta cells and the development of resistance to insulin in peripheral tissues (Vaidya, 2002). Obesity is another major etiological factor, as 80% of type 2 DM patients are obese. Sahaja or Beeja-dosha type of diabetes was said to be quiet recalcitrant (Asadhya). The obese patients were managed by langhana-fasting (calorie restriction) and the lean by additional nutrition (calorie supplementation and nutrients). Apathya nimittaja or aberrant lifestyle, as well as obesity, are managed by correcting the lifestyle (diet, exercise, and rest), samshodhana (Panchakarma procedures), and samshamana (medications) (Singh, 1998).

According to classic Ayurvedic texts, DM and all pramehas (urinary disorders) start with the derangement of kapha that spreads throughout the body and mixes with fat (Meda) that is similar in physical properties to kapha (mucus). Kapha mixed with fat passes into the urinary system, thereby interfering with normal urine excretion. Vitiated pitta, vata, and other body fluids (malas) may also be involved in this blockade. This blockade is believed to be the cause of frequent urination observed in DM. Pramehas left untreated may lead to deranged development of the bone marrow, body tissues, nutritional materials (fat, proteins, and carbohydrates), and hormones (ojas). The incurable stage of pramehas is madhumeha, which is insulin-dependent DM. Madhumeha may not be described precisely in Ayurveda, but it points in the direction of the current knowledge we have about the disease with respect to neurological damage and insulin (ojas) malfunctioning at the production (degeneration of islets of Langerhans in the pancreas) or at the utilization levels. The involvement of tissues (dushyas) leading to blood vessels, kidney, eye, and nerve damage is also described in Ayurveda as major complications. DM is described not only as a condition of madhumeha (sugar loss in urine) but also as a condition of ojameha (immunity and hormone loss) in Ayurveda for the purpose of treatment.

According to classical Ayurveda, all pramehas have the potential to become incurable (madhumeha) if left untreated. The kaphaja urinary disorders (pramehas) are curable because the causative dosha and the affected tissues (dushya) have the same properties, thus requiring the same type of therapy. Although the pittaja urinary disorders are controllable (palliative), the resulting disorder may persist for life because the causative dosha is pitta, but the tissues and waste products (dushya) are different, requiring a different type of therapy. Vataja urinary disorders are considered incurable because tissues (dhatus) and hormones (ojas) undergo deterioration. Recent studies have observed a relationship between the body constitution and relative amounts of hyperglycemia and insulinemia consistent with the Ayurvedic prognosis (Bharti, 1995; Chandola, 1994; Kar, 1997). Kapha constitution patients showed the highest level of insulinemia and the lowest levels of fasting blood sugar (FBS) and postprandial blood sugar (PPBS).

Vata patients showed the lowest level of insulinemia and the highest levels of FBS and PPBS. Pitta patients were in the middle. Further studies are necessary to confirm these findings. In Ayurveda, the major complications of kaphaja urinary disorders are believed to be poor digestion, anorexia, vomiting, drowsiness, and coughing. Pittaja urinary disorder patients tend to exhibit a pricking pain in the urinary bladder, penis, and scrotum, as well as fever, burning sensations, thirst, sourness of the throat, fainting, and loose bowel movements. Vata urinary disorders (diabetes) patients often experience tremors, pain in the cardiac region, abdominal tenderness, insomnia, and dryness of the mouth. The major complications of vata DM most commonly include ulcers (eruptions) over joints, muscles, skin, blood vessels, as well as damage to the kidney and the retina. Historically, Ayurveda diagnosis of DM was primarily based on the sweetness of urine that was identified by a swarm of flies and ants over the urine. Ayurvedic physicians currently use urine, blood sugar, and glycohemoglobin (HbA1c) levels to confirm the diagnosis. Ancient Ayurvedic texts give the following signs and symptoms of kaphaja, pittaja, and vataja pramehas for diagnosis. Recently, however, Ayurvedic doctors' diagnostic tools evolved to more modern clinical and laboratory methods consistent with those of Western medicine.

15.8 MODERN HERBAL-BASED ANTIDIABETIC THERAPY

The management of diabetes without any side effects is still a challenge in the medical field, as presently available drugs for diabetes have one or more adverse effects (Bohannon, 2002). Since the existing drugs for the treatment of DM do not satisfy our need completely, the search for new drugs continues. In recent years, herbal remedies for the unsolved medical problems have been gaining importance in the research field. Apart from the currently available therapeutic options, many herbal medicines have been recommended for the treatment of diabetes. Herbal drugs are prescribed widely because of their effectiveness, fewer side effects, and relatively low cost (Venkatesh et al., 2003; Devaki et al., 2011).

Plants have always been an exemplary source of drugs and many of the currently available drugs have been derived directly or indirectly from them. The ethnobotanical information reports about 800 plants that may possess antidiabetic potential (Alarcon-Aguilara et al., 1998). Several such herbs have shown antidiabetic activity when assessed using presently available experimental techniques (Jafri et al., 2000). India has a rich history of using various potent herbs and herbal preparations for treating diabetes. In India, indigenous remedies have been used in the treatment of diabetes since the time of Charaka and Sushrutha (Grover et al., 2001). There have been several reviews on the hypoglycemic medicinal plants more particularly use of Indian botanicals for hypoglycemic activity (Saxena and Vikram, 2004; Sudha et al., 2011). Many Indian plants have been investigated for their beneficial use in different types of diabetes and are reported in numerous scientific journals (Joy and Kuttan, 1999; Nagarajan et al., 2005; Verma et al., 2010). To date, over 400 traditional plant treatments for diabetes have been reported in India (Modak et al., 2007). The use of medicinal plants in modern medicine suffers from the fact that though hundreds of plants are used in the world to prevent or to cure diseases, scientific evidence in terms of modern medicine is lacking in most cases. However, today it is necessary to provide scientific proof to justify the use of the plant as well as its active principles. A survey of the literature has revealed that a large variety of compounds obtained from several plant families were found to be responsible for the hypoglycemic action (Table 15.3).

TABLE 15.3 Indian Medicinal Plants with Antidiabetic and Related Beneficial Properties.

Plant name	Pharmacological effects
Annona squamosa	Hypoglycemic and antihyperglycemic activities of ethanolic leaf-extract, increased plasma insulin level
Artemisia pallens	Hypoglycemic, increases peripheral glucose utilization or inhibits glucose reabsorption
Areca catechu	Hypoglycemic
Beta vulgaris	Increases glucose tolerance in OGTT
Boerhavia diffusa	Increase in hexokinase activity, increase plasma insulin level, antioxidant
Bombax ceiba	Hypoglycemic
Butea monosperma	Antihyperglycemic
Camellia sinensis	Antihyperglycemic activity, antioxidant
Capparis decidua	Hypoglycemic, antioxidant, hypolipidaemic
Caesalpinia bonducella	Hypoglycemic, insulin secretagogue, hypolipidemic
Coccinia indica	Hypoglycemic
Emblica officinalis	Decreases lipid peroxidation, antioxidant, hypoglycemic
Eugenia uniflora	Hypoglycemic, inhibits lipase activity
Enicostema littorale	Increase hexokinase activity, dose-dependent hypoglycemic activity
Ficus bengalensis	Hypoglycemic, antioxidant
Gymnema sylvestre	Antihyperglycemic effect, hypolipidemic
Hemidesmus indicus	Anti-snake venom activity, anti-inflammatory
Hibiscus rosa-sinesis	Initiates insulin release from pancreatic beta cells
Ipomoea batatas	Reduces insulin resistance
Momordica cymbalaria	Hypoglycemic, hypolipidemic
Murraya koenigii	Hypoglycemic, increases glycogenesis and decreases gluconeogenesis and glycogenolysis
Musa sapientum	Antihyperglycemic, antioxidant
Phaseolus vulgaris	Hypoglycemic, hypolipidemic, inhibit alpha amylase activity
Punica granatum	Antioxidant, antihyperglycemic effect
Salacia reticulata	Inhibitory activity against sucrase
Scoparia dulcis	Insulin-secretagogue activity, antihyperlipidemic, hypoglycemic, antioxidant
Swertia chirayita	Stimulates insulin release from islets

TABLE 15.3   *(Continued)*

Plant name	Pharmacological effects
Syzygium alternifolium	Hypoglycemic and antihyperglycemic
Terminalia belerica	Antibacterial, hypoglycemic
Terminalia chebula	Antibacterial, hypoglycemic
Tinospora crispa	Antihyperglycemic, stimulates insulin release from islets
Vinca rosea	Antihyperglycemic
Withania somnifera	Hypoglycemic, diuretic, and hypocholesterolemic

15.9 MODERN HERBAL ANTIDIABETIC MARKETED FORMULATIONS IN INDIAN SUBCONTINENT BASED ON TRADITIONAL AYURVEDIC PRINCIPLES

Diabecon manufactured by "Himalaya" is reported to increase peripheral utilization of glucose, increase hepatic and muscle glucagon contents, promote B cells repair and regeneration and increase peptide level. It has antioxidant properties and protects B cells from oxidative stress. It exerts insulin-like action by reducing the glycated hemoglobin levels, normalizing the microalbuminurea and modulating the lipid profile. It minimizes long-term diabetic complications.

Epinsulin marketed by Swastik formulations, contains epicatechin, a benzopyran, as an active principle. Epicatechin increases the cAMP content of the islet, which is associated with increased insulin release. It plays a role in the conversion of proinsulin to insulin by increasing cathepsin activity. Additionally, it has an insulin-mimetic effect on osmotic fragility of human erythrocytes and it inhibits Na/K ATPase activity from patient's erythrocytes. It corrects the neuropathy, retinopathy, and disturbed metabolism of glucose and lipids. It maintains the integrity of all organ systems affected by the disease. It is reported to be curative for diabetes, Non-Insulin-Dependent DM (NIDDM) and a good adjuvant for Insulin-Dependent DM (IDDM), in order to reduce the amount of needed insulin. It is advised along with existing oral hypoglycemic drugs and is known to prevent diabetic complication. It has gentle hypoglycemic activity and hence induces no risk of being hypoglycemic.

Pancreatic Tonic (Ayurvedic herbal supplement): Pancreas Tonic is a botanical mixture of traditional Indian Ayurvedic herbs currently available as a dietary supplement.

Bitter gourd powder marketed by Garry and Sun, it lowers blood and urine sugar levels. It increases the body's resistance to infections and purifies the blood. Bitter gourd has excellent medicinal virtues. It is anti-dotal, antipyretic tonic, appetizing, stomachic, antibilious, and laxative. The bitter gourd is also used in native medicines of Asia and Africa. The bitter gourd is specifically used as a folk medicine for diabetes. It contains compounds like bitter glycosides, saponins, alkaloids, reducing sugars, phenolics, oils, free acids, polypeptides, sterols, 17-amino acids including methionine and a crystalline product named p-insulin. It is reported to have hypoglycemic activity in addition to being antihemorrhoidal, astringent, stomachic, anthelmintic, and blood purifier.

Dia-Care manufactured by Admark Herbals Ltd. is claimed to be effective for both Type 1, Type 2 diabetes within 90 days of treatment and cures within 18 months. Persons taking insulin will eventually be liberated from the dependence on it. The whole treatment completes in 6 phases, each phase being of 90 days. Approx. 5 g (1 teaspoon) powder is mixed with 1/2 glass of water, stirred properly and kept overnight. Only the water and not the sediment must be taken in the morning on empty stomach. To the remaining medicine fresh water is added and kept for the whole day and is consumed half an hour before dinner. It is a pure herbal formula without any side effects.

Diabetes Daily Care manufactured by Nature's Health Supply is a unique natural formula, which effectively and safely improves sugar metabolism. Diabetes Daily Care was formulated for type 2 diabetics and contains all natural ingredients listed in Table 15.4 below in the proportion optimal for the body's use.

Gurmar powder manufactured by Garry and Sun is an antidiabetic drug, which suppresses the intestinal absorption of saccharides, which prevents blood sugar fluctuations. It also correlates the metabolic activities of liver, kidney, and muscles. Gurmar stimulates insulin secretion and has blood sugar reducing properties. It blocks sweet taste receptors when applied to tongue in diabetes to remove glycosuria. It deadens taste of sweets and bitter things like quinine (effects lasts for 1–2 h). Besides having these properties, it is a cardiac stimulant and diuretic and corrects metabolic activities of liver, kidney, and muscles.

DIABETA, a formulation of Ayurvedic Cure, available in the capsule form is antidiabetic with a combination of proven antidiabetic fortified with potent immunomodulators, anti-hyperlipidemics, anti-stress, and hepatoprotective of plant origin. The formulation of DIABETA is based on ancient Ayurvedic references, further corroborated through modern research and clinical trials. It acts on different sites in differing ways to effectively control factors and pathways leading to DM. It attacks the various factors, which precipitate the diabetic condition, and corrects the degenerative complications, which result because of diabetes. It is safe and effective in managing DM as a single agent supplement to synthetic antidiabetic drugs. It helps overcome resistance to oral hypoglycemic drugs when used as an adjuvant to cases of uncontrolled diabetes. It confers a sense of well-being in patients and promotes symptomatic relief of complaints like weakness giddiness, pain in legs, body ache, polyuria, and pruritis.

Syndrex, manufactured by Plethico Laboratory contains extracts of germinated fenugreek seed. Fenugreek is used as an ingredient of traditional formulations over 1000 years. The current study is based on the mechanism of this antidiabetic drug using animal model on one hand and cultured islet cells on the other. Thus, many different plants have been used for the treatment of diabetes and its complications. One of the major problems with this herbal formulation is that the active ingredients are not well defined. It is important to know the active component and molecular interaction, which help to analyze the therapeutic efficacy of the product and also to standardize the product. Efforts are being made to investigate the mechanism of action of these plants using model systems.

TABLE 15.4 Antidiabetic Herbal Products Marketed in Indian Subcontinent.

Drug	Company	Ingredients
Diabecon	Himalaya	*Gymnema sylvestre, Pterocarpus marsupium, Glycyrrhiza glabra, Casearia esculenta, Syzygium cumini, Asparagus racemosus, Boerhavia diffusa, Sphaeranthus indicus, Tinospora cordifolia, Swertia chirata, Tribulus terrestris, Phyllanthus amarus, Gmelina arborea, Gossypium herbaceum, Berberis aristata, Aloe vera,* Triphala, *Commiphora wightii,* shilajeet, *Momordica charantia, Piper nigrum, Ocimum sanctum, Abutilon indicum, Curcuma longa, Rumex maritimus*

TABLE 15.4 *(Continued)*

Drug	Company	Ingredients
Diasulin	Himalaya	*Cassia auriculata, Coccinia indica, Curcuma longa, Emblica officinalis, Gymnema sylvestre, Momordica charantia, Scoparia dulcis, Syzygium cumini, Tinospora cordifolia, Trigonella foenum graecum*
Pancreatic tonic 180 cp	Ayurvedic herbal Supplement	*Pterocarpus marsupium, Gymnema sylvestre, Momordica charantia, Syzygium cumini, Trigonella foenum graceum, Azadirachta indica, Ficus racemosa, Aegle marmelos, Cinnamomum tamala*
Ayurveda alternative herbal formula to Diabetes	Chakrapani Ayurveda	Gurmar (*Gymnema sylvestre*) Karela (*Momordica charantia*) Pushkarmool (*Inula racemosa*) Jamun Gutli (*Syzygium cumini*) Neem (*Azadirachta indica*) Methika (*Trigonella foenum gracecum*) Guduchi (*Tinospora cordifolia*)
Bitter gourd powder	Garry and Sun Natural Remedies	Bitter gourd (*Momordica charantia*)
Dia-care	Admark Herbals Limited	Sanjeevan Mool; Himej, Jambu beej, Kadu, Namejav, Neem chal.
Diabetes-Daily care	Nature's Health Supply	Alpha Lipoic Acid, Cinnamon 4% Extract, Chromax, Vanadium, Fenugreek 50% extract, *Gymnema sylvestre* 25% extract Momordica 7% extract, Licorice Root 20% extract
Gurmar powder	Garry and Sun Natural Remedies	Gurmar (*Gymnema sylvestre*)
Epinsulin	Swastik Formulations	Vijaysar (*Pterocarpus marsupium*)
Diabecure	Nature beaute sante	*Juglans regia, Berberis vulgaris, Erytherea centaurium*, Millefolium, Taraxacum
Diabeta	Ayurvedic cure Ayurvedic Herbal Health Products	*Gymnema sylvestre, Vinca rosea* (Periwinkle), *Curcuma longa* (Turmeric), *Azadirachta indica* (Neem), *Pterocarpus marsupium* (Kino Tree), *Momordica charantia* (Bitter Gourd), *Syzygiumcumini* (Black Plum), *Acacia arabica* (Black Babhul), *Tinospora cordifolia, Zingiber officinale* (Ginger)
Syndrex	Plethico Laboretaries	Germinated Fenugreek seed extract

TABLE 15.4 *(Continued)*

Drug	Company	Ingredients
Diabecure	Nature beaute sante	*Berberis vulgaris*, Millefolium, *Juglans regia, Erytherea centaurium*, Taraxacum
Epinsulin	Swastik Formulations	Vijaysar (*Pterocarpus marsupium*)
Madhumeha Kusumakara Rasa	Shree Dhoothapapeshwar Limited	Vasant Kusumakar Rasa (Suvarnayukta), Mamajjaka ghana (Dried Aq. extract of *Enicostemma littorale*), Haridra (*Curcuma longa*), Amalaki *(Emblica officinalis)*, Shuddha Shilajatu (Processed asphaltum), Guduchi (*Tinospora cordifolia*), Yashada bhasma (*Zinc bhasma*), Bilva patra swaras (*Aegle marmelos),* Asana kwath (*Pterocarpus marsupium*)
Zpter	Om Pharmaceuticals Limited	Vijayasara, Dalchini, Haridra, Haritaki, Bibhitaki, Amalaki, Chtrak, Jasad Bhasma, Guduchi (*Tinospora cordifolia*) and Madhunashini (*Gymnema sylvestre*).
Hyponidd	Charak Pharma	Yashad Bhasma (Zinc Calx), Shilajit (Purified Asphaltum), Karela (*Momordica charantia*, bitter gourd), Haridra (*Curcuma longa*, turmeric), Tarwar (*Cassia auriculata,* Avarakkai, Indian broad-beans), Amalaki (Amla, Indian Gooseberry, *Emblica officinalis*), Raja Jambu (*Eugenia jambolana*), Mamejavo (*Enicostemma littorale*), Meshashringi (*Gymnema sylvestre*), Vijaysaar (*Pterocarpus marsupium*), Guduchi (*Tinospora cordifolia*), Neem (*Melia azadirachta*), Kirat Tikta (*Swertia chirata*)
Dabur Madhu Rakshak	Dabur	Amla (*phyllanthus emblica*), Tejpatra (*Cinnamomum tamala*), Vijaysar (*Pterocarpus marsupium*), Gurmar (*Gymnema sylvestre*), Jamum seed (*Eugenia jambolana*), Kali marich (*piper nigrum*), Neem leaves (*azadiracheta indiaca*), Methi (*trigonella foenum-graecum*), Bahera (*Terminalia belerica*), Bhavana Dravyas, Shudh Shilajit, karela fruit (*momordica charantia*), Hareetaki (*Terminalia chebula*)

TABLE 15.4   *(Continued)*

Drug	Company	Ingredients
Ojamin	Tates remedies	*Aegle Marmelos, Trigonella Foenum Graecum, Carum Carvi, Emblica Offcinails, Terminalia Chebula, Terminalia Belarica, Swertia Chirata, Tinospora Cordifolia, Eugenia Jambolana, Picrorhiza Kurroa, Gymnema Sylvestre, Salacia Chinensis* Linn, *Curcuma Longa, Melia Azadirachta*
Madhumehari granules	Baidyanath	Gudmar (*Gymnema sylvestre*), Jamun guthali (*Syzygium cumini*), Gulvel (*Tinospora cordifolia*), Kkarela Beej (*Momordica charantia*), Khadir Chuma (*Acacla Catechu*), Haldi (*Curcuma longa*), Amia (*Emblica officinalis*), vijay-sar (*Pterocarpus marsupium*), Tejpatra (*Cinnamomum tamala*), Shilajit (Asphaltum), Gularphal Chuma (*Ficus glomerata*), Kutki (*Picrorhiza kurroa*), Chitrak (*Plumbago zeylanica*), Methi (*Trigonella-foenum graecum*), Bhavna of Neem Patti (*Azadirachta indica*), Bilwa Patra (*Aegle marmelos)*
Glucomap tablet	Maharishi Ayurved	*Enicostemma littorale, Phyllanthus niruri, Eugenia jambolana* (leaf), *Eugenia jambolana* (seed), *Azadirachta indica, Terminalia arjuna, Aegle marmelos, Asphaltum,* Processed in the aqueous extract of Bilva *(Aegle marmelos),* Karavellaka *(Momordica cherantia)* and Salsaradigan.

15.10   CONCLUSION

The chapter highlighted the hypoglycemic potentials of various antidia-betic Indian plants and numerous products such as Diabecon, Diabecure, Dia-care, Diabeta, Hyponidd, Ojamin, Syndrex, Zpter, and so on which work on the traditional principles of Ayurveda that correlates in modern medicine by modulating several biological molecular targets such as peroxisome proliferator-activated receptor-γ (PPAR-γ), dipeptidyl pepti-dase-4 (DPP-4), α-glucosidase, aldose reductase (ALR), protein tyrosine phosphatase-1B (PTP1B), and so on. The chapter will provide information of the antidiabetic plant extracts and products utilizing both modern approach and inspiration from the traditional Ayurvedic principles.

KEYWORDS

- hypoglycemic
- antihyperglycemic
- Ayurveda
- traditional knowledge
- pharmaceutical products
- plant extracts
- traditional medicine

REFERENCES

Agarwal, S. P.; Khanna, R.; Karmarkar, R; Anwer, M. K., Khar, R. K. Shilajit: A Review. *Phytother. Res.* **2007,** *21* (5), 401–415.

Ahamad, J.; Amin, S.; Mir, S. R. Development and Validation of HPTLC Densitometric Method for Estimation of Charantin in *Momordica charantia* Fruits and Herbal Formulation. *J. Pharmacogn. Phytochem.* **2014,** *2* (5), 172–176.

Ahamad, J.; Amin, S.; Mir, S. R. Simultaneous Quantification of Gymnemic Acid as Gymnemagenin and Charantin as β-Sitosterol Using Validated HPTLC Densitometric Method. *J. Chromatogr. Sci.* **2015,** *53* (7), 1203–1209.

Ahmad, J.; Muneer, A. M.; Mohd, A.; Rauf, R.; Rafiq, A.; Ashfaq, A.; Sheikh, D. Prevalence of DM and its Associated Risk Factors in Age Group of 20 Years and above in Kashmir. *Al. Ameen J. Med. Sci.* **2011,** *4* (1), 38–44.

Ahmed, A. B; Rao, A. S.; Rao, M. V.; Taha, R. M. HPTLC/HPLC and Gravimetric Methodology for the Identification and Quantification of Gymnemic Acid from *Gymnema sylvestre* Methanolic Extracts. *Acta Chromatographica.* **2013,** *25* (2), 1–23.

Ajgaonkar, S. S. Herbal Drugs in the Treatment of Diabetes. *Int. Diabetes Federation Bulletin.* **1979,** *24,* 10–17.

Alarcon, F. J.; Jimenez, M.; Reyes, R. Hypoglycemic Effects of Extracts and Fractions from Psacalium Decompositum in Healthy and Alloxan Diabetic Mice. *J. Ethnopharmacol.* **2000,** *72,* 21–27.

Alarcon-Aguilara, F. J.; Roman-Ramos, R.; Perez-Gutierrez, S.; Aguilar-Contreras, A.; Contreras-Weber, C. C.; Flores-Saenz, J. L. Study of the Antihyperglycemic Effect of Plants used as Anti-Diabetics. *J. Ethnopharmacol.* **1998,** *61,* 101–110.

Alberti, G. Non Communicable Diseases Tomorrows Pandemic. *Bulletin World Health Organ.* **2001,** *79* (10), 907.

American Diabetes Association-2011. Standards of Medical Care in Diabetes—2011. *Diabetes Care* **2011**, *34*, Supplement 1, S11–S61.

Anand, A. V.; Divya, N.; Kotti, P. P. An Updated Review of Terminalia Catappa. *Pharmacogn. Rev.* **2015**, *9* (18), 93–98.

Anandharajan, R.; Jaiganesh, S.; Shankernarayanan, N. P.; Viswakarma, R. A.; Balakrishnan, A. In vitro glucose uptake activity of *Aegles marmelos* and *Syzygium cumini* by activation of Glut-4, PI3 kinase and PPARgamma in L6 myotubes. *Phytomedicine* **2006**, *13* (6), 434–441.

Aparajeya, P.; Jena, S.; Sahu, P. K.; Nayak, S.; Padhi, P. Effect of Polyherbal Mixtures on the Treatment of Diabetes. *Endocrinology 2013*, 934797, 5.

Arlan, R.; Janet, H. S. Type 2 Diabetes in Children and Adolescents: A Clinician's Guide to Diagnosis, Epidemiology, Pathogenesis, Prevention, and Treatment. American Diabetes Association, U. S. A. 2003.

Ashtang Hradayam, Srikanthamurthy K. Krishnadas Academy, Varanasi, U. P. India, 1998; pp 479–484.

Ashtang Hridayam Sarwanga Sundar Vyakhya; Vaidya, P. H., Ed.; Krishnadas Academy: Varanasi, Reprint 2000; p 504.

Aswal, B. S.; Goel, A. K; Kulshrestha, D. K.; Mehrotra, B. N.; Patnaik, G. K. *Indian J. Exp. Biol.* **1996**, *34*, 444.

Aulton, M. E. *Pharmaceutics: The Science of Dosage Form Design*, 2nd ed.; Churchill Livingstone: London, 2002.

Ayurveda Sarsangrah. 20th ed.; Shri Baidhnath Ayurveda Bhawan Ltd.: Nagpur, 2000; pp 1–131.

Ayurvedia Dravyaguna Vidnyan (Tr). The Team Bhartiya Vidya Bhawan's Swami Prakashananda Ayurveda Research Centre, 2000; p 524.

Ayurvedic Pharmacopoeia of India, Part I. Government of India, Ministry of Health and Family Welfare, Department of Indian Systems of Medicine and Homoeopathy: New Delhi, India, 2001; Vol. I.

Ayurvedic Pharmacopoeia of India, Part I. Government of India, Ministry of Health and Family Welfare, Department of Indian Systems of Medicine and Homoeopathy: New Delhi, India, 2001a; Vol. II.

Babish, J. G.; Pacioretty, L. M.; Bland, J. S.; Minich, D. M.; Hu, J.; Tripp, M. L. Anti-Diabetic Screening of Commercial Botanical Products in 3T3-L1 Adipocytes and db/db Mice. *J. Med. Food* **2010**, *13* (3), 535–547.

Badole, S. L; Shah, S. N.; Patel, N. M.; Thakurdesai, P. A.; Bodhankar, S. L. Hypoglycemic Activity of Aqueous Extract of Pleurotus pulmonarius in Alloxan- Induced Diabetic Mice. *Pharm. Biol.* **2006**, *44*, 421–425.

Bailey, C. J.; Day, C. Traditional Plant Medicines as Treatments for Diabetes. *Diabetes Care* **1989**, *12*, 553–564.

Baliga, M. S.; Fernandes, S.; Thilakchand, K. R.; D'souza, P.; Rao, S. Scientific Validation of the Anti-Diabetic Effects of Syzygium jambolanum DC (Black Plum), a Traditional Medicinal Plant of India. *J. Altern. Complement. Med.* **2013**, *19* (3), 191–197.

Banga, K.; Rajbir, S.; Anitha, K.; Navjot, K. Efficiency of Chromium Supplementation and Nutrition Counseling on the Anthropometric Profile of NIDDM Subjects. *Indian J. Nutr. Diet.* **2005**, *42*, 549–555.

Bastaki, S. Review: DM and its Treatment. *Int. J. Diabetes Metab.* **2005**, *13*, 111–134.

Belapurkar, P.; Goyal, P.; Tiwari-Barua, P. Immunomodulatory Effects of Triphala and its Individual Constituents: A Review. *Indian J. Pharm. Sci.* **2014,** *76* (6), 467–475.

Bellamy, I. J. *The Infra Red Spectra of Complex Molecules*; John Willey and Sons, Inc.: New York, 1962; p 398.

Bhaisajyaratnavali. 2nd ed.; Chowkhamba Sanskrit Series office: Varanasi, 1961, sloke no.149–150, p 163.

Bhaishajya Ratnawali. Shashtri, R. D., Ed.; Choukhamba Sanskrit Sansthan Varanasi, 1985.

Bharti, M. S; Singh, R. H. Constitutional Study of Patients of DM visà- vis Madhumeha. *Ancient Sci. Life.* **1995,** *15* (1), 35.

Bhatt, A. D.; Bhatt, N. S. Indigenous Drugs and Liver Disease. *Indian J. Gastroenterol.* **1996,** *15*, 63.

Bhattacharjee, S. No One Can Eat Just One Diet, Diseases and the Media in a Consumerist Society. *J. Indian Med. Assoc.* **2004,** *102* (8), 457.

Bhope, S. G.; Dheeraj, H.; Nagore, T.; Vinod, V.; Kuber, L.; Gupta, P. K.; Patil, M. J. Design and Development of a Stable Polyherbal Formulation Based on the Results of Compatibility Studies. *Pharmacog. Res.* **2011,** *3* (2), 122–129.

Bisht, S.; Sisodia, S. S. Assessment of Anti-Diabetic Potential of Cinnamomum tamala Leaves Extract in Streptozotocin Induced Diabetic Rats. *Indian J. Pharmacol.* **2011,** *43* (5), 582–585.

Bohannon, N. J. V. Treating Dual Defects in Diabetes: Insulin Resistance and Insulin Secretion. *Am. J. Health Syst. Pharm.* **2002,** *59,* S9–S13.

Burnett, A.; McKoy, M. L.; Singh, P. Investigation of the Blood Glucose Lowering Potential of the Jamaican Momordica charantia (Cerasee) Fruit in Sprague-Dawley Rats. *West Indian Med J.* **2015,** *64* (4), 315–319.

Chandaraju, A. Follow the Golden Mean, The Hindu, (Magazine) 2005 (Nov.20), p 7.

Chandel H. S; Pathak, A. K.; Tailang, M. Standardization of Some Herbal Anti-Diabetic Drugs in Polyherbal Formulation. *Pharmacogn. Res.* **2011,** *3* (1), 49–56.

Chandola, H. M.; Tripathi, S. N.; Udupa, K. N. Variations in the Progression of Maturity Onset Diabetes According to Body Constitution. *Ancient Sci. Life.* **1994,** *13* (3–4), 293.

Chen, H.; Guo, J.; Pang, B.; Zhao, L.; Tong, X. Application of Herbal Medicines with Bitter Flavor and Cold Property on Treating DM. *Evid Based Complement Alternat. Med.* **2015,** *2015*, 529491.

Choudhary, B. The New International Seed Treaty: Promises and Prospects for Food Security. *Curr. Sci.* **2002,** *83*, 366–369.

Costa, P. Lobo Sousa JM. Modeling and Comparison of Dissolution Profile. *Eur. J. Pharm. Sci.* **2001,** *13*, 123–133.

Crawford, J. M; Cotran, R. S. The Pancreas, in Robins Pathological Basis of Disease; Cotran, R. S., Kumar, V., Collins, T., Eds.; W.B. Saunders: New York, 1999; p 20.

Dallaqua, B.; Saito, F. H.; Rodrigues, T.; Calderon, I. M.; Rudge, M. V.; Herrera, E.; Damasceno, D. C. Treatment with Azadirachta indica in Diabetic Pregnant Rats: Negative Effects on Maternal Outcome. *J. Ethnopharmacol.* **2012,** *143* (3), 805–811.

Dandagi, P. M.; Patil, M. B.; Mastiholimath, V. S.; Gadad, A. P.; Dhumansure, R. H. Development and Evaluation of Hepatoprotective Polyherbal Formulation Containing Some Indigenous Medicinal Plants. *Indian J. Pharm. Sci.* **2008,** *70* (2), 265–268.

Dev, S. Ancient-Modern Concordance in Ayurvedic Plants: Some Examples. *Environ. Health Perspect.* **1999,** *107*, 783–789.

Devaki, K.; Beulah, U.; Akila, G.; Narmadha, R.; Gopalakrishnan, V. K. Glucose Lowering Effect of Aqueous Extract of Bauhinia tomentosa L. on Alloxan Induced Type 2 DM in Wistar Albino Rats. *J. Basic Clin. Pharm.* **2011**, *2*, 167–174.

Devaraj, V. C.; Gopala Krishna, B.; Viswanatha, G. L.; Jagadish Kamath, V.; Sanjay Kumar. Hepatoprotective Activity of Hepax-A polyherbal Formulation. *Asian Pac. J. Trop. Biomed.* **2011**, *1* (2), 142–146.

Dhanukar, R. A.; Kulkarni, R. A; Rege, N. N. Pharmacology of Medicinal Plants and Natural Products. *Indian J. Pharmacol.* **2000**, *32*, S81.

Dhanukar, S., and Thatte U.M., Ayurveda revisited. 3rd ed. Popular Prakashan, Mumbai, 2000.

Donald, M. M.; Arthur, P. G. Botanical Medicines the Need for New Regulations. *New Eng. J. Med.* **2002**, *347* (25), 2073–2076.

Dong, M. W. Practical HPLC for Practicing Scientists, Wiley-Inters Science, 2001; 5–7, 16–39.

D'souza, J. J.; D'souza, P. P.; Fazal, F.; Kumar, A.; Bhat, H. P.; Baliga, M. S. Anti-Diabetic Effects of the Indian Indigenous Fruit Emblica officinalis Gaertn: Active Constituents and Modes of Action. *Food Funct.* **2014**, *5* (4), 635–644.

Dubey, N. K.; Rajeshkumar, T. P. Global Promotion of Herbal Medicine: India's Opportunity. *Curr. Sci.* **2004**, *86*, 37–41.

Duraiswamy, A.; Shanmugasundaram, D.; Sasikumar, C. S.; Cherian, S. M.; Cherian, K. M. Development of an Anti-Diabetic Formulation (ADJ6) and its Inhibitoryactivity Against a-Amylase and a-Glucosidase. *J. Tradit. Complement Med.* **2016**, *6* (3), 204–208.

Dwivedi, G.; Dwivedi, S. History of Medicine: Sushruta—the Clinician—Teacher Par Excellence. *Indian J. Chest. Dis. Allied Sci.* **2007**, *49*, 243–244.

Elamthuruthy, A. T.; Shah, C. R.; Khan, T. A.; Tatke, P. A.; Gabhe, S. Y. Standardization of Marketed Kumariasava—An Ayurvedic Aloe Vera Product. *J. Pharm. Biomed. Anal.* **2005**, *29*, *37* (5), 937–941.

Elder, C. Ayurveda for DM: A Review of the Biomedical Literature. *Altern. Ther. Health Med.* **2004**, *10* (11), 44–50.

Elizabeth, A M.; Makol, N. Diabetes-The Silent Killer Disease. *Health Action* **2005**, *18*, 4–7.

ESCOP (European Scientific Cooperative on Phytotherapy), The Scientific Foundation for Herbal Medicinal Products, completely revised and expanded, 2nd ed.; Georg Thieme Verlag: Germany, 2003.

Fan, T. Y.; Wall, G. M.; Sternitzke, K.; Bass, L.; Morton, A. B.; Muegge, E. Improved High Performance Liquid Chromatographic Determination of Pilocarpine and its Degradation Products in Ophthalmic Solutions Importance of Octadecylsilane Column Choice. *J. Chromatogr. A* **1996**, *740*, 289–295.

Fernandes, N. P.; Lagishetty, C. V.; Panda, V. S.; Naik, S. R. An Experimental Evaluation of the Anti-Diabetic and Antilipidemic Properties of a Standardized Momordica Charantia Fruit Extract. *BMC Complement Altern. Med.* **2007**, *24*, 7–29.

Fowler, M. J. Microvascular and Macrovascular Complications of Diabetes. *Clin. Diabetes* **2008**, *26*, 77–82.

Frank, L.; Engelgace, M. M.; Thompson, T. J.; Smith, P. J.; Herman, W. H.; Gunter, E. W. Screening for DM in Adults: The Utility Of Random Capillary Blood Glucose Measurements. *Diabetes Care* **2003**, *18*, 463–466.

Frode, T. S.; Medeiros, Y. S. Animal Models to Test Drugs with Potential Anti-Diabetic Activity. *J. Ethnopharmacol.* **2008,** *115* (2), 173–183.

Furniss, B. S., et al. Vogel's "Textbook of Practical Organic Chemistry", 5th ed; Pearson Education, 2004; pp 256.

Galani, V. J.; Patel, B. G.; Rana, D. G. *Sphaeranthus indicus* Linn.: A Phytopharmacological Review. *Int. J. Ayurveda Res.* **2010,** *1* (4), 247–253.

Geevarghese, P. J. *A Hand Book Of Diabetes*, Chapters 2–9; KM Varghese Co: Bombay, 1976; pp 3–43.

Ghaisas, M.; Zope, V.; Takawale, A.; Navghare, V.; Tanwar, M.; Deshpande, A. Preventive Effect of *Sphaeranthus indicus* During Progression of Glucocorticoid-Induced Insulin Resistance in Mice. *Pharm. Biol.* **2010,** *48* (12), 1371–1375.

Gibson, M. Pharmaceutical Preformulation and Formulation: A Practical Guide from Candidate Drug Selection to Commercial Dosage Form; CRC Press: Boca Raton, 2001.

Green, K. H.; Aubert, R.; Herman, W. Prevalence, Numerical Estimates and Projections, Diabetes Research and Clinical Practice. *Global Burd. 1995-2005.* **2003,** *59,* 37–42.

Grover, J. K.; Vats, V.; Rathi, S. S. Amelioration of Experimental Diabetic Neuropathy and Gastropathy in Rats Following Oral Administration of Plants (*Eugenia jambolana, Mucuna Purines* and *Tinospora cardifolia*) Extracts. *Ind. J. Exp. Bio.* **2002,** *40* (3), 273–276.

Grover, J. K.; Vats, V.; Rathi, S. S.; Dawar, R. Traditional Indian Anti-Diabetic Plants Attenuate Renal Hypertrophy, Urine Volume and Albuminuria in Streptozotocin Induced Diabetic Mice. *J. Ethnopharmacol.* **2001,** *76,* 233–238.

Grover, J. K.; Yadav, S.; Vats, V. Medicinal Plants of INDIA with Anti-Diabetic Potential. *J. Ethnopharmacol.* **2002,** *81* (1), 81–100.

Gubbannavar, J. S.; Chandola, H.; Harisha, C. R.; Kalyani, R.; Shukla, V. J. Analytical Profile of Brahmi Ghrita: A Polyherbal Ayurvedic Formulation. *J. Ayu.* **2012,** *33* (2), 289–293.

Gupta, S. P.; Garg, G. Quantitative Estimation of Gallic Acid and Tannic Acid in Bhuvnesvara Vati by RP-HPLC. *Pharm. Lett.* **2014,** *6* (2), 31–36.

Gupta, S. S. Prospects and Perspectives of Natural Plants Products in Medicine. *Indian J. Pharmacol.* **1994,** *26* (1), 1–12.

Hankey, A. The Scientific Value of Ayurveda. *J. Altern. Complement. Med.* **2005,** *11* (2), 221–225.

Hilarg. Asian Diabetes Prevalence. *Am. Diabetes Assoc.* **2003,** *98,* 121–122.

Hoffman, E. *Thin Layer Chromatography.* 2nd ed.; 1966, p 165.

Hossain, M. D.; Sarwar, M. S.; Dewan, S. M.; Hossain, M. S.; Shahid-Ud-Daula, A.; Islam, M. S. Investigation of Total Phenolic Content and Antioxidant Activities of Azadirachta Indica Roots. *Avicenna J. Phytomed.* **2014,** *4* (2), 97–102.

Humber, J. M. The Role of Complementary and Alternative Medicine: Accommodating Pluralism. *J. Am. Med. Assoc.* **2002,** *288,* 1655–1656.

ICH 2005 Validation of Analytical Procedures: Text and Methodology. ICH-Q2 (R1), International Conference on Harmonization: Geneva.

ICH Guidelines (1993). Stability Testing of New Drug Substances and Products, 27th October, 1993.

ICH Topic Q 2 (R1) International Conference on Harmonisation. Validation of Analytical Procedures: Text and Methodology. http://www.ich.org.

IDF. International Diabetes Federation, Diabetes Atlas, 4th ed.; Belgium, 2009, pp 1–105. www.diabetesatlas.org.

Indian Herbal Pharmacopoeia. Regional Research Laboratory, Jammu and Indian Drug Manufacturers' Assn.: Mumbai, 1998; Vol. I and II.

Irwin, N.; Clarke, G. C.; Green, B. D.; Greer, B.; Harriot, P.; Gault, V. A.; et al. Evaluation of the Anti-Diabetic Activity of DPP IV Resistant N-Terminally Modified Versus Mid-Chain Acylated Analogues of Glucose-Dependent Insulinotropic Polypeptide. *Biochem. Pharmacol.* **2006,** *72,* 719–728.

Itankar, P. R.; Sawant, D. B.; Tauqeer, M.; Charde, S. S. High Performance Thin Layer Chromatography Fingerprinting, Phytochemical and Physico-Chemical Studies of Anti-Diabetic Herbal Extracts. *AYU* **2015,** *36* (2), 188–195.

Ivorra, M. D.; Payaa, M.; Villarb, A. A Review of Natural Products and Plants as Potential Hypoglycemic Drugs. *J. Ethnopharmacol.* **1989,** *27,* 243–275.

Jafri, M. A.; Aslam, M.; Javed, K.; Singh, S. Effect of Punica granatum Linn. (Flowers) on Blood Glucose Level in Normal and Alloxan Induced Diabetic Rats. *J. Ethnopharmacol.* **2000,** *70,* 309–314.

Jafri, M. A.; Aslam, M.; Javed, K.; Singh, S. Effect of *Punica granatum* Linn. (Flowers) on Blood Glucose Level in Normal and Alloxan Induced Diabetic Rats. *J. Ethnopharmacol.* **2000,** *70,* 309–314.

Jain, S.; Koka, S.; Gupta, A.; Barik, R.; Malviya, N. Standardization of "Chopchiniyadi Churna": An Ayurvedic Polyherbal Formulation. *Phcog. J.* **2010,** *2* (5), 1–5.

Jalpa, J.; Desai, P.; Desai, V. HPTLC and Bioautography Analysis of *Casuarina equisetifolia* L. and *Sphaeranthus indicus* Extracts Against Salmonella spp. *Biotec. Res. J.* **2015,** *1* (2), 132–134.

Jayakumar, R. V.; Nisha, B. Prevention of DM. *Health Action* **2005,** *18* (6), 19–25.

John, E. B. Miscellaneous Mycoses and Algal Infections. In *Harrisons Principles of Internal Medicine*; 16th ed., Mc Graw-Hill publications, 2004; pp 1180–1181.

Joshi, N.; Caputo, M. G.; Weitekamp, R. M.; Karchmer, A. W. Infections in Patients with DM. *New Engl. J. Med.* **1999,** *341,* 1906–1912.

Joy, K. L.; Kuttan, R. Anti-Diabetic Activity of *Picrorrhiza kurroa* Extract. *J. Ethnopharmacol.* **1999,** *167,* 143–148.

Jude, E.; Okokon, B.; Antia, S.; John Udobang, A. Anti-diabetic Activities of Ethanolic Extract and Fraction of Anthocleista Djalonensis. *Asian Pac. J. Trop. Biomed.* **2012,** *2* (6), 461–464.

Kajaria, D. K.; Gangwar, M.; Kumar, D.; Kumar Sharma, A.; Tilak, R.; Nath, G., Tripathi, Y. B.; Tripathi, J. S.; Tiwari, S. K. Evaluation of Antimicrobial Activity and Bronchodialator Effect of a Polyherbal Drug-Shrishadi. *Asian Pac. J. Trop. Biomed.* **2012,** *2* (11), 905–909.

Kalaiselvan, V.; Shah, A. K.; Patel, F. B.; Shah, C. N.; Kalaivani, M.; Rajasekaran, A. Quality Assessment of Different Marketed Brands of Dasamoolaristam, an Ayurvedic formulation. *Int. J. Ayurveda Res.* **2010,** *1* (1), 10–13.

Kamalakkannan, N.; Mainzen, S.; Prince, P. Effect of *Aegle marmelos* Correa. (Bael) Fruit Extract on Tissue Antioxidants in Streptozotocindiabetic Rats. *Indian J. Exp. Biol.* **2003,** *41* (11), 1285–1288.

Kar, A.; Choudhary, B. K.; Bandyopadhyay, N. G. Comparative Evaluation of Hypoglycaemic Activity of Some Indian Medicinal Plants in Alloxandiabetic Rats. *J. Ethnopharmacol.* **2003**, *84* (1), 105–108.

Kar, C. A.; Upadhyay, B. N.; Ojha, D. Prognosis of Prameha on the Basis of Insulin Level. *Anc. Sci. Life* **1997**, *16*, 277–281.

Kellar, M. C.; J. D., Keith, H.; John, P. D. Depression Increases Diabetes Symptoms by Complicating Patients Self-Care Adherence. *Diabetes Educ.* **2004**, *30*, 485–492.

Khandal, S. Rasa Bhaisajya Kalpana Vigyan, 7th ed; Publication Scheme: Jaipur, 2006, 409.

Kokate, C. K. *Practical Pharmacognosy*; Vallabh Prakashan: New Delhi, *1994*, 107–113.

Kompoti, M. Diabetic Foot Infections: Risk Factors and Microbiological Spectrum. *Eur. Soc. Clin. Microbiol. Infect. Dis.* **2004**, *902*, 1441.

Krithika, R.; Verma, R. J.; Shrivastav, P. S.; Suguna, L. Phyllanthin of Standardized Phyllanthus amarus Extract Attenuates Liver Oxidative Stress in Mice and Exerts Cytoprotective Activity on Human Hepatoma Cell Line. *J. Clin. Exp. Hepatol.* **2011**, *1* (2), 57–67.

Kumar, G. V.; Kalia, A. N. Development of Polyherbal Anti-Diabetic Formulation Encapsulated in the Phospholipids Vesicle System. *J. Adv. Pharm. Technol. Res.* **2013**, *4* (2), 108–117.

Kumar, V.; Bhandari, U.; Tripathi, C. D.; Khanna, G. Protective Effect of Gymnema Sylvestre Ethanol Extracts on High Fat Diet-Induced Obese Diabetic Wistar Rats. *Indian J. Pharm. Sci.* **2014**, *76* (4), 315–322.

Kurian, G. A.; Manjusha, V.; Nair, S. S.; Varghese, T. P. *J. Nutr.* **2014**, *30* (10), 1158–1164.

Kuzuya, T.; Stoichi, N.; Jo, S.; Yasunori, K.; Yasuhiko, I.; Masashi, K.; Kishio, N.; Akira, S.; Yutaka, S. Report of the Committee on the Classification and Diagnostic Criteria of DM. *Diabetes Res. Clin. Pract.* **2002**, *55*, 65–85.

Lachman, L.; Liberman, H. A.; Kanig, J. L. *The Theory and Practice of Industrial Pharmacy*, 3rd ed.; Varghese publishing House: Bombay, 1999; pp 443–453.

Lad, V. S. *Fundamental Principles of Ayurveda*; The Ayurvedic Press: Albuquerque, New Mexico, 2002; pp 25–29.

Ladva, B. J.; Mahida, V. M.; Kantaria, U. D.; Gokani, R. H. Marker Based Standardization of Polyherbal Formulation (SJT-DI-02) by High Performance Thin Layer Chromatography Method. *J. Pharm. Bioallied. Sci.* **2014**, *6* (3), 213–219.

Lanjhiyana, S.; Patra, K. C.; Ahirwar, D.; Rana, A. C.; Lanjhiyana, S. K. A Validated HPTLC Method for Simultaneous Estimation of Two Marker Compounds in *Aegle marmelos* (L.) Corr., (Rutaceae) Root Bark. *Pharm. Lettre.* **2012**, *4* (1), 92–97.

Lazarowych, N. J.; Pekos, P. Use of Fingerprinting and Marker Compounds for Identification and Standardization of Botanical Drugs: Strategies for Applying Pharmaceutical HPLC Analysis to Herbal Products. *Drug Inf. J.* **1998**, *32*, 497–512.

Makhija, I. K.; Shreedhara, C. S.; Ram, H. H. Physico-Chemical Standardization of Sitopaladi Churna. *Anc. Sci. Life* **2012**, *31* (3), 107–116.

Manik, S.; Gauttam, V.; Kalia, A. N. Anti-Diabetic and Anti-Hyperlipidemic Effect of Allopolyherbal Formulation in OGTT and STZ-Induced Diabetic Rat Model. *Indian J. Exp. Biol.* **2013**, *51* (9), 702–708.

McNeill, J. H. *Experimental Models of Diabetes*; CRC Press: United States of America, 1999; p 2–5.

Mishra, A.; Srivastava, R.; Srivastava, S. P.; Gautam, S.; Tamrakar, A. K.; Maurya, R.; Srivastava, A. K. Anti-Diabetic Activity of Heart Wood of Pterocarpus marsupium Roxb. and Analysis of Phytoconstituents. *Indian J. Exp. Biol.* **2013**, *51* (5), 363–374.

Mishra, L. C.; Adra, T. DM (Madhumeha). In *Scientific Basis for Ayurvedic Therapies;* Mishra, L. C., Ed.; CRC Press: Boca Raton, 2004; pp 101–131.

Mithal, B. M. A Textbook of Forensic Pharmacy, 10th ed.; Vallabh Prakashan: Delhi, 2002; pp 186–187.

Modak, M.; Dixit, P.; Londhe, J.; Ghaskadbi, S.; Devasagayam, T. P. Indian Herbs and Herbal Drugs used for the Treatment of Diabetes. *J. Clin. Biochem. Nutr.* **2007**, *40* (3), 163–173.

Mohan, V.; Gundu, H. R.; Rao, P. *Type 2 Diabetes in South Asians: Epidemiology, Risk Factors and Prevention*; Jaypee Brothers Medical Publishers: New Delhi, 2007; pp 138–152.

Mopuri, R.; Ganjayi, M.; Banavathy, K. S.; Parim, B. N.; Meriga, B. Evaluation of Anti-Obesity Activities of Ethanolic Extract of Terminalia paniculata Bark on High Fat Diet-Induced Obese Rats. *BMC Complement Altern. Med.* **2015**, *24* (15), 76.

Moran, A. Type 1 Diabetes CME, Diabetes, University of Minnesota, 2009, (www.cme.umn.edu/cme/ online/diabetes /posttest).

Kunga, M. R.; Pachamuthu, V.; Chindambaram, U.; Natarajan, S.; Elango, B.; Jaiganesh, S. Anti-Diabetic Activity of Alcoholic Stem Extracts of Gymnema montanum in Streptozotocin Induced Diabetic Rats. *Food Chem. Technol.* **2011**, *49* (12), 3390–3394.

Mukherjee, P. K. Evaluation of Indian Traditional Medicine. *Drug Inf. J.* **2001**, *35*, 631–640.

Mukherjee, P. K; Maiti, K.; Mukherjee, K.; Houghton, P. J. Leads from Indian Medicinal Plants with Hypoglycemic Potentials. *J Ethnopharmacol.* **2006**, *106* (1), 1–28.

Mukherjee, P. K.; Wahile, A. Integrated Approaches Towards Drug Development from Ayurveda and other Indian System of Medicines. *J. Etheanpharmacol.* **2006**, *103* (1), 25–35.

Mukherjee, P. K. Marker Analysis of Polyherbal Formulation, Triphala—a Well Known Indian Traditional Medicine. *Indian J. Tradit. Knowl.* **2008**, *7* (3), 379–383.

Mukhtar, H. M.; Ansari, S. H.; Ali, M.; Bhat, Z. A.; Naved, T. Effect of Aqueous Extract of *Pterocarpus marsupium* Wood on Alloxan-Induced Diabetic Rats. *Pharmazie* **2005**, *60* (6), 478–479.

Nagappa, A. N; Thakurdesai, P. A.; Venkat Rao, N.; Singh, J. Anti-Diabetic Activity of *Terminalia Catappa* Linn Fruit. *J. Ethnopharmacol.* **2003**, *88*, 45–50.

Nagarajan, N. S.; Murugesh, N.; Thirupathy, K. P.; Radha, N.; Murali, A. Anti-Diabetic and Antihyhyperlipidemic Effects of *Cleome feline. Fitoterapia* **2005**, *76*, 310–315.

Neeraj, K.; Sriwastava, C. S.; Shreedhara, H. N. Aswatha Ram Standardization of Ajmodadi Churna, a Polyherbal Formulation. *Pharmacog Res.* **2010**, *2* (2), 98–101.

Nkobole, N.; Houghton, P. J.; Hussein, A.; Lall, N. Anti-Diabetic Activity of Terminalia Sericea Constituents. *Nat. Prod. Commun.* **2011**, *6* (11), 1585–1588.

Ornish, D. Prevalence of DM. *Am. J. Clin. Nutr.* **2004**, *49*, 9–10.

Patel, D. K.; Prasad, S. K; Kumar, R.; Hemalatha, S. An Overview on Anti-Diabetic Medicinal Plants having Insulin Mimetic Property. *Asian Pac. J. Trop. Biomed.* **2012**, *2* (4), 320–330.

Patwardhan, B. Ayurveda for All: 11 Action Points for 2011. *J. Ayurveda Integr. Med.* **2010**, *1* (4), 237–239.

Patwardhan, B.; Vaidya, A.; Chorghade, M. Ayurveda and Natural Products Drug Discovery. *Curr. Sci.* **2004**, *86* (6), 789–799.

Paulose, K. P. Control of DM. *Health Action* **2005**, *18* (6), 15–18.

Pelczar, J. R.; Chan, E.; Krieg, N. *Microbiology*, 5th ed.; Tata Mcgraw Hills: New Delhi, 1987, p 598.

Podsedek, A. Natural Antioxidants and Antioxidant Capacity of Brassica Vegetables: A Review. *Food Sci. Tech.* **2007**, *40* (1), 1–11.

Ponnusamy, S.; Haldar, S.; Mulani, F.; Zinjarde, S.; Thulasiram, H.; RaviKumar, A. Gedunin and Azadiradione: Human Pancreatic Alpha-Amylase Inhibiting Limonoids from Neem (Azadirachta indica) as Anti-Diabetic Agents. *PLoS One.* **2015**, *10* (10), 0140113.

Portha, B., J.; Movassat, C.; Cuzin-Tourrel, D.; et al. The Neonatally Streptozotocin Induced (n-STZ) Rat Model of Type 2 Diabetes. Several Variants with Multiple and Complementary Talents. In *Animal Models of Diabetes*; Shafrir, E., Ed.; Taylor and Francis: London, 2007; pp 221–248 (b).

Pradeepa, R.; Mohan, V. The Changing Scenario of the Diabetes-Epidemic Implications for India. *Indian J. Med. Res.* **2002**, *116*, 121–132.

Prasad, C. V. R. *Diabetes And Heart Diseases*; The Hindu, 2002; p 7.

Preston, A. M. Modification of Streptozotocin Induced Diabetes by Protective Agents. *Nutr Res.* **1985**, *5*, 435–446.

Pushpalatha, H. B.; Kumar, P.; Devanathan, R.; Sundaram R. Use of Bergenin as an Analytical Marker for Standardization of the Polyherbal Formulation Containing *Saxifraga ligulata*. *Pharmacogn. Mag.* **2015**, *11* (Suppl 1), S60–S65.

Shanmugapriya, R.; Poornima, S. Detection of Charantin in the Leaves and Fruits of *Momoridca tuberosa* (Cogn) Roxb and *Momordica dioica* (Roxb Ex Wild) by Analytical HPTLC. *Int. J. Sci. Res.* **2014**, *4* (6), 1–8.

Rahman, A. U; Zaman, K. Medicinal Plants with Hypoglycemic Activity. *J. Ethnopharmacol.* **1989**, *26*, 1–55.

Raina, M. K. Quality Control of Herbal and Herbo-Mineral Formulations. *Indian J. Nat. Prod.* **2003**, *19* (1), 11–15.

Ramachandran, S. Review on *Sphaeranthus indicus* Linn. (Koṭṭaikkarantai). *Pharmacogn. Rev.* **2013**, *7* (14), 157–169.

Ramesh, P. R.; Vijaya, C.; Parasuraman, S. Anti-Diabetic Activity of Polyherbal Formulation in Streptozotocin—Nicotinamide Induced Diabetic Wistar Rats. *J. Tradit. Complement Med.* **2014**, *4* (2), 108–117.

Rao, S. S; Najam, R. Efficacy of Combination Herbal Product (*Curcuma longa* and *Eugenia jambolana*) used for DM. *Pak. J. Pharm. Sci.* **2016**, *29* (1), 201–204.

Rastogi, S. B.; Govindarajan, R.; Shukla, M.; Rawat, A. K. S.; Mehrotra, S. Quantitative HPLC Analysis of Amino Acids in Chyavanprash: A well known Ayurvedic Formulation. *Indian J. Pharm. Sci.* **2004**, *66*, 753–757.

Remington. *The Science and Practice of Pharmacy*, 20th ed.; Vol. I, pp 590–592.

RSSDI-35th Annual Scientific Meeting of the Research Society for the Study of Diabetes in India (RSSDI) 2007, November 23, 24 and 25, Science City, Kolkata.

Sabu, M. C.; Ramadasan, K. Anti-Diabetic Activity of *Aegele marmelos* and its Relationship with its Antioxidant Properties. *Indian J. Physiol. Pharmacol.* **2004**, *48* (1), 81–88.

Sabu, M. C.; Kuttan, R. Anti-Diabetic Activity of Medicinal Plants and its Relationship with their Antioxidant Property. *J. Ethnopharmacol.* **2002**, *81* (2), 155–160.

Sahoo, H. B; Nandy, S.; Senapati, A. K; Sarangi, A. K.; Sahoo S. K. Aphrodisiac Activity of Polyherbal Formulation in Experimental Models on Male Rats. *Pharmacogn. Res.* **2014**, *6* (2), 120–126.

Samarakoon, S. M. S.; Chandola, H. M.; Shukla, V. J. Evaluation of Antioxidant Potential of Amalakayas Rasayana: A polyherbal Ayurvedic formulation. *Int. J. Ayurveda Res.* **2011**, *2* (1), 23–28.

Satyanarayana, K.; Sravanthi, K.; Shaker, I. A.; Ponnulakshmi, R. Molecular Approach to Identify Anti-Diabetic Potential of Azadirachta Indica. *J. Ayurveda Integr. Med.* 2015, *6* (3), 165–174.

Satyavati, G.; Tandon, N.; Sharma, M. Indigenous Plant Drugs for DM. *Diabetes Bulletin* **1989**, *9* (4), 181–211.

Saxena, A.; Vikram, N. K. Role of Selected Indian Plants in Management of Type 2 Diabetes: A Review. *J. Alt. Comp. Med.* **2004**, *10*, 369–378.

Sharma P. Caraka Samhita, 4th ed., Chaukhambha Orientalia, Varanasi, India, 1998, 120, 55-59.

Shaw, J. E; Sicree, R.; Zimmet, P. Z. Global Estimates of the Prevalence of Diabetes for 2010 and 2030. *Diabetes Res. Clin. Prac.* 2010, *87*, 4–14.

Shetti, A. A.; Sanakal, R. D.; Kaliwal, B. B. Anti-Diabetic Effect of Ethanolic Leaf Extract of hyllanthus amarus in alloxan Induced Diabetic Mice. *Asian J. Plant Science Res.* **2012**, *2*, (1), 11–15.

Shukla, K.; Saraf, S.; Saraf, S. Development of Quality Control Parameters of Bhaskar Lavan Churna: A Ayurvedic formulation. *Taiwan Pharm. J.* **2007**, *59*, 47–56.

Silverstein, R. M.; Webster, F. X. "Spectrometric Identification of Organic Compounds", 6th ed.; John Willey and Sons, Inc.: New York, 2002; p 71.

Singh, B. V. *Chemistry of Milk and Milk Products*; Asian publisher: Muzaffarnagar, 1965; p 143.

Singh, H; Mishra, S. K.; Pande, M. Standardization of Arjunarishta Formulation By TLC Method. *Int. J. Pharm. Sci. Rev. Res.* **2010**, *2* (1), 25–28.

Singh, R. K; Mehta, S.; Jaiswal, D.; Rai, P. K.; Watal, G. Anti-Diabetic Effect of Ficus Bengalensis Aerial Roots in Experimental Animals. *J. Ethnopharmacol.* **2009**, *123* (1), 110–114.

Singh, R. *The Holistic Principles of Ayurvedic Medicine*; Vedic life Sciences: Mumbai, 1998.

Sinko, P. J. *Martin's Physical Pharmacy and Pharmaceutical Sciences*, 5th ed., Indian ed., 2006.

Skoog, D. A., Hollar, J. F.; Nieman, T. A. *Principles of Instrumental Analysis*, 4th ed., 2003.

Skoog, D. A.; Holler, F. J.; Nieman, T. A. *Principles of Instrumental Analysis*; Thomson Brook, 2005.

Snyder, L. R.; Kirkland, J. J.; Glajch, L. J. *Practical HPLC Method Development*; John Wiley and Sons, INC., 1997.

Sridhar, G. R.; Venkaa, P. Sleep and Body Weight in DM: A Large Retrospective Analysis from South India. *Diabetes Res. Clin. Pract.* **2005**, *72* (2), 209–211.

Standard Nomenclature of Ayurvedic Medicinal Plants. Central Council for Research in Ayurveda and Siddha (CCRAS): New Delhi, 2009.

Subbalakshmi, G.; Naik, M. Indigenous Foods in the Treatment of DM. *Bombay Hosp. J.* **2001,** *43* (4), 548–561.

Subrahmanyam. CVS. *Text Book of Physical Pharmaceutics*, 2nd ed.; Vallabh Prakashan: New Delhi, 2001.

Sudha, P.; Zinjarde, S. S.; Bhargava, Y. S.; Kumar, R. A. Potent α-Amylase Inhibitory Activity of Indian Ayurvedic Medicinal Plants. *BMC Compl. Alt. Med.* **2011,** *11*, 1–10.

Tatiya, A. U.; Surana, S. J.; Sutar, M. P.; Gamit, N. H. Hepatoprotective Effect of Poly Herbal Formulation against Various Hepatotoxic Agents in Rats. *Pharmacogn. Res.* **2012,** *4* (1), 50–56.

Thakkar Nima, V.; Jagruti Patel, A. Pharmacological Evaluation of "Glyoherb": A Polyherbal Formulation on Streptozotocin-Induced Diabetic Rats. *Int. J. Diabetes Dev. Ctries.* **2010,** *30* (1), 1–7.

The Ayurvedic Formulary of India, Part I, 1st ed. Govt. of India, Ministry of Health and Family Planning, Dept. of Health: Delhi, 2003; pp 381–398.

The Ayurvedic Formulary of India, Part I, 2nd ed. Govt. of India, Ministry of Health and Family Planning, Dept. of Health: Delhi, 2003; p 110.

The Ayurvedic Formulary of India, Part II, 1st ed. Govt. of India, Ministry of Health and Family Planning, Dept. of Health: Delhi, 2000; p 178.

The Ayurvedic Formulary of India, Part II, 1st ed. Govt. of India, Ministry of Health and Family Planning, Dept. of Health: Delhi, 2000a; p 177.

The Ayurvedic Formulary of India, Part II, 1st ed.; Govt. of India, Ministry of Health and Family Planning, Dept. of Health, Delhi, 2000b; p 177.

The Ayurvedic Formulary of India, Part II, 1st ed.; Govt. of India, Ministry of Health and Family Planning, Dept. of Health: Delhi, 2000; pp 385–413.

The Ayurvedic Pharmacopoeia of India, Part II (Formulations), 1st ed.; Appendices 1 to 5; Government, of India Ministry of Health and Family Welfare Department of Ayurveda, Yoga Naturopathy, Unani, Siddha and Homoeopathy: New Delhi, 2008; Vol. II.

The Ayurvedic Pharmacopoeia of India, Part I. (API); Ministry of Health, Govt. of India: New Delhi, 2004; Vol. I to IV.

The Ayurvedic Pharmacopoeia of India, 1st ed.; Ministry of Health and Family Welfare, Government of India, Department of Health: New Delhi, 1986, Vol. I., pp 31–32.

The Ayurvedic Pharmacopoeia of India, 1st ed.; Ministry of Health and Family Welfare, Government of India, Department of Health: New Delhi, 1986a, Vol I., pp 33–34.

The Complete German Commission E Monographs, American Botanical Council, Austin, 1998.

The Hindu. *Diabetic Population Highest in India*; Atlas Hindu, 2006; p 20.

The Pharmacopoeia of India, 2nd ed.; Manager of publications, Govt. of India: Delhi, 1966, Appendix XXXI, XXXII 971–985.

Tierney, L. M.; McPhee, S. J.; Papadakis, M. A. *Current Medical Diagnosis and Treatment*; International edition, Lange Medical Books/McGraw-Hill: New York, 2002.

Tiwari, P.; Mishra, B. N.; Sangwan, N. S. Phytochemical and Pharmacological Properties of Gymnema Sylvestre: An Important Medicinal Plant. *Biomed. Res. Int.* **2014,** *2014*, 830285.

Tripathi, A. K.; Kohli, S. Pharmacognostical Standardization and Anti-Diabetic Activity of Syzygium Cumini (Linn.) Barks (Myrtaceae) on Streptozotocin-Induced Diabetic Rats. *J. Complement. Integr. Med.* **2014**, *11* (2), 71–81.

Uma, L. R.; Tripathi, S. M.; Jachak, S. M.; Bhutani, K. K.; Singh, I. P. HPLC Analysis and Standardization of Arjunarishta—An Ayurvedic Cardioprotective Formulation. *Sci. Pharm.* **2009**, *77*, 605–616.

Upreti, J.; Ali, S.; Basir, S. F. Effect of Lower Doses of Vanadate in Combination with Azadirachta indica Leaf Extract on Hepatic and Renal Antioxidant Enzymes in Streptozotocin-Induced Diabetic Rats. *Biol. Trace Elem. Res.* **2013**, *156* (1–3), 202–209.

Vaidya, A.; Pandya, S. The Golden Age of Indian Medicine. *Bombay Hosp. J.* **1971**, *3*, 95.

Vaidya, A.; Antarkar, D.; Joshi, B. Traditional Remedies for DM: Trails, Trials and Trilateral Quest. *Diabetes Bulletin.* **1989**, *14*, 186–199.

Vaidya, A.; Vaidya, R.; Nagral, S. Ayurveda and a Different Kind of Evidence: From Lord Macaulay to Lord Walton (1835 to 2001 AD). *J. Assoc. Phy. India.* **2001**, *49*, 534–537.

Vaidya, A.; Vaidya, R.; Shah, S.; et al. Current Status of Indigeneous Drugs and Alternative Medicine in the Management of DM. In *Textbook of DM*, 2nd ed.; Tripathy, B. B., Chandelia, H. B., Das, A. K., Rao, P. V., Madhu, S. V., Mohan, V., Eds.; Chapter 47, 2008.

Vaidya, A.; Vaidya, R.; Joshi, V. D. Obesity (Medoraoga). In *Scientific Basis for Ayurvedic Therapies;* Mishra, L.C., Ed.; CRC Press: Boca Raton, 2004.

Vaidya, A. We Can Still Learn from Indian Medicine. *CIBA-GEIGY J.* 1979.

Vaidya, A. B.; Antarkar, V. D. S. New Drugs from Medicinal Plants and Approaches. *J. Assoc. Phys. India* **1994**, *42*, 221.

Vaidya, A. B. The Status and Scope of Indian Medicinal Plants Acting on Central Nervous System. *Indian J. Pharmacol.* **1997**, *29*, 340–343.

Vaidya, R.; Vaidya, A.; Talwalkar, S.; et al. Clinical Endocrine and Metabolic Studies in the Kindred of Familial Partial Lipodystrophy—a Syndrome of Insulin Resistance. *J. Assoc. Physicians India.* **2002**, *50*, 773–776.

Valentao, P.; Andrade, P. B.; Areias, F.; Ferreres, F.; Seabra, R. M. Analysis of Vervain Flavonoids by HPLC/Diode Array Dector Method. Its Application to Quality Control. *J. Agric. Food Chem.* **1999**, *47*, 4579.

Venkatesh, S.; Reddy, G. D.; Reddy, B. M.; Ramesh, M.; Rao, A. V. N. Antihyperglycemic Activity of *Caralluma attenuate. Fitoterapia* **2003**, *74*, 274–279.

Verma, L.; Khatri, A.; Kaushik, B.; Patil, K. U.; Pawar, S. R. Anti-Diabetic Activity of Cassia Occidentalis (Linn) in Normal and Alloxan Induced Diabetic Rats. *Indian J. Pharmacol.* **2010**, *42*, 224–228.

Verpoorte, R. In *Bioassay Methods in Natural Product Research and Drug Development*; Kulwar Academic Publishers: Dordrecht, Netherlands, 1999; 43, p 11

Viswanathan, V.; Kesavan, R.; Kavitha, K. V.; Kumpatla, S. A Pilot Study on the Effects of a Polyherbal Formulation Cream on Diabetic Foot Ulcers. *Indian J. Med. Res.* **2011**, *134* (2), 168–173.

Wadkarm, K. A.; Magdum, C. S.; Patil, S. S.; Naikwade, N. S. Anti-Diabetic Potential and Indian Medicinal Plants. *J. Herb. Med. Toxicol.* **2008**, *2* (1), 45–50.

Wallis, T. E. *Text Book of Pharmacognosy.* 5th ed.; J and A Churchill Ltd: London, 1967.

WHO. Monographs on Selected Medicinal Plants. *1, 2, 3,* (Website).

WHO. *The Use of Traditional Medicine in Primary Health Care;* AITBS Publisher and Distributor: Delhi, 2004; p 40.

WHO. *The Use of Traditional Medicine in Primary Health Care;* AITBS Publisher and Distributor: Delhi, 2004a; p 86.

WHO. *The Use of Traditional Medicine in Primary Health Care;* AITBS Publisher and Distributor: Delhi, 2004b; p 3.

WHO. *The Use of Traditional Medicine in Primary Health Care;* AITBS Publisher and Distributor: Delhi, 2004c; p 90.

WHO. *The Use of Traditional Medicine in Primary Health Care;* AITBS Publisher and Distributor: Delhi, 2004d; p 66.

WHO. *The Use of Traditional Medicine in Primary Health Care;* AITBS Publisher and Distributor: Delhi, 2004e; p 67.

WHO. *The Use of Traditional Medicine in Primary Health Care;* AITBS Publisher and Distributor: Delhi, 2004f; p 88.

WHO. The Use of Traditional Medicine in Primary Health Care; AITBS Publisher and Distributor: Delhi, 2004g; p 98.

WHO. WHO Traditional Medicine Strategy 2002–2005.World Health Organization, Geneva, 2005.

World Health Organisation. Report of the Expert Committee on the Diagnosis and Classification of DM. *Diabetes Care* **1997,** *20,* 1183–1197.

World Health Organisation. WHO Prevention of DM; Geneva, WHO, 2005; pp 11–17.

World Health Organization. Quality Control Methods for Medicinal Plants Materials; Geneva, 1998; pp 1–115.

Yadav, D.; Chaudhary, A. A; Garg, V.; Anwar, M. F.; Rahman, M. M.; Jamil, S. S; Khan, H. A.; Asif, M. In Vitro Toxicity and Anti-Diabetic Activity of a Newly Developed Polyherbal Formulation (MAC-ST/001) in Streptozotocin-Induced Diabetic Wistar Rats. *Protoplasma* **2013,** *250* (3), 741–749.

Yogendra, K.; Badar, V.; Hardas, M. Efficacy and Safety of Livwin (polyherbal formulation) in Patients with Acute Viral Hepatitis: A Randomized Double-Blind Placebo-Controlled Clinical Trial. *Int. J. Ayurveda Res.* **2010,** *1* (4), 216–219.

Yoshiharu, A. Diabetes Research and Clinical Practice. *WHO Collab. Centre Diabetes Treat. Educ.* **1994,** *24,* S331–S333.

Zar, C. T.; Das, S. Potential Effect of Herbs on Diabetic Hypertension: Alternative Medicine Treatment Modalities. *Clin. Ter.* **2013,** *164* (6), 529–535.

Zhang, F.; Lin, L.; Xie, J. A Mini-Review of Chemical and Biological Properties of Polysaccharides from Momordica charantia. *Int. J. Biol. Macromol.* **2016,** *S0141–8130* (16), 30696–1.

INDEX